Your Brain, Your Body, Your *Blueprint*

The Brain Plate is more than just a cookbook – it's a guide to nourishing your mind through the power of food. In order to get the most out of it, you need to know:

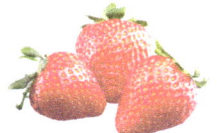

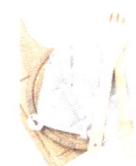

Which **nutrients** and **supplements** are important for you?

What **cooking strategies** are best for your lifestyle?

What **common blocks** get in the way of your success?

Start by taking our free 2-minute quiz at TheBrainPlate.com/Quiz

Scan the QR code to take the quiz and unlock your personalized plan

Brought to you by two registered dietitians – one a licensed therapist and the other a certified intuitive eating counselor.

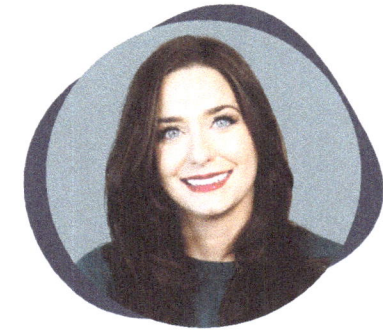

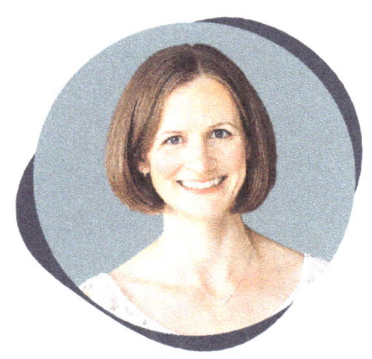

Amanda Ashcraft, MS LPC, RD
NutriMind.org

Ann Kent, MS, RD, CDCES, CIEC
PeasAndHoppiness.com

The Brain Plate

The Brain Plate

Cookbook, Meal Plan, and Supplement Guide for Mental Health

By Amanda Ashcraft and Ann Kent

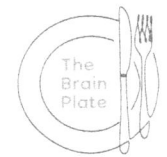

The Brain Plate
Fort Collins, Colorado

Edited by: Jennifer Kent, Savannah Scheufler, Rebecca Martin
Published by: The Brain Plate, Fort Collins, Colorado
Cover Design by: Nicole Hart, Supernova Creative Inc., www.supernovasites.com
Interior Layout by: Ann Kent

ISBN: 979-8-218-69022-9
Library of Congress Control Number: 2025910515

This publication is intended for educational purposes only and is not a substitute for professional medical advice, diagnosis, or treatment. It is not intended to take the place of a treatment plan for mental health. Always seek the advice of a qualified healthcare provider with any questions you may have regarding a medical condition. The publisher and authors disclaim any liability arising directly or indirectly from the use of this book. No legal responsibility will be accepted for any damages incurred, whether directly or indirectly, due to the use of this information.

A big thank you to my family for supporting me in this out-of-the-box endeavor from my usual one-on-one client work and allowing time to stretch my writing skills. I want to thank my parents for encouraging me to pursue my additional education and combining my skills to help people in a new way. Then, last but not least, to my co-author, Ann, for being patient and encouraging as our project grew and my life was in ever-changing cycles. I would not have done this without you.

-Amanda Ashcraft

Special thanks to my husband Patrick, who kept our household running while I finished this project, and who often believes in me more than I do myself. Thanks also to my parents, especially my mom – who not only taught me how to cook, but also helped test, taste, and critique so many of the recipes I've written. Additionally, a huge thanks goes to both of my sisters-in-law, Dr. Aunt Jen and Sister Savvy, and my dear friend Dr. Becca, who graciously spent their time, expertise, and editing skills to review this book.

-Ann Kent

Table of Contents

Table of Contents

Nutrition Matters

Introduction: Nutrition Matters

"You are what you eat." This common phrase holds more truth than you might think. Unlike plants, humans cannot grow or obtain energy from carbon dioxide and sunlight, so we have to eat our nutrients instead. Our bodies use these nutrients to make everything from nerve cells to hormones.

The Brain Plate is rooted in scientific research that shows that the foods we eat are the building blocks for our bodies and brain. If you don't eat enough of the nutrients you need, your body simply won't be able to function at its best. When you understand how the brain and body work and respond to foods, you will have the power to change your diet, which can then support your physical and mental health.

While learning about the ways in which food and supplements affect your body is important, this knowledge alone isn't enough. Your mindset and approach to food choices is also integral to your mental health. As dietitians who celebrate all foods and the nutrients they provide, we know foods nourish our bodies as well as our souls. In addition to education, you'll find a blueprint in these pages to translate this information; it will help you make choices about the foods you eat and the supplements you take.

This method is not about restrictive diets or quick fixes. Instead of focusing on nutrients to cut out, we take the opposite approach. You'll learn how to <u>add in</u> important nutrients using a simple, practical meal-planning approach to support your mental health. Each sample meal is balanced with the macronutrients, including carbohydrates, protein, and fat, to give you optimal blood glucose and energy levels. We emphasize micronutrients like folate and magnesium, which play crucial roles in neurotransmitter synthesis and mood regulation.

Sometimes it's difficult to obtain all the nutrients you need from food. Dietary supplements can serve as a bridge to fill this gap. In addition to a nutritional foundation from food, our supplement guide will help you decide which kinds of macronutrients, micronutrients, and herbal supplements you may wish to add.

From finding time and energy to cook, to navigating food intolerances, changing your eating pattern can be tough. Perhaps you struggle with eating too much or too little at times – or eating to soothe emotions rather than physical hunger. That's why in addition to a meal plan and recipes, we've also provided a troubleshooting guide where you'll find solutions to common barriers. We refer to these barriers as blocks because they can get in the way of meal planning and cooking. Spend as much – or as little – time as you need in each section, focusing on your specific mental health needs.

Introduction: Nutrition Matters

Section 1: Nutrition and Brain Health

We begin our conversation by providing you with a basic understanding of how nutrition impacts the brain and body to support mental health. Here you'll find definitions of terms used throughout the book.

Section 2: Meal Planning for Mental Health

In Section 2, you'll learn to make a non-diet meal plan, navigating busy schedules and mental health challenges in a way designed for those new to meal planning. You'll also get practical tips to make grocery shopping easier.

Section 3: Your 4-Week Meal Plan and Recipes

Here you'll discover four weeks of seasonal meals and recipes that highlight nutrients to support mental health. Each meal plan is designed to meet nutrient needs over the course of a week, with the understanding that there is normal variance from meal to meal. Each meal plan and recipe include adjustments for gluten-free, dairy-free, vegetarian, and vegan needs.

Section 4: Nutrient and Supplement Guide for Mental Health

In this section you'll learn how macronutrients, micronutrients, and dietary supplements function in the brain, and discover which may be helpful for your unique needs. We encourage you to focus on food first, then use this information to decide where you may have nutritional gaps to fill. The dietary supplement fact sheets provide accurate information about the options on the market. You can use these in conversations with your mental health team to determine which, if any, may be beneficial for you.

Section 5: Troubleshooting Guide for Common Challenges in Mental Health

Education is only part of the equation. You also need the skills to implement this knowledge in a way that is realistic and sustainable for your life. This section walks you through the most common blocks for different mental health and lifestyle challenges. Choose the sections to read based on your specific needs.

Introduction: Nutrition Matters

While nutrition is a basic component of a healthy brain and body, it's not the only thing that matters. We believe in a holistic approach to mental health. Nutrition is not meant to be used by itself. Instead, we encourage you to build on your nutrition foundation with mindfulness practices, quality sleep, stress management, talk therapy, movement, community engagement, social interaction, and medication when needed.

Our advice in this book is not a substitute for medical care and does not constitute medical advice. Rather, our goal is to empower you to ask questions of your mental health team. We believe a team approach to mental health works best. Your team might include a licensed therapist, a prescribing psychiatric provider, and other ancillary team members, such as an occupational therapist or registered dietitian.

Look for providers who specialize in your specific mental health needs and use a collaborative approach. Including additional types of treatment, such as alternative medicine or meditation, may be beneficial in conjunction with your primary mental health team. We encourage you to find healthcare providers who will listen to your concerns, provide a safe place to process your experiences, and give you clear, evidenced-based recommendations for treatment. Find recommended resources on page 272.

Your Mental Health Team May Include

Licensed Therapist:
- Licensed Practicing Counselor (LPC)
- Licensed Clinical Social Worker (LCSW)
- Licensed Marriage and Family Therapist (LMFT)
- Licensed Psychologist (PsyD or PhD level in a psychology degree)

Prescribing Psychiatric Provider:
- Psychiatrist (MD or DO)
- Medical Doctor (MD)
- Doctor of Osteopathy (DO)
- Nurse Practitioner (NP)
- Physician Assistant (PA-C)

Ancillary Team Members:
- Registered Dietitian (RD or RDN)
- Occupational Therapist (OT)
- Physical Therapist (PT)
- Certified Personal Trainer (CPT)
- Speech Language Pathologist (SLP)

Nutrition and Brain Health

Whole Body *Wellness*

A healthy brain starts with a healthy body. Your mental health is intricately connected with and deeply influenced by all the systems in your body. This includes cardiovascular health, blood glucose (aka blood sugar) balance, hormone regulation, and gut health. Consistent nutrition and rest help stabilize your hormone levels. With more stable hormones, you have better sleep. Better sleep helps improve mood, energy, and blood glucose levels. A healthy cardiovascular system transports nutrients and oxygen more effectively to the brain. When you support one system, you support your whole body.

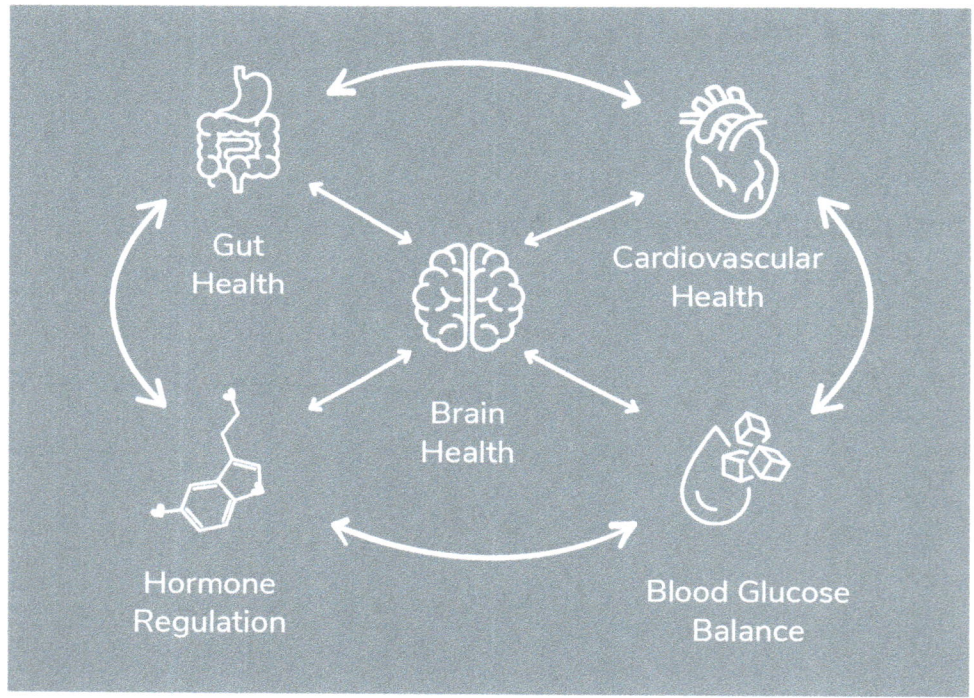

The systems in the body work together to maintain all internal conditions in homeostasis, a state of balance that ensures metabolic reactions can take place and nutrients are available when and where they are needed. A few of the internal conditions the body regulates include temperature, pH, oxygen, blood glucose, electrolytes, and blood pressure among many others. See the example on the next page for a visual representation of how the body maintains homeostasis.

Whole Body *Wellness*

In homeostasis, fluctuations are normal, but levels are kept within a range for optimal health (area shaded green). For example, blood glucose levels are maintained within a tight range so that all parts of your body have access to energy when they need it.

If levels shift abnormally low or too high (the area shaded red), this can cause severe health symptoms. Sometimes they are acute and life-threatening, such as if blood glucose levels drop too low. Other symptoms are not immediately life-threatening, but can cause long-term complications if not corrected, such as with high blood glucose levels in uncontrolled diabetes.

Homeostasis in the Body

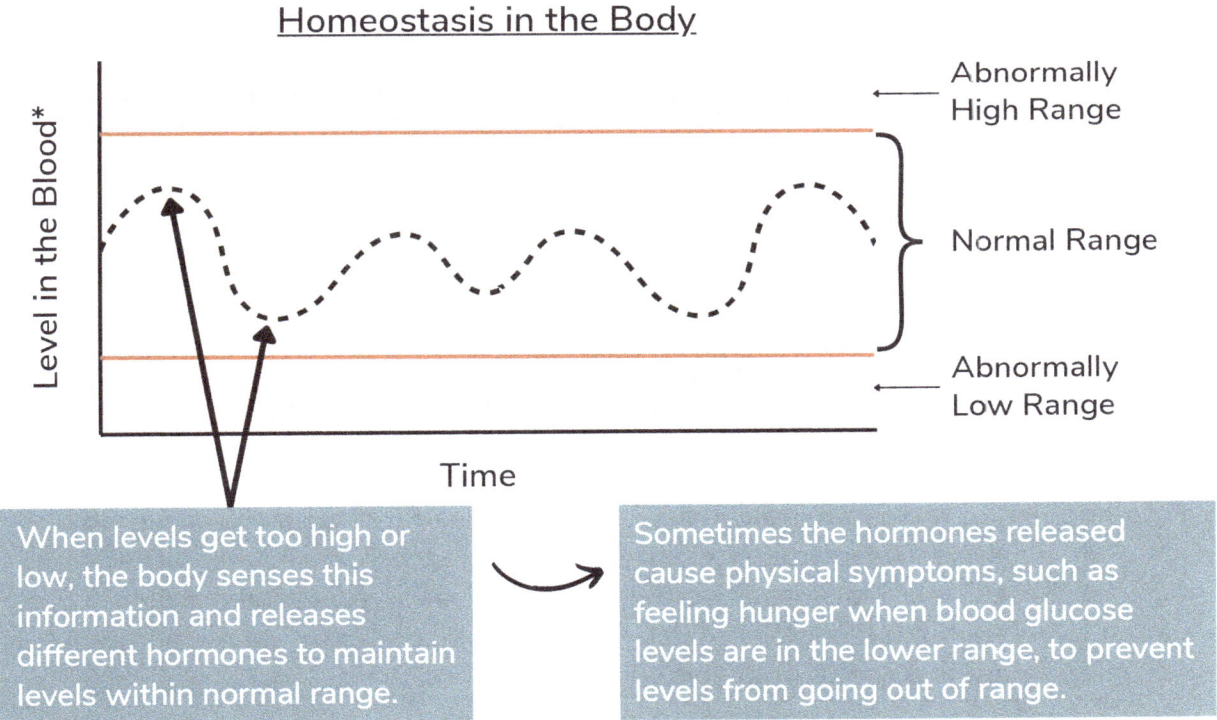

When levels get too high or low, the body senses this information and releases different hormones to maintain levels within normal range.

Sometimes the hormones released cause physical symptoms, such as feeling hunger when blood glucose levels are in the lower range, to prevent levels from going out of range.

*The body works hard to maintain everything in balance. Essentially everything we can measure in the body, such as pH, temperature, blood glucose, oxygen, hormones, electrolytes, and so many more, are all meant to be within particular ranges to promote optimal functioning of each system and the body as a whole.

Whole Body *Wellness*

Hormones are one of the key mechanisms the body uses to maintain homeostasis. These are chemical messengers released by internal organs into the bloodstream. When released, hormones communicate instructions to various cells and organs to help the body return to homeostasis. Examples of hormones include cortisol, epinephrine (ie adrenaline), dopamine, serotonin, and insulin, among many others.

Blood glucose levels are one of the internal conditions the body maintains in a tight range. When blood glucose levels drop to a low-normal level, you may feel symptoms of irritability or brain fog because glucose is the primary energy source for the brain and muscles. On the other end of the spectrum, consistently high blood glucose levels above the normal range (like those observed with uncontrolled diabetes) can cause excess glucose molecules to stick to proteins, a process called glycosylation. This leads to increased oxidative stress in the body. Long-term oxidative stress is a significant risk factor for Alzheimer's disease and cognitive decline, among other damage it does to the body – particularly in the cardiovascular system.

The cardiovascular system is made up of your heart, arteries, and veins, which carry blood, and thus oxygen and nutrients, throughout your body. Maintaining cholesterol and blood pressure within the normal range reduces the risk for cognitive decline because a healthy cardiovascular system can more effectively deliver nutrients to cells. It also improves nerve responses, hormone production, blood glucose absorption, energy, and blood glucose concentration in the brain, nerves, and gastrointestinal system, ie your gut.

The gastrointestinal system breaks down and digests the food you eat, absorbs nutrients from food, and eliminates waste products. It involves many organs, including the stomach, small and large intestines, liver, gallbladder, and pancreas. Additionally, a key component of the gastrointestinal system is made of the naturally-occurring microorganisms that live in your intestines, primarily in the colon in your large intestine. These live organisms in the intestines are collectively called the gut microbiota. A healthy gut microbiota has been linked to better digestion, hormone production, immunity, health of the nervous system, and more.

 Have you noticed that your stomach feels upset when you're under stress? This is because of the intricate connection between the brain and the gastrointestinal tract via the enteric nervous system. They are so highly interconnected that the gut is sometimes referred to as the "second brain."

Whole Body *Wellness*

The term "second brain" describes the connection between the gut and brain via the enteric nervous system. This system of nerves communicates between the digestive tract and central nervous system. Stress impairs digestion by keeping the body in the sympathetic "fight or flight" state and inhibiting digestive processes. When this happens, the digestive system is not as effective in breaking down food into the building blocks needed for your body, including neurochemicals for the brain. In fact, over 90% of the body's serotonin is produced in the gut, which is one of the most well-known neurotransmitters involved in mood. Our emotional and digestive health are intricately connected.

On a larger scale, each body system affects the other. Nutrition is essential for these systems as a foundation for the health of your brain, starting in your body.

 What's the deal with Cortisol?

We can't talk about stress without talking about cortisol. The media uses cortisol as a common scapegoat for inflammation and undesirable weight distribution. However, cortisol serves many important functions in the body, including playing a role in immune function, the sleep-wake cycle, and metabolism, among others. Its levels fluctuate normally throughout the day, rising in the morning and falling in the evening.

During stress or with a traumatic event, cortisol rises quickly to a high-normal level to help the body stay on high alert. It increases blood pressure, appetite, and blood glucose, so you have enough nutrients and oxygen to escape danger. After stress subsides, cortisol levels return to baseline. This response is helpful for short-term stress, but repeated activation increases the risk of some diseases.

Abnormally high cortisol levels are caused by Cushing syndrome, high doses of corticosteroid medications, or certain types of tumors. Low levels of cortisol can be life-threatening, as seen with untreated Addison's disease (ie primary adrenal insufficiency, not to be confused with the common term "adrenal fatigue"). We recommend working with an endocrinologist if you have concerns about your cortisol levels.

Whole Body *Wellness*

Physical Health	Mental Health Relationship	Nutritional Support
Gut Health	The gastrointestinal system digests food, absorbs nutrients, and gets rid of waste. It involves many organs and includes the gut microbiota, the living organisms in your intestines that affect health. The enteric nervous system is impacted by the microbiome.	Including a variety of fiber-rich, fermented, and prebiotic foods in your diet feeds gut bacteria and can improve gut health.
Cardio-vascular Health	Your cardiovascular system is made of arteries, veins, and the heart. This system transports nutrients and oxygen to all the cells in your body, including your brain.	Eating a balance of healthy fat, increasing fiber-rich foods, and including colorful fruits and vegetables supports cardiovascular health.
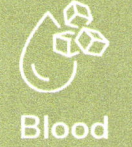 Blood Glucose Balance	The body transports glucose, or sugar, in the blood to all parts of the body so it can use it as energy. Stable blood glucose levels provide stable energy for your body and brain.	To prevent spikes and drops in blood glucose levels, eat fat, protein, and fiber alongside carbohydrates. Spacing meals and snacks evenly throughout the day provides you with consistent energy.
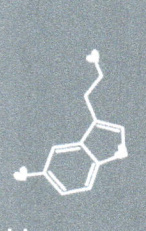 Hormone Regulation	Hormones act as messengers to instruct cells and organs to take action. They are involved in growth, metabolism, sexual function, mood, stress, inflammation, and more. Hormones are highly intertwined and work interdependently with each other to regulate various systems.	Fat and protein are the building blocks of hormones, so you need to eat adequate amounts for hormonal health. Many factors affect hormonal balance, such as sleep, stress, age, timing of food intake, body composition, weight, medications, genetics, and hormone-disrupting chemicals.

Food as a **Building Block**

Food is more than just calories. The nutrients in food make up the anatomy of the brain and nervous system, as well as neurotransmitters, hormones, and cells that affect mood, focus, sleep, and emotional balance. Nutrients like amino acids, fatty acids, vitamins, and minerals come from the food you eat. If key nutrients are missing from your diet, or if digestion is impaired and you're unable to effectively get nutrients from food, mental health symptoms can worsen or become harder to manage.

 The nutrients in food are the building blocks for everything in the body, including the brain, nervous system, neurotransmitters, hormones, and more. Restrictive diets may limit the intake of critical nutrients, such as omega-3 fatty acids or certain vitamins and minerals, which can worsen the symptoms of various mental health conditions.

Carbohydrates break down into glucose, which fuels your brain. Proteins become amino acids, which help you build neurotransmitters. Fats make up 60% of the brain, insulate it, form cell membranes, serve as a building block of many hormones, and help absorb the fat-soluble vitamins A, D, E, and K – each of which play a role in regulating mood and neurological function. Restrictive diets may unintentionally limit access to these crucial nutrients that are necessary to support mental health.

As an example, phospholipids are a type of fat that have a wide variety of functions in the body. Related to mental health, several different types of phospholipids make up the lining of neurons, or nerve cells. This phospholipid lining is critical for cell-to-cell communication and without it, brain function lacks structure and substance. Nutrients such as omega-3 fatty acids and choline are essential components of these phospholipids, and without enough of them, phospholipid integrity decreases. This has been linked to major depression and mood disorder, pointing to the importance of nutrition for brain health. You'll find examples like this in every system within the body.

Different parts of the brain and hormones impact different mental health conditions. Each of these components of the brain and their related neurotransmitters benefit by focusing on specific nutrients to support the related anatomy. For example, dopamine and norepinephrine are important neurotransmitters that are involved in many of the body's responses to the environment. Nutrients that support these neurotransmitters can be helpful to manage the body's reward response, regulate mood, and increase alertness.

Food as a **Building Block**

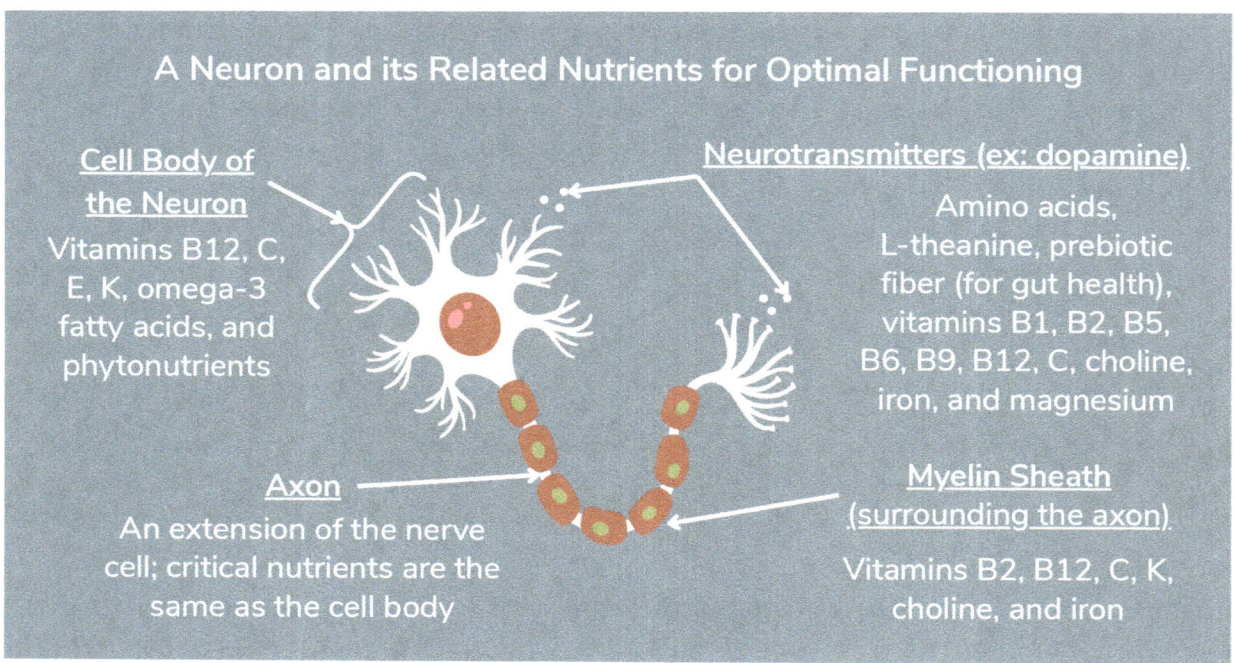

A Neuron and its Related Nutrients for Optimal Functioning

Cell Body of the Neuron

Vitamins B12, C, E, K, omega-3 fatty acids, and phytonutrients

Neurotransmitters (ex: dopamine)

Amino acids, L-theanine, prebiotic fiber (for gut health), vitamins B1, B2, B5, B6, B9, B12, C, choline, iron, and magnesium

Axon

An extension of the nerve cell; critical nutrients are the same as the cell body

Myelin Sheath (surrounding the axon)

Vitamins B2, B12, C, K, choline, and iron

 Find more in-depth information about how each nutrient and dietary supplement affect mental health in Section 4. Look for critical nutrients and easy food additions for mental health conditions in Section 5.

To aid in our discussion, it's helpful to have a basic working knowledge of the brain and nervous system anatomy and physiology. In the following pages, you'll find definitions of different parts of the brain, neurotransmitters, and hormones discussed in the book, giving you a foundation to understand how nutrients and supplements work in mental health.

Additionally, we provide definitions of common terms related to nutrition. While food is part of our everyday life, some of the phrases used in discussing nutrition are not. To better understand how food, nutrients, and dietary supplements work in the body, you should refer to these definitions.

We encourage you to briefly read through these definitions to help the rest of the sections in the book make more sense, then reference these pages as needed.

Brain and Nervous System *Anatomy*

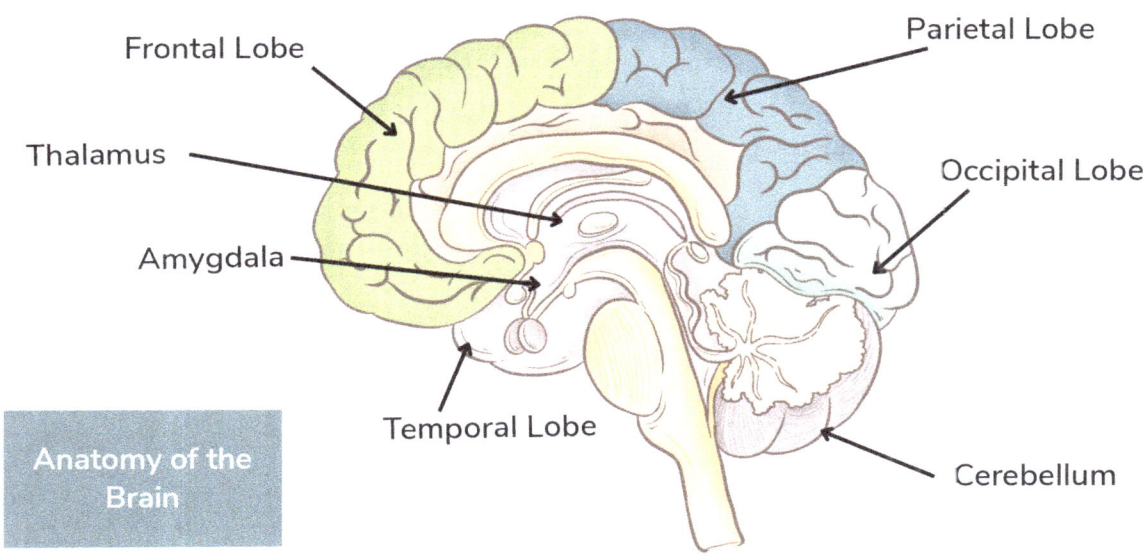

Frontal Lobe

Parietal Lobe

Thalamus

Occipital Lobe

Amygdala

Temporal Lobe

Cerebellum

Anatomy of the Brain

Amygdala: is a component of the limbic system, and is responsible for emotional processing, especially fear and anxiety. It initiates the stress response.

Cerebellum: coordinates movement, balance, and motor learning.

Frontal Lobe: controls decision-making, problem-solving, impulse control, and motor function. It is not fully developed until around age 25.

Occipital Lobe: handles visual processing and interpretation.

Parietal Lobe: processes sensory information, spatial awareness, and coordination.

Temporal Lobe: is involved in memory, language processing, and auditory interpretation. It contains the amygdala and hippocampus.

Thalamus: relays incoming motor and sensory information to the brain, including hearing, taste, sight and touch (but not smell, which goes to the olfactory bulb).

Brain and Nervous System *Anatomy*

Neurons: are also called nerve cells. These are the fundamental cells of the brain and nervous system. They are responsible for receiving sensory input from the external world, sending motor commands to our muscles, and transforming and relaying the electrical signals in between.

Neural Synapse: is the space in between neurons. It requires an electrical signal or chemical messenger called a neurotransmitter to send information across the space to allow neurons to communicate.

Axon: is the long, threadlike extension of a neuron's cell body that transmits impulses from the neuron to other cells. It's protected by the myelin sheath.

Myelin Sheath: is a protective, insulating cover surrounding the axon, composed of layers of fats and proteins. It prevents signal leakage and speeds the transmission of nerve impulses by allowing them to "jump" from one gap to the next.

Vagus Nerve: is also known as the vagal nerve. It is the main connection between the enteric nervous system and the central nervous system and is involved in digestion, heart rate, and immune function.

Hypothalamic-Pituitary-Adrenal Axis (HPA Axis): is a complex communication system between the hypothalamus, pituitary gland, and adrenal glands that regulates part of the body's stress response.

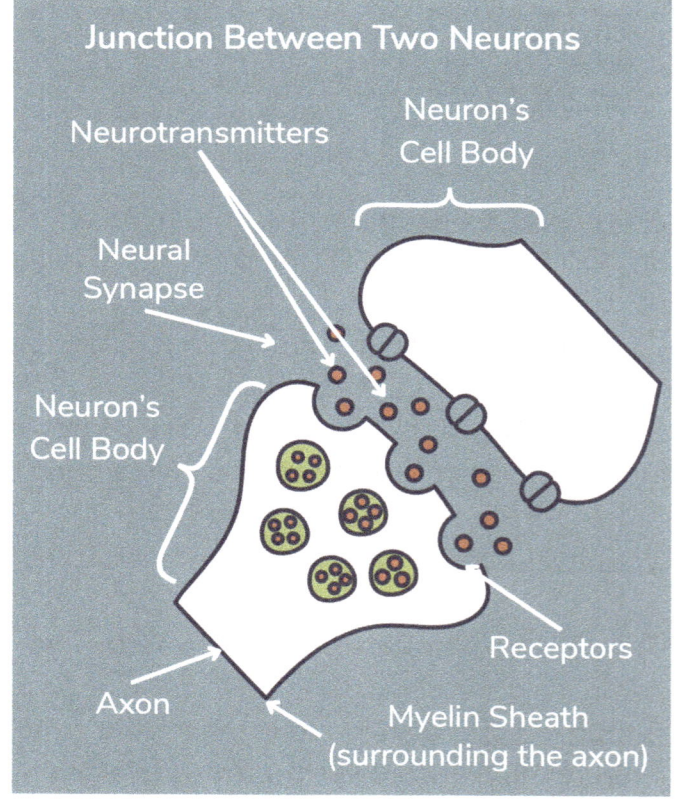

N-Methyl-D-Aspartate Receptor (NMDA): is a receptor in the brain activated by glutamate and glycine and is responsible for learning, memory, and the ability of the brain to form and modify connections between neurons (synaptic plasticity).

Nervous System *Branches*

Central Nervous System: is the part of the nervous system made up of the brain and spinal cord. The brain controls how we think, move, learn, and feel. The spinal cord carries messages to and from nerves in the body to the brain.

Peripheral Nervous System: is the part of the nervous system that includes the nerves that run throughout your body that are not in your brain or spinal cord. These nerves carry messages to and from your brain and spinal cord to the rest of the body.

Somatic Nervous System: is a component of the peripheral nervous system. It includes nerves that control voluntary muscle movements and sensory nerves that carry information from the skin, muscles, and joints back to the brain. The sensory information these nerves carry include sound, smell, taste, and touch, but do not include vision because the optic nerves are part of the brain.

Autonomic Nervous System: is the component of the nervous system that operates outside of our conscious control. This system is responsible for breathing, heart rate, pupil changes, epinephrine (adrenaline) release, and other physical responses you don't think about consciously. It includes the sympathetic, parasympathetic, and enteric nervous system.

Enteric Nervous System: is a component of the autonomic nervous system. It consists of a complex network of neurons within the gastrointestinal tract that controls various digestive functions. The enteric nervous system communicates with, but can operate independently of, the central nervous system. For this reason it's often called the "second brain." It includes the vagus nerve.

Parasympathetic Nervous System: is a component of the autonomic nervous system. It works in opposition to the sympathetic nervous system to maintain the body's homeostasis. It's commonly referred to as the "rest and digest" nervous system because its main purpose is to conserve energy that can be used later and to regulate bodily functions like digestion. Acetylcholine is the primary neurotransmitter released when the parasympathetic nervous system is activated.

Sympathetic Nervous System: is a component of the autonomic nervous system that works in opposition with the parasympathetic nervous system to maintain the body's homeostasis. It prepares your body to be on alert for intense physical activity, involved in the "fight or flight" response. Norepinephrine is the primary neurotransmitter released when the parasympathetic nervous system is activated.

Nervous System *Branches*

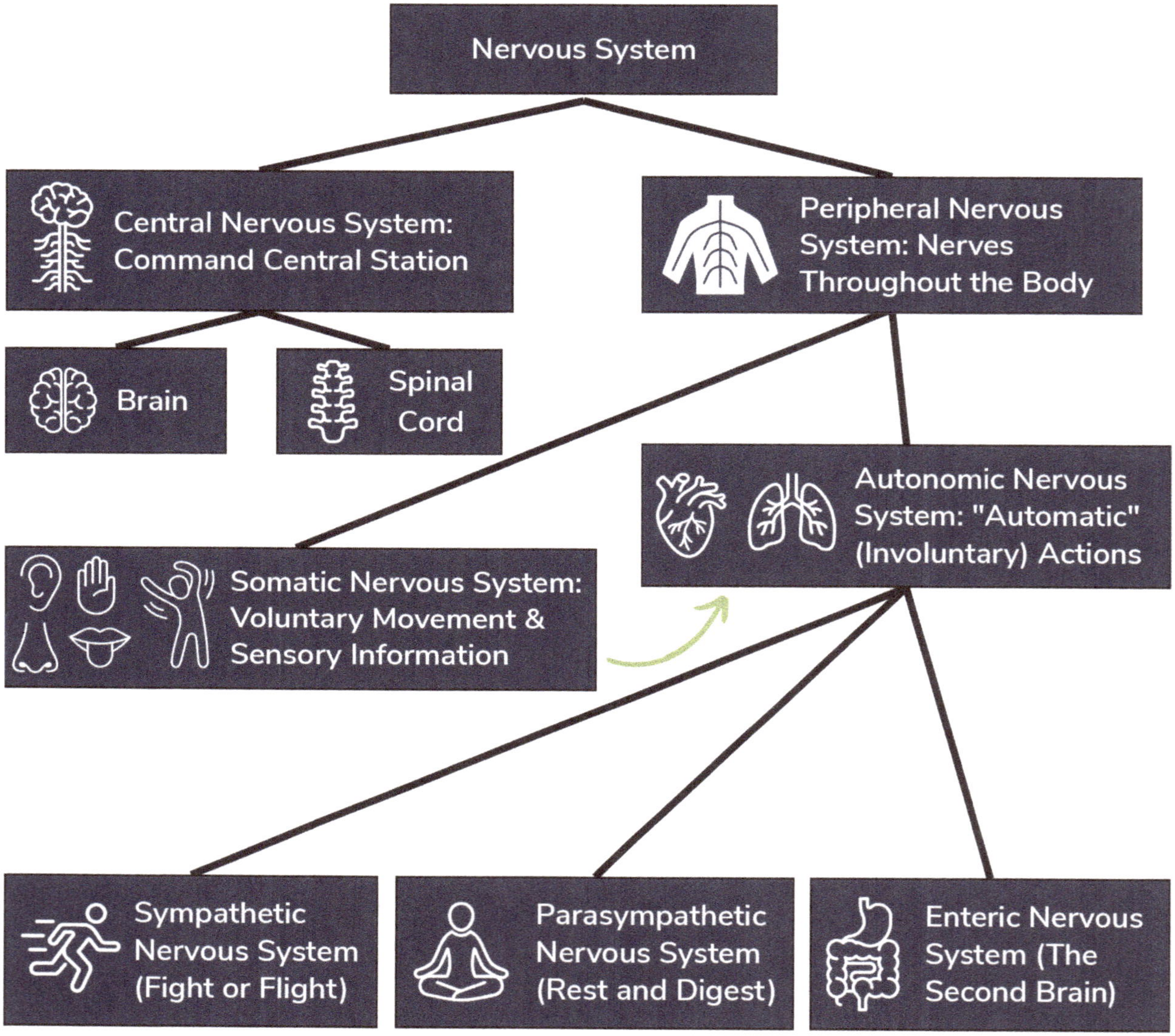

Nervous System

Central Nervous System: Command Central Station

- **Brain**
- **Spinal Cord**

Peripheral Nervous System: Nerves Throughout the Body

Somatic Nervous System: Voluntary Movement & Sensory Information

Autonomic Nervous System: "Automatic" (Involuntary) Actions

Sympathetic Nervous System (Fight or Flight)

Parasympathetic Nervous System (Rest and Digest)

Enteric Nervous System (The Second Brain)

 You can impact the autonomic nervous system by using muscles under voluntary control to affect involuntary actions. For example, deep breathing can shift the autonomic nervous system activation from sympathetic to parasympathetic.

Brain and Nervous System *Messengers*

Acetylcholine: is an excitatory neurotransmitter that enhances messages sent between neurons and plays a role in muscle movement, memory, and attention. It is the main neurotransmitter released in the parasympathetic nervous system response.

Adaptogen: is an umbrella term for compounds that increase or decrease chemical reactions or hormones in the body to help it return to homeostasis.

Brain-Derived Neurotrophic Factor (BDNF): is a protein found primarily in the brain and spinal cord that is essential for learning and memory due to its role in neuronal plasticity (the ability to modify the strength of connections between neurons). BDNF also plays a role in nerve cell survival and growth, regulates glucose and energy metabolism, and protects insulin-producing beta cells in the pancreas.

Cyclic Adenosine Monophosphate (cAMP): is a molecule that acts as a secondary messenger. It takes messages from hormones like epinephrine and glucagon, which cannot enter the cell, and delivers their messages through the cell membrane. It also helps initiate a variety of other metabolic reactions in the body.

Cortisol: is a hormone that regulates how your body uses glucose for energy, decreases inflammation, regulates blood pressure, and controls your sleep-wake cycle. It's also released after initial "fight or flight" stress hormones like epinephrine, in response to acute, chronic, or traumatic stress, to help the body remain on high alert.

Dopamine: is a hormone that plays a role in your body's positive responses to the environment. It helps you feel pleasure, increases arousal, and helps with learning. Dopamine also helps with focus, concentration, memory, sleep, mood, and motivation.

Endorphins: are hormones that act as your body's natural pain reliever by playing a role in your perception of pain and increasing positive feelings.

Epinephrine: is also called adrenaline. It is a hormone released during the sympathetic nervous system's initial "fight or flight" acute stress response to increase blood pressure and heart rate and suppress digestion. It affects metabolism, attention, focus, panic, and excitement.

Glutamate: is the most abundant excitatory neurotransmitter in the brain, enhancing communication between neurons for learning and memory. It's a precursor to GABA.

Gamma-Aminobutyric Acid (GABA): is an inhibitory neurotransmitter produced from glutamate that blocks signals between neurons to prevent overstimulation. It helps to calm the nervous system, reduce nerve activity during rest to promote sleep, and helps regulate blood pressure.

Brain and Nervous System *Messengers*

<u>Histamine:</u> is a naturally-occurring compound produced by the body, found in food, and in the environment, that acts as a chemical messenger in the brain to regulate body functions like wakefulness, immune response, feeding behavior, and motivation.

<u>Homeostasis:</u> is a state of balance among the systems in the body, which is necessary for survival. It includes maintenance of pH levels, hormone levels, blood glucose levels, oxygen, electrolytes, and temperature regulation, among many other factors.
See page 7 for a visual representation.

<u>Hormones:</u> are chemical messengers released by internal organs into the bloodstream that communicate instructions to various cells and organs to help the body maintain homeostasis. Examples of hormones include cortisol, epinephrine (ie adrenaline), dopamine, serotonin, and insulin, among many others. Hormone levels fluctuate normally throughout the day but are maintained within a normal range. Levels outside of normal can be serious and life-threatening in either the short- or long-term.

<u>Insulin:</u> is a hormone that plays an important role in blood glucose management by acting as a "key" to unlock cells in the body, allowing glucose to move from the blood stream into muscle and fat cells where it can be used as energy. Stable blood glucose levels are a prerequisite for stable mood, energy, and cognitive function.

<u>Limbic System:</u> is a system in the brain that includes the hippocampus, amygdala, hypothalamus, and thalamus. It regulates emotions, memory, and hormone control.

<u>Neurotransmitters:</u> are any chemical messenger in the brain that transmit signals across neural synapses to allow neurons to communicate with each other. Examples include dopamine, acetylcholine, epinephrine, and GABA, among many others.

<u>Norepinephrine:</u> is also called noradrenaline. This hormone is released as one of the initial "fight or flight" stress hormones in response to acute, chronic, or traumatic stress. It increases blood pressure and affects alertness, arousal, decision-making, attention, and focus. It is the main neurotransmitter released in the sympathetic nervous system response

<u>Oxytocin:</u> is often called "the love hormone." Oxytocin enhances human relationship behaviors, such as sexual arousal, recognition, trust, romantic attachment, and parent-infant bonding. It also plays a key role in labor, delivery, and lactation.

<u>Serotonin:</u> is an inhibitory neurotransmitter that helps to reduce overstimulation and regulate mood, sleep patterns, sexuality, anxiety, appetite, and pain.

Nutrition and Brain Health

Nutrition *Definitions*

Anti-Inflammatory: describes compounds that reduce chronic inflammation processes in the body. This promotes health, reduces pain, and lowers the risk of disease.

Antioxidants: are bioactive compounds that control or eliminate free radicals from the body to prevent or reduce the damage from oxidation. Vitamins C and E are antioxidants, as are a number of phytonutrients found in plant foods.

Bioavailability: describes the amount of a nutrient that is absorbed and used by the body. Different forms of nutrients or their combination with other substances can increase or decrease the amount that is available for the body to use.

Co-Enzyme A (CoA): is a cofactor essential in metabolic pathways and energy production, helping enzymes to create and break down fatty acids and carbohydrates to use as energy.

Essential Nutrients: are compounds the body requires to function but is not able to produce, or does not produce in sufficient quantities, and so must be consumed in food. Examples include vitamins, minerals, and omega-3 fatty acids, among others.

Food and Drug Administration (FDA): is a federal agency in the United States that oversees safety and efficacy of food, drugs, medical devices, cosmetics, and more. Dietary supplements are regulated as a food, rather than a drug like pharmaceutical medications.

Free Radicals: are atoms or molecules in the body with an unpaired electron, making them highly reactive with other compounds in the body. They are formed on exposure to smog, ozone, certain chemicals, drugs, or during the body's natural defense process against microbes or other foreign substances, among other causes. Free radicals take electrons from cell parts and proteins, which damages their components, including DNA and cell membranes. The result is called oxidative damage, or oxidation.

Generally Recognized As Safe (GRAS): is a designation by the FDA for food additives and ingredients that have been determined to meet safety standards showing reasonable certainty that the substance will not cause harm to consumers.

Macronutrients: are the large parts of food, sometimes referred to as "macros," and include carbohydrates, protein, and fat.

Micronutrients: are naturally-occurring small, essential parts of food, including vitamins, minerals, and phytonutrients.

Nutrition *Definitions*

Microbiome: refers to a community of microorganisms and the environment in the human body in which they live. The gut microbiome includes the microbiota and the digestive tract, specifically the colon in the large intestine, where microorganisms live.

Microbiota: refers to the microorganisms living in a specific area in the human body. The gut microbiota includes primarily bacteria and yeast, but can also include viruses, fungi, and mold, which consume prebiotic fiber and produce a number of bioactive substances called postbiotics.

Minerals: are naturally-occurring inorganic elements needed in small quantities by the body. They are used as components of cells and in metabolic reactions.

Oxidative Stress: is an imbalance in the body between free radicals and antioxidants, causing damage to cells, DNA, and tissues. Chronic oxidative stress is linked to a higher risk of many diseases, including cancer, Alzheimer's disease, and heart disease.

Phytonutrients: are sometimes called "phytochemicals." These are compounds produced by plants that influence the colors you see in fruits and vegetables. They have a wide variety of actions in the human body, including antioxidant and anti-inflammatory properties.

Postbiotics: are metabolites and byproducts of bacteria in the gut, many of which appear to have a positive impact on health. Postbiotic supplements also sometimes contain inactivated microorganisms and cell components.

Prebiotics: are nondigestible carbohydrates that are consumed by bacteria in the large intestine. These are necessary for a healthy gut microbiota.

Probiotics: are live microorganisms found in fermented foods and dietary supplements that can repopulate the gut microbiota.

Tolerable Upper Intake Level (UL or upper limit): is the maximum daily intake of a nutrient that can be consumed on an ongoing basis without adverse events for the general population. This book will use the common term "upper limit" when referring to this value.

Vitamins: are naturally-occurring essential nutrients needed in small quantities by the body that are used in various metabolic reactions and cell functions.

Meal Planning
for Mental Health

Meal Planning *Without Restriction*

Choosing foods to nourish your brain and body is important to mental health, but the way you approach eating matters just as much. Food is more than its individual nutrients. It holds memories, helps us celebrate, and is an expression of culture. That's why we believe a balanced approach to eating is more effective for long-term health than restricting food groups or avoiding certain ingredients.

Restrictive dieting often cuts out essential nutrients, like fats or carbohydrates, and can cause insufficient intake of vitamins, minerals, or amino acids. When the brain isn't properly fueled, higher-level thinking suffers and could lead to difficulty concentrating, brain fog, forgetfulness, and poor decision-making. These symptoms are especially problematic for people with ADHD, depression, or anxiety disorders who already struggle with executive functions such as time management and working memory.

Additionally, a large body of evidence shows that restrictive diets often cause long-term challenges with healthy eating, including increased risk for eating disorders and future weight gain. Many diets disconnect you from your hunger cues, lead to distrust of your body, and depress your metabolism. Avoiding certain foods can trigger a psychological fear of restriction that can cause out-of-control eating and a rebound effect if any weight was lost initially. Despite what the weight loss industry might tell you, the answer is not working harder to follow another diet.

 Restrictive diets often backfire in the long-term and can cause disordered eating patterns. Instead, we encourage you to use a non-restrictive approach and focus on adding nutrients rather than taking foods out.

We're using a non-restrictive meal planning approach to building a healthy plate and nourishing your mind. Our goal is to help you move the control around food from external food rules back to your body's internal wisdom. Instead of telling you exactly what or how much to eat, we provide guidance around the balance of nutrients. Rather than measuring, weighing, or tracking every nutrient, we encourage you to listen to your internal hunger and fullness cues to know how much and when to eat.

Our approach focuses on what to add to your diet instead of instructions on what to remove. You don't have to deprive yourself in order to feel your best. In fact, research shows you are more likely to achieve your best health when you feel satisfied and enjoy the food you eat. We include all types of food in our meal plans – yes, even sugar – because we know giving yourself unconditional permission to eat all food is important to avoid the psychological trap of the restriction-binge cycle.

Meal Planning *Without Restriction*

If you find that building a healthy meal plan makes you feel anxious or nervous that you won't be able to eat what you love, you may need to pause here and first work through your fears around food on a more personal level. A dietitian who incorporates mindful eating can help you reconnect with your body and feel confident in your choices. See page 272 to find resources for more support.

As you embrace a non-restrictive approach to eating, reframing the language you use to talk about food can be a powerful way to shift your mindset. Instead of using words that promote restriction or poor body image, using affirmations and simple language shifts can help you transition to a nourishing, loving approach to caring for your body. Here are some ways to change your self-talk and mindset around food.

Meet Your Basic Needs First

Behaviors are your best attempt to get your needs met. If you frequently struggle with cravings or eating past fullness, this may be a signal you have an underlying need that's not being met. Ask yourself: Are you hungry? Tired? Stressed? Do you feel safe? Food can be a helpful coping mechanism, but it's important to first make sure you're meeting your needs. If this feels hard, work with your mental health team and find resources on page 272 to help you along your personal journey.

Learn to Cope With Emotions in Healthy Ways

Food is one of the most common and socially acceptable coping mechanisms in our culture — we eat ice cream when we're sad, and we eat birthday cake when we celebrate. As with most coping skills, eating food for comfort is not harmful if done in moderation and with awareness. If you find yourself constantly feeling and coping with emotions using food, it may be a sign that you need to address an underlying cause for this feeling and incorporate other coping mechanisms. Talking with a licensed therapist may be beneficial to identify your needs and create a comprehensive plan of care. See pages 267–270 for more tips.

Meal Planning *Without Restriction*

Focus on Pleasure

Pleasure is an important part of nourishing your body because when you are truly tuned into what makes you feel your best, it will be easier to eat what you need. Practicing mindful eating can enhance the pleasure of food – slow down and notice flavors, textures, sights, sounds, and smells of foods when you eat.

Allow Flexibility

Some days you'll eat more foods from home-cooked foods and others you'll eat more foods for convenience. Some days you'll be hungrier and others you won't need to eat as much. This variation is normal. Embrace it and continue to tune into your needs.

Approach With Curiosity Instead of Judgment

While healing your relationship with food you'll experience "ups" and "downs." Practice curiosity when things don't go as planned to help reduce your guilt and shame. If these feelings come up, ask questions to help you focus on problem-solving instead of judgment. What is your underlying need? Was there a trigger for this event? Who were you with? Where were you when this happened? Noticing patterns can help you better meet your needs.

Rather than striving for the elusive "perfect diet," focus instead on balance and satisfaction with eating. Meal planning is a tool for healthy eating and is meant to serve you – you are not meant to serve your meal plan. Rather than giving you rigid food rules, the meal planning process in this section will guide you through creating a plan that works holistically for your life. Focus on addition rather than restriction as you shift your eating pattern towards a healthier plate for mental health.

Most importantly, remember that food is more than nutrients. The joy, community, and culture food fosters is just as important to your mental health as the nutrients we explore in this guide.

Building a Positive Food and Body Relationship for Kids and Young Adults

Building a healthy relationship with food is even more important if you have children or young adults in your life. In a world filled with poor body image and damaging messages around food, you can provide a solid foundation to protect your children from disordered eating patterns. It starts with your own relationship with food and the language you use.

Practice using neutral language around food, focusing on the function of your body rather than the appearance, and having fun with physical activity rather than using it as a punishment for eating.

DON'T	DO
Restrict your eating in front of your child	Model balanced eating
Pressure your child to eat or make comments about how much they eat	Encourage listening to your body's hunger and fullness cues
Moralize food or label it as "good" or "bad"	Use neutral language around food
Restrict or ban certain foods	Enjoy special foods as a part of celebrations and culture
Compare your child's body to others	Foster body acceptance
Reward or punish with food (such as withholding dessert, bribing with candy)	Involve kids in food prep
Use exercise to "make up" for eating	Promote physical activity for joy
Eat with distractions or stress	Create a positive mealtime atmosphere
Make negative comments about your own body or your child's body	Avoid commenting on any bodies including your child's body
Focus on body weight	Focus on food's function
Ignore emotional eating	Teach emotional intelligence and healthy coping skills

How to Create Your Meal Plan

Knowing how to nourish your body and mind is a powerful tool, but only when you are able to put this knowledge into action will you see true benefits. The key to long-term success is learning how to include the nutrients you need in foods you love, in a way that works with your schedule and doesn't leave you spending hours in the kitchen when you would rather be doing something else. Structure and routine can be powerful tools to help support your nutrition journey when you have mental health challenges, such as ADHD, anxiety, or depression.

Meal planning can save you time, money, energy, and stress – when it's done right. Knowing which recipes you're making for the week allows you to write a specific shopping list and reduce food waste. Instead of making last-minute decisions about what's for dinner – particularly stressful if you struggle with decision paralysis – you think about it once and can avoid the "5-o'clock dinner time panic." If you struggle with fatigue, planning meals ahead of time helps space out energy-consuming tasks so you can follow through with cooking. Section 5 provides specific recommendations for how to overcome common blocks you might experience.

If you've tried meal planning before and it hasn't worked, you're not alone. There are so many meal plans, apps, templates, systems, and online tools out there for meal planning. If you've tried some of these options and found yourself frustrated, it's not because you're doing anything wrong. It's likely because you haven't found the right system for you.

 The number 1 reason most meal plans don't work is because they don't take into account YOUR life!

For a meal planning system to work, it needs to work <u>for you</u> – for your time, schedule, unique mental health challenges, taste preferences, and cooking ability. The biggest mistake with meal planning is starting with a meal plan and then trying to adjust your life around it, instead of the other way around. Rather than giving you a rigid meal plan that tells you what time of day to eat or when to prep your meals during the week, this easy 3-step meal planning process starts with <u>your</u> schedule. Work backward from there to make a plan that will fit your life.

While planning out the recipes you want to cook is important, we also recommend scheduling the days you plan to eat out or order take-out, so you can include this in your food budget. This will help you enjoy going out to eat instead of using it as a last-minute dinner option.

How to Create Your Meal Plan

To help you answer the "What's for dinner?" question, Section 3 provides you a 4-week meal plan to give you inspiration and examples of foods you can plug into your meal plan to support your mental and physical health. These are designed to meet your nutrient needs for mental health over the course of a week, so don't worry if each meal isn't perfect or if you want to substitute a few meals. Pick and choose the recipes that work for you rather than try and follow the plan exactly.

Tips for Successful Meal Planning

DON'T	DO
✕ **Try to fit your schedule around a meal plan:** you have to plan for your busy life if you want this to work!	✓ **Start with your schedule:** this is the #1 tip for success! We teach you how to do this in step 1 on page 30.
✕ **Make yourself eat meals you don't enjoy:** this can backfire and you end up going out to eat more than planned.	✓ **Pick foods that sound good to you:** include foods you're craving, favorite meals, and cuisines.
✕ **Over-plan:** it's better to only cook a few times per week than toss ingredients because you didn't use them.	✓ **Consider your time and cooking skills:** meals don't need to be "gourmet" to be delicious and nourishing.

To make sure your meals provide adequate nutrition for your body and mind, the meals are balanced using the "Healthy Plate" method, modeled after MyPlate from the Dietary Guidelines for Americans (www.myplate.gov). Instead of counting calories or macronutrients, use this method and focus on responding to your hunger and fullness cues. The Healthy Plate is made of 1/2 fruits and veggies, 1/4 protein, and 1/4 starch. Add fat to the meal in cooking or as a condiment, focusing on heart-healthy options.

How to Create Your Meal Plan

In addition to the meals we've included in the meal plan, we encourage you to continue serving meals your family loves. Use the "Healthy Plate" method to add in nutrients that might be missing. For example, if your family loves spaghetti, make sure to include a protein and vegetables with the meal. The "Quick Options to Build a Healthy Plate" on page 38 will help with inspiration.

 Try to include something from each of these categories to make sure your meal is nutritionally-balanced and will keep you full.

Healthy Plate Method

Fruit Provides:

- Carbs
- Fiber
- Vitamins and minerals
- Phytonutrients

Protein Provides:

- Protein
- Often contains fat
- Vitamins and minerals

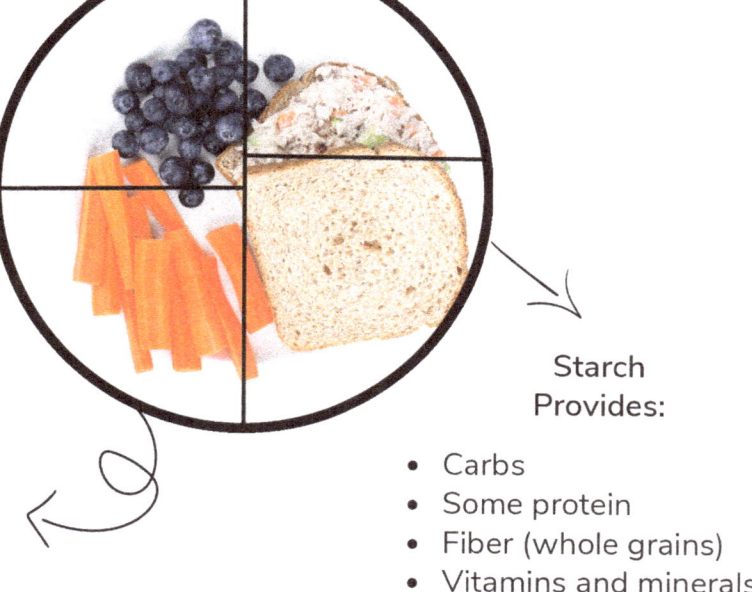

Non-Starchy Veggies Provide:

- Fiber
- Water
- Vitamins and minerals
- Phytonutrients

Starch Provides:

- Carbs
- Some protein
- Fiber (whole grains)
- Vitamins and minerals

How to Create Your Meal Plan

   Our biggest tip for successful meal planning is to schedule time with yourself to make your meal plan. Set aside time before grocery shopping each week to walk through the meal planning process explained on the following pages and watch how much of a difference it makes to have confidence in your plan.

   To get started, scan the QR code or go to thebrainplate.com/resources to download our meal planning template. Our process has three steps to help you create a realistic plan that will work with your lifestyle: Step 1) Plan Your Week; Step 2) Plan Your Meals; Step 3) Make Your Shopping List.

In Step 1 you'll add in everything on your schedule & figure out how many people you're feeding each day.

In Step 2 you'll decide when and what to cook, based on your schedule and number of eaters.

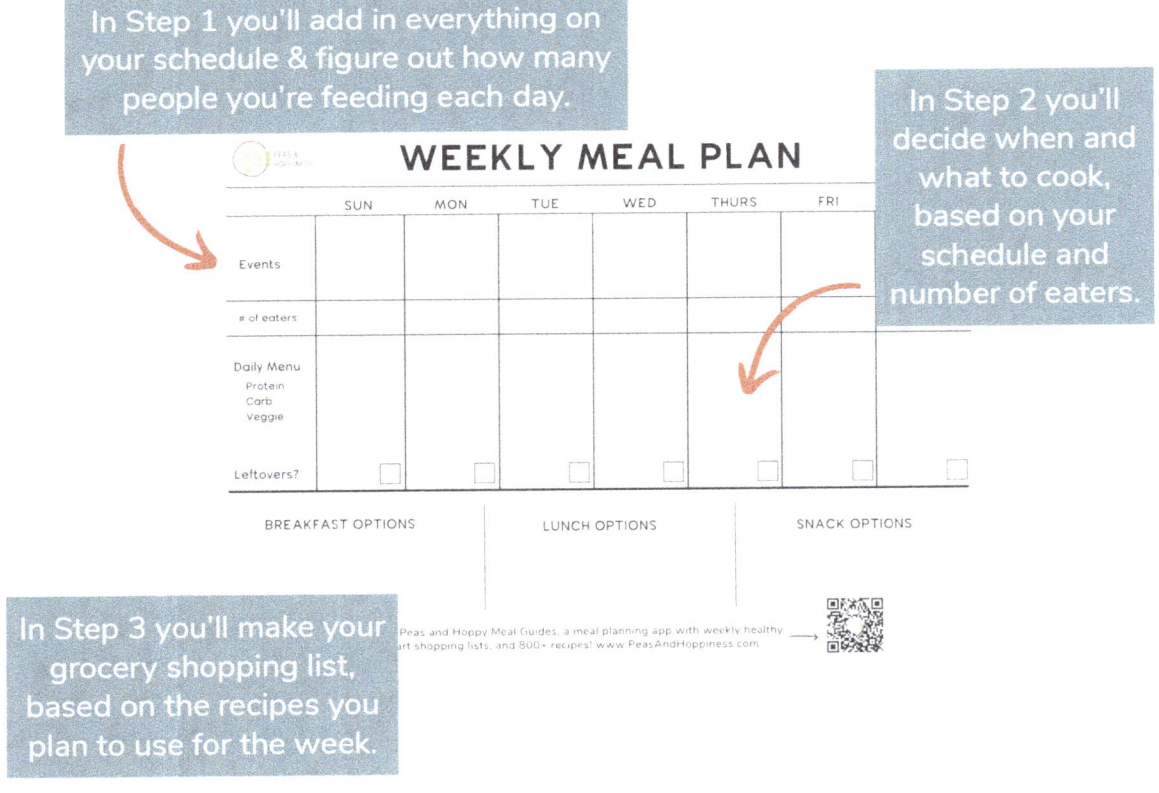

In Step 3 you'll make your grocery shopping list, based on the recipes you plan to use for the week.

Step 1: Plan Your Week

In Step 1 of our meal planning process, the goal is to get everything you can think of down on paper for your weekly schedule. This will help you visualize how much time and energy you have to cook, so you can create a realistic meal plan for your life.

Print out a hard copy of the meal planning template (follow the QR code on page 29 if you missed it) and grab your calendar. On your meal planning template, write down everything on your schedule for that week under the space for "events." This includes your meetings, your kids' practices, or when you plan to have date night with your partner.

> Add everything to your meal plan that's going on during the week. Bonus – this helps with managing busy schedules, too!

Step 1: Example

	SUN	MON	TUE	WED	THURS
Events	Family Night		7pm - Basketball Game	6pm - Mom at a meeting	
# of eaters	5	4	0	3	
Daily Menu					

> Once you have all the events on your meal plan, use this to figure out how many people you'll be feeding each day.

Once you have all your weekly events on the meal plan, think through how many people will be at home for dinner each night, and write down how many people you're feeding each day. For example, if everyone is out at meetings and practices, the number could be zero and you might choose not to cook that night. This will help you decide how often you need to cook and manage your inventory to prevent food waste.

Step 2: Plan Your Meals

Now that you can see your schedule for the week and how many people you're feeding, it's time to decide when and what to cook. To answer the question of <u>when</u> to cook, first decide <u>how often</u> you need or want to cook.

You don't need to cook every day of the week to have a healthy lifestyle. Instead of cooking every day, schedule in purposefully unplanned days (with no cooking scheduled) for leftovers, take-out, or meals out to eat. It's better to start with smaller goals and focus on realistic changes rather than burn yourself out.

If you're not sure how many meals to plan for the week, think about how often you cook at home now. Then, ask these questions to decide if your cooking frequency is right for you.

- **Is your budget tight and you'd like to save some money?** Cooking at home is typically more affordable, and so you may want to set a goal to increase how often you cook at home.
- **Do you often feel burned out by cooking?** It may be helpful to choose recipes that make leftovers, so you don't have to cook as often.
- **Do you frequently find yourself throwing out leftovers or ingredients you didn't use?** You may need to cut back on the number of meals you plan to cook in a week so that it's more realistic for your lifestyle.

"How often should I cook?"

If you're not sure how many meals to plan for the week, start with where you are now. How many times per week do you usually cook? If you want to cook at home more often, use this formula to decide how many meals to plan in a given week:

[Times per week you cook now] plus [ONE] = [Cooked meals on your plan]

For example, if you cook once or twice per week and you want to cook more often at home, this means you should aim to cook two or three times per week to start.

To decide which recipes to make on the days you've planned to cook, think about the amount of time and energy you will have each day. Based on this assessment, consider which days you need or want to cook and what types of recipes to use. The meal plans include different meal types to meet your needs for different days.

Step 2: Plan Your Meals

30-Minute Meals

Designed to get dinner on the table quickly, these recipes should take 30 minutes from start to finish. If you're new to cooking, these may take slightly longer than the recipe notes. Consider buying pre-chopped vegetables or prepping parts of the recipe ahead of time to save time during cooking. These meal types may be helpful if you struggle with low energy or time management.

Slow-Cooker Meals

Slow-cooker recipes are typically easy to make, and they often provide excellent leftovers. Some have longer cooking times and it works best to put them together in the morning, so you can return home to a hot, fresh meal at the end of the day. This may be helpful if you struggle with decision fatigue or executive functions such as working memory in the evening. If you have events in the evening or everyone is eating at different times, consider a slow-cooker option. These recipes will stay warm and fresh for several hours to accommodate different schedules.

Vegetarian Meals

Plant proteins are often less expensive than animal proteins, so learning how to incorporate these into your meal plan can help reduce your food spending and stretch your food budget. When balanced appropriately, plant-based meals have plenty of protein, healthier fats, and more fiber and phytonutrients to support your mental health.

Challenge Meals

These meals are designed to improve your cooking ability and introduce you to new foods or cooking techniques. They may take longer than the other meal types, so plan these meals for a day when you have more time and energy to devote to cooking. If you're struggling with boredom with meals or feeling disinterested in food, these may bring fun, new variety to your rotation. If you don't like cooking or struggle with feeling overwhelmed, you don't need to use these meals at all.

Step 2: Plan Your Meals

After adding your cooked meals to your meal plan, put a checkmark in the "leftover" box on the days your meal will make more than you need. Planning one or two large meals that will make leftovers can save you from cooking every night. Decide if you want to eat leftovers for lunch or use them on a different night for dinner. Make note of when you'll eat leftovers to make sure they don't go to waste – which is particularly helpful if you struggle to remember leftovers because they are "out of sight, out of mind."

In addition to the cooked meals on each meal plan, we also provide ideas for Grab & Go Meals, breakfast, and snacks. You may have a few go-to options, but these recipes will give you more variety and ensure your meals are balanced.

Grab & Go Meals

These are super-easy meals for you to either prep ahead and have ready to go, or that you can make simply by putting together ready-to-eat ingredients from your refrigerator. You don't have to cook in order to have a healthy meal – use these meals as inspiration when you need something very easy. These may be especially helpful on days when time management is challenging, if you find yourself overscheduled, or if you have less energy than you thought you would.

Breakfast

Each week you'll find a savory and a sweet option for breakfast to balance your blood glucose levels, give you variety, and enhance your nutrition for the day. It is important to fuel your brain starting early in the day, even if you have a reduced appetite. Intense cravings or extreme hunger in the afternoon and evening are signs you might not be eating enough in the morning.

Snacks

If your meals are spaced more than 4-5 hours apart, you may benefit from adding a snack to balance your blood glucose and energy levels. Snacks can also be a great opportunity to add in easy foods containing critical nutrients you need for various mental health conditions. Use the savory and sweet ideas on each meal plan for inspiration. Find ideas specific to your mental health needs in Section 5.

Step 2: Plan Your Meals

 We recommend not to cook multistep meals more than once per day – this can lead to burnout and feeling overwhelmed. Instead, jot down quick ideas for breakfast, lunch, and snacks at the bottom of the meal planning template.

Step 2: Example

Schedule slightly more complicated meals on days when you have more time and energy.

Intentionally leave some days unplanned or go out to eat when you're really busy or your schedule is unknown.

	SUN	MON	TUE	WED
Events	Family Night		7pm - Basketball Game	6pm - Mom at a meeting
# of eaters	5	4	0	3
Daily Menu Protein Carb Veggie	Pork Chops, Potatoes, Brussels Sprouts (Double Portion)	Easy Pasta Primavera	Take-Out / Eat at the Game	Slow-Cooker Spicy Lentil Chili
Leftovers?	☒	☐	☐	☒

BREAKFAST OPTIONS
Oatmeal;
Yogurt & Granola;
Blueberry Breakfast Bars

LUNCH OPTIONS
Salmon Avocado Boats;
Leftover Pork Chops

Include family favorites for breakfast, lunch, and snacks or use the inspiration on the meal guides if you want more variety.

Make a note of meals that provide leftovers to help manage food inventory and prevent waste.

Step 3: Make Your Shopping List

The final step of meal planning is to make your grocery list. This is key to saving time and money at the store and avoiding multiple grocery store runs per week. There's just no such thing as a "quick" grocery store run in our experience. The fewer trips, the better! See the QR code on page 29 to download the blank list included with the meal planning template.

To make your shopping list, review each recipe on your meal plan and write down what you need. Next, add your family's "staple" grocery items — things like milk, apples, or spices you use often. Lastly, add any ingredients you need to keep on hand for super-easy last-minute meals, such as frozen vegetables, peanut butter, or canned soup.

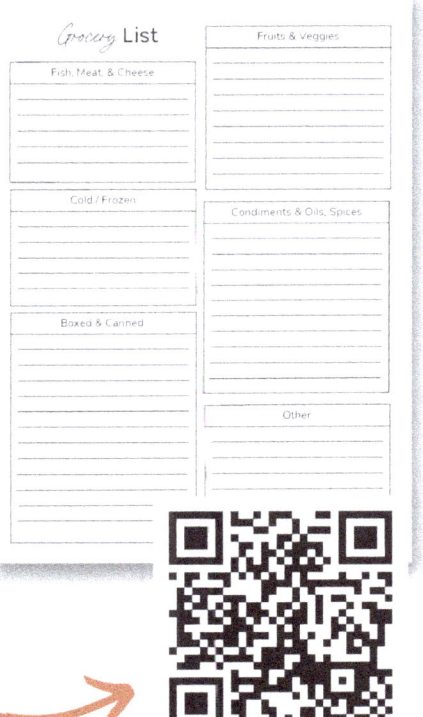

 Would you prefer to make your list digitally? Scan the QR code or go to the website PeasAndHoppiness.com to download the Peas and Hoppy Meal Guides app. You will find the meal plans already uploaded. Delete recipes you don't need, then flip to the ready-made shopping list and add your "staple" grocery items. Take your phone to the store, or sync with Instacart for grocery delivery. Use the code BRAINPLATE for 3 months of complimentary premium access.

Shopping List Tips

- **Double check** if you already have ingredients before you go to the store to save money and prevent food waste.
- **Organize ingredients by the section** of the store to save time when shopping.
- **Cross off the items** as you put them in your cart so you don't miss any.

If grocery shopping feels overwhelming, see tips on page 240 for additional strategies to use, such as shopping online or using meal delivery kits instead.

Adjusting Your Meal Plan

Congratulations on making your first meal plan! Now get ready to change it. No matter how perfect the original meal plan might be, sometimes it just doesn't work out – plans change, meetings run late, and coaches move practice at the last minute. The most successful meal planners are those who learn how to adjust their meal plan for last-minute needs. See this example for how to adjust your meal plan due to schedule changes.

An Example of Changing Your Plan

Reschedule the slow cooker meal to the night when everyone will be home at different times so that food will be available all evening.

	SUN	MON	TUE	WED
Events	Family Night	Extra Bball Practice; Mom Works Late	7pm - Basketball Game	6pm - Mom at a meeting
# of eaters	5	✗ 0	0	3
Daily Menu Protein Carb Veggie	Pork Chops, Potatoes, Brussels Sprouts (Double Portion)	Leftovers from yesterday Easy Pasta Primavera	Take-Out / Eat at Game Slow-Cooker Spicy Lentil Chili	Slow-Cooker Spicy Lentil Chili Dad cooks - Pasta Primavera
Leftovers?	☒	☐	☒	☒

Use leftovers or one of your Grab & Go Meals if you need to cancel your original meal plan.

NS

LUNCH OPTIONS

Yogurt & Granola
Blueberry Breakfast Bars

Ask your family to be part of the team to help with meals, including your partner or older children.

Adjusting Your Meal Plan

Most importantly, when you're new to meal planning and changing your eating habits, remember that it's more important to make progress than it is to be perfect. Incorporate these tips to keep you on track when unexpected challenges come up.

 Keep frozen or canned fruits and veggies on hand so you always have an option without an extra trip to the store.

 Use foods that have a long shelf life to reduce food waste from spoilage. Examples include frozen meat, canned tuna or beans, whole blocks of cheese, tortillas, rice, or crackers.

 Make "snack dinner" using ready-to-eat foods that don't need to be cooked. Use the "Healthy Plate" method and choose proteins, starches, fruits, and vegetables to balance your plate. See the Grab & Go Meals in section 3 and ideas on page 38 for examples.

 Substitute other fruits and veggies in recipes and snacks based on what's in season or what you have on hand. See the "Pro Tip" in each recipe for substitution suggestions.

 Use different types of recipes in your meal plan such as Slow-Cooker, 30-Minute, and Grab & Go Meals to allow you flexibility to swap around within your plan if the timing around meals changes.

 Remember the mantra – _progress over perfection._ Things in life rarely go as planned, and that's okay! Focus on the big journey and make small changes rather than worrying if things don't go perfectly.

Quick Options to Build a Healthy Plate

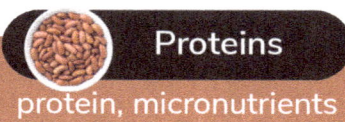 **Proteins**
protein, micronutrients

- **Canned beans***: black, pinto, kidney, red, black eyed peas, navy, etc.
- **Lentils**, split peas, or pea milk
- **Eggs, cheese**, cottage cheese
- **Milk***, Greek or regular yogurt*
- **Deli meat**, rotisserie chicken
- **Peanut butter** or other nut butters
- **Nuts**: almonds, cashews, walnuts
- **Seeds**: hemp, sunflower, flax, pumpkin
- **Canned tuna**, salmon, or chicken
- **Edamame**, tofu, tempeh, or soymilk
- **Frozen meat**: chicken strips, fish fillets, ready-to-eat meats, hamburgers

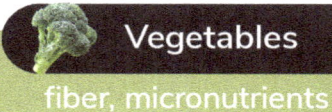 **Vegetables**
fiber, micronutrients

- **Fresh veggies** dipped in salad dressing, buffalo sauce, or hummus: cucumbers, bell peppers, carrots, radishes, snap peas, grape tomatoes, broccoli, cauliflower, celery
- **Frozen or pre-cut veggies** (steam, roast, or sauté): green beans, asparagus, broccoli, Brussels sprouts, baby carrots, mushrooms
- **Pre-made salad** or coleslaw mix
- **Canned veggies**: green beans, beets, carrots, baby corn, bean sprouts, water chestnuts

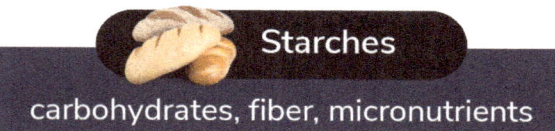 **Starches**
carbohydrates, fiber, micronutrients

- Corn or flour **tortillas**
- **Whole grain bread**, bagel
- **Milk***, yogurt,* oat milk
- **Canned beans***: black, pinto, kidney, red, black eyed peas, navy, etc.
- **Corn**, peas, or potatoes
- Tortilla or potato **chips**
- Whole grain **crackers**
- **Pasta**, cous cous, rice, or quinoa
- **Cereal**, oatmeal, or grits
- **Pancake**, waffle, muffin
- **Sweets**: cookies, candy, ice cream

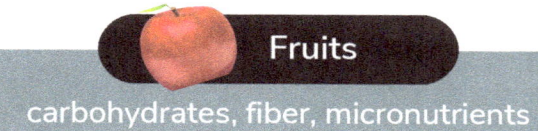 **Fruits**
carbohydrates, fiber, micronutrients

- **Whole fruit**: apples, apricots, bananas, clementines, kiwis, oranges, pears, peaches, nectarines
- **Fruit canned in juice** or rinsed: pineapple, peaches, pears, grapes, mandarin oranges
- **Fresh or frozen berries**, mango, pineapple, or cherries
- **Pre-cut watermelon**, cantaloupe, or honeydew
- **Dried fruit**: raisins, cranberries, blueberries, cherries, mangos, dates

*These foods contain both protein and carbohydrates.

Your 4-Week Meal Plan and Recipes

Winter/Spring Meal Plan: Week 1

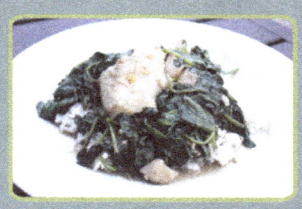
30-Minute Meal 1: Coconut Cod & Spinach Over Coconut Rice

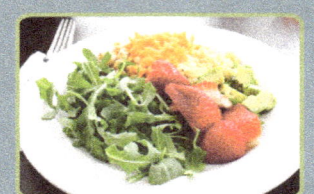
30-Minute Meal 2: Springtime Greens & Grain Bowls With Easy Lemon Pepper Chicken

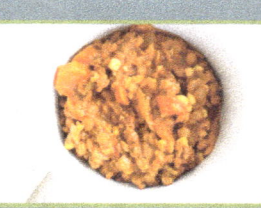
Slow-Cooker: Spicy Lentil Chili With Crusty Bread

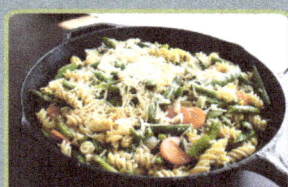
Vegetarian: Easy Pasta Primavera

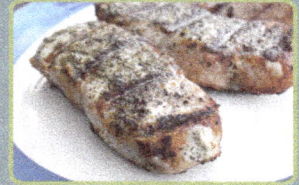
Challenge: Oven Baked Pork Chops With Buttery Potatoes & Roasted Brussels Sprouts

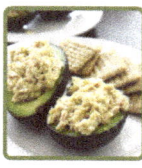
Savory Grab & Go: Salmon Stuffed Avocado Boats With Crackers

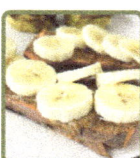
Sweet Grab & Go: Peanut Butter & Banana Sweet Potato Toast and Greek Yogurt

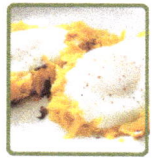
Savory Breakfast: Eggs in a Butternut Squash Nest

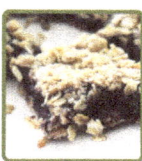
Sweet Breakfast: Blueberry Breakfast Bars & Glass of Milk

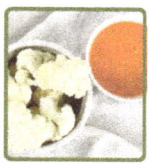
Savory Snack: Cauliflower With Buffalo Sauce

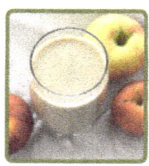
Sweet Snack: Apple Pie Smoothie

Winter/Spring Meal Plan: Week 1

30-Minute Meal 1

Coconut Cod & Spinach Over Coconut Rice

✓ Dairy-Free

Whole Meal Total Time: 25 Min | Prep Time: 10 Min | Cook Time: 10-15 Min

Recommended order of prep:
1. Make recipe for <u>Coconut Rice</u>.
2. While rice cooks, make recipe for <u>Coconut Cod & Spinach</u>.
3. Serve Coconut Cod & Spinach over Coconut Rice.

Pro Tip: Keep coconut milk, frozen cod fillets, and frozen spinach on hand to make this meal as a back-up option when you need something quick without going to the store.

Dietary Adjustments

Gluten-Free: Use gluten-free soy sauce or sub Tamari in Coconut Cod & Spinach.

Vegetarian / Vegan: Sub recipe for <u>Coconut Tofu & Spinach</u> in place of Coconut Cod & Spinach.

 Nutrition facts are available to download for each recipe. Scan the QR code or go to <u>TheBrainPlate.com/resources</u>

Coconut Cod & Spinach

Prep Time: 5 Min | Cook Time: 15 Min   Serves: 4

Ingredients

- 1 tbsp Fresh ginger (minced)
- 1 tbsp Coconut oil
- 1 3/4 cup Coconut milk (about 14.5 oz can)
- 3 tbsp Soy sauce (sub Tamari for gluten-free or coconut aminos for soy free)
- 2 tbsp Rice vinegar
- 1 1/2 lb Cod fillets
- 10 oz Spinach (fresh or frozen whole leaves; about 7–8 cups fresh leaves)

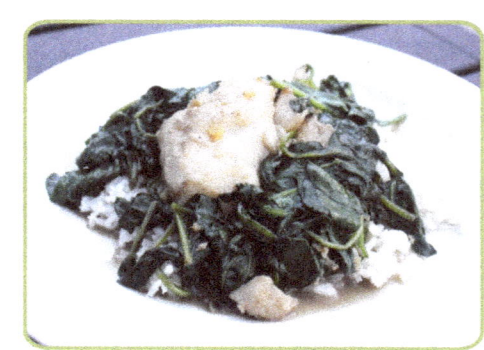

Instructions

1. Mince ginger and set aside. In a large sauté pan, melt coconut oil. Once hot, add ginger and cook about 30 seconds until fragrant, being careful not to overcook and burn ginger.
2. To the pan with ginger, add coconut milk, soy sauce, and rice vinegar. Stir to combine and bring to a boil, then reduce heat to a simmer. If time allows, simmer for 5–10 minutes to allow flavors to combine and to reduce liquid.
3. Add cod fillets to pan, making sure they are submerged under the sauce. Cook about 8 minutes to an internal temperature of 145° Fahrenheit, until flesh is opaque and flakes easily with a fork. Turn the fish once to ensure sauce evenly flavors the meat.
4. Remove fish from the sauce and set aside. Add whole spinach leaves to sauce, stirring them into sauce as they cook down. Once all spinach has been added, continue to cook 2–3 minutes until it has wilted, then remove from heat. Serve the fish and sauce over coconut rice.

Pro Tip: No rice vinegar on hand? Sub apple cider vinegar instead. Try this dish with baby Bok choy or broccolini in place of spinach for variety; cook an additional 2–3 minutes as these vegetables take longer to wilt.

Picky Eater Tips: Serve a small piece of cod plain without sauce, and offer a dip like ranch or ketchup for comfort. Serve spinach and sauce separately. Serve with "safe food" options such as plain rice, fruit, and a protein they like, such as string cheese.

Leftovers: Store in an airtight container for 3–5 days. Freeze for up to 1 month.

Coconut Rice

Prep Time: 5 Min | Cook Time: 25 Min   Serves: 4

Ingredients
- 1 cup Jasmine rice (dry, rinsed)
- 1 tbsp Coconut oil
- 2 cup Water
- 1/4 tsp Salt

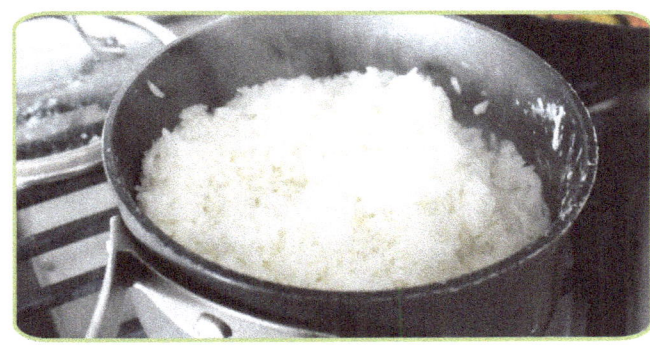

Instructions
1. Rinse jasmine rice and set aside: place rice in a large bowl and add water to completely submerge rice. Stir the rice around with your hand or a spoon, then drain it through a colander or mesh sieve. Repeat once or twice until water is clear when drained.
2. Melt coconut oil in a small saucepan over medium heat. Add jasmine rice and sauté 3–4 minutes, stirring frequently.
3. Add water and salt to saucepan with rice. Turn up heat to bring to a boil, then reduce heat, cover, and simmer 10–15 minutes until all water has been absorbed.
4. Turn off heat and let rice sit another 10 minutes, then fluff with a fork and serve.

Pro Tip: Use coconut milk instead of water for added flavor, fat, and calories. If you're missing a veggie in your meal, this a veggie side instead by substituting cauliflower rice in place of jasmine rice and water.

Picky Eater Tips: Coconut rice can be a great way to add fat and calories for picky eaters who enjoy it, especially if you make this with coconut milk instead of water. If coconut flavor is new, try mixing a bit of plain rice in to soften the taste and help with acceptance. Serve a second carbohydrate option if they don't like this, such as plain rice, bread, or crackers.

Leftovers: Refrigerate in an airtight container for up to 5 days, or freeze for up to 3 months.

Coconut Tofu & Spinach

Prep Time: 15 Min | Cook Time: 15 Min   Serves: 4

Ingredients

- 28 oz Extra firm tofu (about 2 packages; cut into 1-inch cubes, liquid pressed)
- 1 tbsp Fresh ginger (minced)
- 1 tbsp Coconut oil
- 1 3/4 cup Coconut milk (14.5 oz can)
- 3 tbsp Soy sauce (sub Tamari for gluten-free)
- 2 tbsp Rice vinegar
- 10 oz Spinach (fresh or frozen whole leaves; about 7–8 cups fresh leaves)

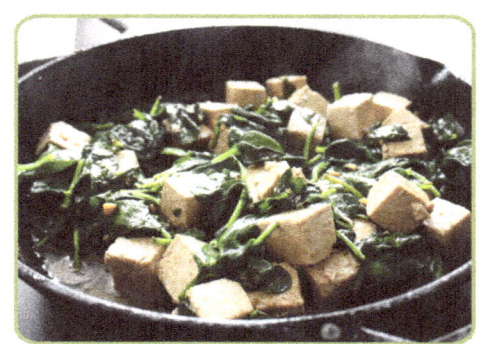

Instructions

1. Press liquid from tofu: drain liquid from tofu, cut into 1-inch cubes, and place between two clean towels. Using hands, press on tofu to remove as much liquid as possible.
2. Mince ginger and set aside. In a large sauté pan, melt coconut oil. Once hot, add ginger and cook about 30 seconds until fragrant, being careful not to overcook and burn ginger.
3. To the pan with ginger, add coconut milk, soy sauce, and rice vinegar. Stir to combine and bring to a boil, then reduce heat to a simmer. Add pressed tofu cubes and simmer 10–15 minutes to allow flavors to combine and to reduce liquid.
4. Add whole spinach leaves to sauce, stirring them into sauce as they cook down. Once all spinach has been added, continue to cook 2–3 minutes until wilted, then remove from heat. Serve tofu, spinach and sauce over coconut rice.

Pro Tip: No rice vinegar on hand? Sub apple cider vinegar instead. Cook tofu in sauce longer for a richer flavor or make coconut milk sauce and marinate tofu in it overnight.

Picky Eater Tips: For a texture variation, pan-fry a few tofu cubes and set aside apart from the sauce. Because tofu is very bland, it can be a good option for picky eaters. Set aside some plain, uncooked cubes to dip in the sauce or choose other sauce to serve, such as teriyaki or soy sauce. Offer spinach raw or sautéed on the side, and include a familiar carb like rice or bread, as well as fruit, if they don't eat the spinach.

Leftovers: Refrigerate in airtight container up to 5 days. Not recommended to freeze.

Winter/Spring Meal Plan: Week 1

30-Minute Meal 2

Springtime Greens & Grain Bowls With Easy Lemon Pepper Chicken

✓ Gluten-Free   ✓ Dairy-Free

Whole Meal Total Time: 30-35 Min | Prep Time: 20 Min | Cook Time: 10-15 Min

Recommended order of prep:
1. Make recipe for <u>Easy Lemon Pepper Chicken</u>.
2. While chicken cooks, make recipe for <u>Springtime Greens & Grains Bowls</u>.
3. Slice Lemon Pepper Chicken and serve on top of Greens & Grains Bowls.

Pro Tip: Try other types of protein to serve with this salad, such as shrimp, salmon, steak, or pan-fried tofu or tempeh. Substitute different types of greens as desired, such as spinach or romaine.

Dietary Adjustments

Vegetarian / Vegan: Sub recipe for <u>Crispy Pan-Fried Tempeh</u> in place of Easy Lemon Pepper Chicken.

Easy Lemon Pepper Chicken

Prep Time: 5 Min | Cook Time: 15 Min   Serves: 4

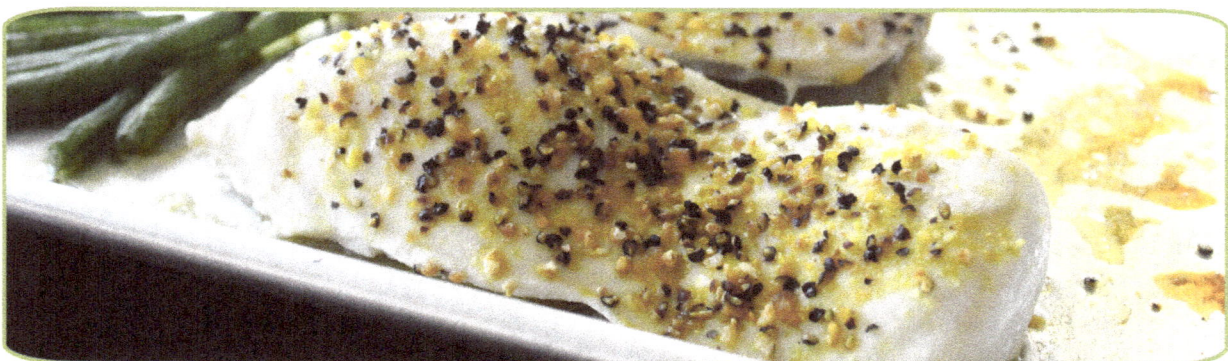

Ingredients
- 1 1/2 lb Boneless, skinless chicken thighs
- 2 tsp Lemon pepper
- 1/2 tsp Salt

Instructions
1. Preheat the oven to 400° Fahrenheit and prepare a baking sheet or baking dish by spraying with cooking spray.
2. Arrange chicken thighs on baking sheet, lying flat with space in between. Sprinkle chicken evenly with lemon pepper and salt.
3. Bake 15–20 minutes or until chicken reaches an internal temperature of 165° Fahrenheit.

<u>Pro Tip:</u> Squeeze a fresh lemon over chicken after removing from the oven for an additional burst of flavor. Use a food thermometer for perfectly cooked chicken. Add other seasonings for variety, such as oregano, basil, or additional lemon pepper.

<u>Picky Eater Tips:</u> Omit lemon pepper seasoning for a very plain version. Serve a very small amount on the plate of your picky eater. Offer the chicken with a variety of dipping sauces to add fun, such as ketchup, barbecue sauce, teriyaki sauce, honey mustard, etc. Pair with a safe food such as rice, bread, or fruit, and let your picky eater help plate the meal or choose their portion to reduce pressure.

<u>Leftovers:</u> Refrigerate in an airtight container up to 5 days. Freeze up to 3 months.

Springtime Greens & Grain Bowls

Prep Time: 15 Min | Cook Time: 15 Min   Serves: 4

Quinoa
- 1/2 cup Quinoa (uncooked)
- 1 cup Water
- 1/4 tsp Salt

Dressing
- 1/4 cup Lemon juice (1 medium lemon)
- 2 tbsp Extra virgin olive oil
- 1 tbsp Dijon mustard
- 1 1/2 tsp Sugar
- 1/2 tsp Salt

Salad
- 2 Carrots (medium, shredded)
- 3 1/2 cup Chickpeas (two 14.5 oz cans, drained and rinsed)
- 1 cup Strawberries (halved)
- 1 Avocado (large, cubed, or 2 small avocados)
- 4 cup Arugula (or other greens: baby kale, spinach, or lettuce of choice)

Instructions
1. Add quinoa, water, and salt for quinoa to a small saucepan. Bring to a boil, then reduce heat, cover, and simmer about 15 minutes until liquid has been absorbed. Turn off heat and allow to rest 5 minutes, then fluff with a fork.
2. While quinoa cooks, make dressing. In a separate small mixing bowl or jar add lemon juice, olive oil, Dijon mustard, sugar, and salt. Whisk or shake jar with lid until dressing is smooth and creamy. Set aside.
3. Prep salad components and set aside: peel and shred carrots using a box grater, drain and rinse chickpeas, slice strawberries, cube avocado, and wash arugula.
4. Assemble individual bowls, including 1/2 cup quinoa, 2/3 cup chickpeas, 1 cup arugula, 1/2 cup shredded carrot, 1/4 cup strawberries, 1/2 avocado. Toss with 2 tbsp dressing just before serving.

Pro Tip: Prep these bowls ahead of time into individual servings in mason jars, layering in jar in order: dressing, carrots, chickpeas, avocado, strawberries, cooled quinoa, and arugula. Refrigerate up to 5 days. Shake jar to distribute dressing and pour onto a plate to serve.

Picky Eater Tips: These bowls are easy to customize; let picky eaters choose the ingredients to make their own bowl. Keep greens and dressing separate. Add other familiar ingredient options like cheese, fruit, or rice to make it approachable.

Leftovers: Squeeze lime juice over avocado before storing to prevent from browning. Refrigerate assembled bowls in airtight container up to 3 days. Do not freeze.

Crispy Pan-Fried Tempeh

Prep Time: 20 Min | Cook Time: 10 Min   Serves: 4

Ingredients
- 16 oz Tempeh (cut into 1/2-inch by 3-inch pieces)
- 1 tbsp Canola oil

Marinade
- 1/4 cup Soy sauce (use gluten-free or sub Tamari for gluten-free)
- 1 tbsp Toasted sesame oil
- 1 tbsp Rice vinegar
- 1 tbsp Brown sugar
- 1 tsp Garlic powder

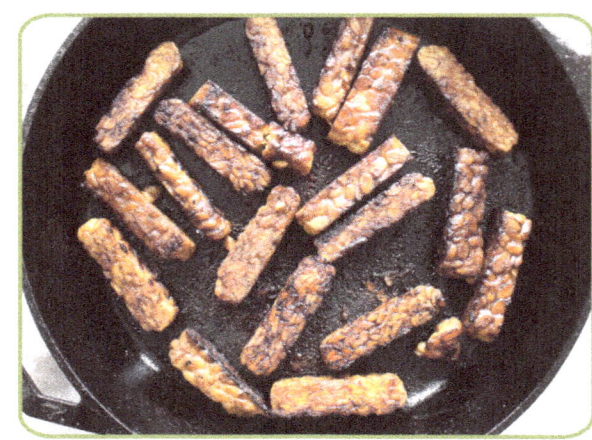

Instructions
1. Slice the tempeh block in half and then into 1/2-inch by 3-inch pieces.
2. In a shallow dish, mix together all marinade ingredients: soy sauce, sesame oil, rice vinegar, brown sugar, and garlic powder. Add tempeh pieces to marinade and turn several times to coat completely. Marinate for 20–30 minutes, or allow to marinate longer for several hours or overnight if possible.
3. For pan-frying: heat canola oil in a large skillet over medium heat. Add marinated tempeh and pan-fry for 10–15 minutes, flipping halfway through. Add remaining marinade at the end of cook time, simmering for 3–4 minutes to evaporate liquid.

Pro Tip: Try air-frying instead of pan-frying: preheat the air fryer to 380° Fahrenheit. Line the basket with parchment paper and cook tempeh for 10–13 minutes, flipping halfway through. If desired, serve tempeh over rice with stir-fry vegetables on the side instead of Greens & Grains Bowls.

Picky Eater Tips: Serve tempeh with a familiar dip like ketchup, barbecue sauce, or honey mustard. Cut it into small, bite-sized pieces for easier tasting. Let your picky eater help flip the pieces in the pan to increase familiarity and engagement. Offer other protein "safe food" options such as plain tofu, chickpeas, or string cheese.

Leftovers: Tempeh is best served fresh, but it can be refrigerated in an airtight container for up to 5 days. Cooked tempeh is not recommended to freeze.

Winter/Spring Meal Plan: Week 1

Slow-Cooker Meal

Spicy Lentil Chili With Crusty Bread

√ Gluten-Free   √ Dairy-Free   √ Vegetarian   √ Vegan

Whole Meal Total Time: 1–10 Hrs | Prep Time: 25–30 Min | Cook Time: 30 Min–10 Hrs

Recommended order of prep:
1. Choose the stovetop, slow cooker, or pressure cooker method in the recipe and make Spicy Lentil Chili.
2. Serve chili with your choice of bread and butter, such as French, sourdough, whole wheat, or breadsticks.

Pro Tip: This recipe works well to start in the slow cooker in the morning and allow to cook all day for a hot meal when you come home. Adjust the amount of chipotle peppers depending on your preferred spice level.

Dietary Adjustments

Gluten-Free: Serve Spicy Lentil Chili with gluten-free bread or crackers.

Spicy Lentil Chili

Prep Time: 30 Min | Cook Time: 30 Min (Stovetop) – 10 Hrs (Slow Cooker)   Serves: 6

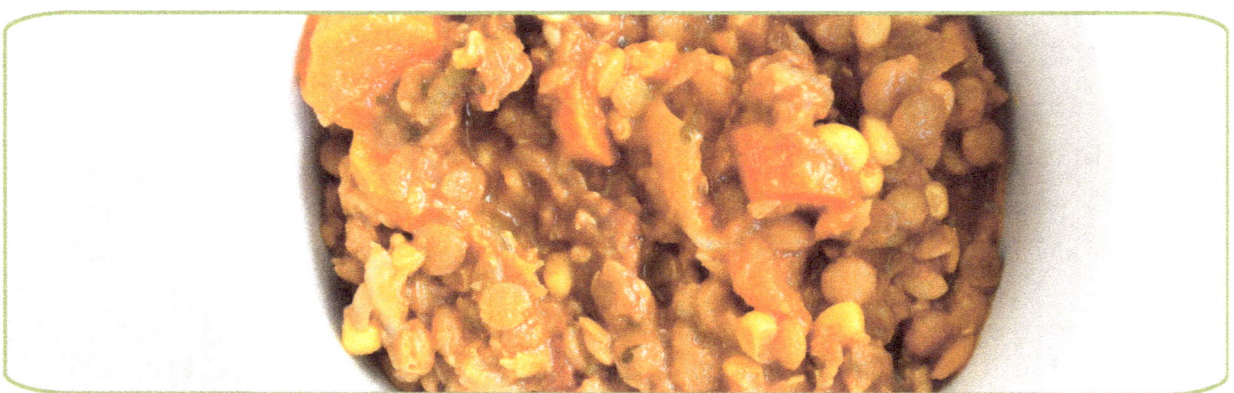

Ingredients

- 1 Yellow onion (medium; diced)
- 3 Carrots (cut into rounds; substitute diced green pepper or celery if desired)
- 3 clove Garlic (minced)
- 2 oz Chipotle peppers in adobo sauce (more for spicier chili; about 4 peppers)
- 2 tbsp Extra virgin olive oil
- 1 1/2 tsp Salt
- 1 tbsp Chili powder
- 2 tsp Cumin
- 1 tsp Paprika
- 1 tsp Oregano
- 1 tsp Cilantro
- 3 1/2 cup Diced tomatoes (two 14.5-oz cans)

- 1 3/4 cup Corn (14.5 oz can)
- 4 oz Diced green chiles
- 1 cup Dry brown lentils
- 4 cup Water (sub unsalted vegetable broth for additional flavor; add more water for a soup with thinner consistency or for longer cooking time)
- 1 tsp Apple cider vinegar (wait to add until finished cooking)
- Toppings for spicy lentil chili as desired: tortilla chips, shredded cheese, sour cream, avocado slices, pickled jalapeños, or fresh cilantro

Instructions

1. Dice onion, cut carrots into rounds, and mince garlic. Coarsely chop chipotle peppers into very small pieces. Wear gloves while handling peppers or wash hands with soap immediately after cutting; avoid touching eyes or other sensitive places.

Spicy Lentil Chili (Continued)

Instructions (Continued)

2. **Stovetop method:** Heat a large pot over medium heat. Once hot, add oil, onion, carrots, and garlic (wait to add chipotle peppers). Sauté until onion becomes translucent and carrots begins to soften, 8–10 minutes. Add salt and spices (chili powder, cumin, paprika, oregano, and cilantro) for the last 1–2 minutes of cooking to allow spices to "bloom" and become fragrant and flavorful. Add all remaining ingredients (including prepared chipotle peppers) to pot except vinegar and toppings. Stir to combine and bring to a boil, then reduce heat and simmer 45–60 minutes until lentils are tender. Cook longer to allow flavors to blend, adding more water if necessary due to evaporation.
3. **Slow cooker method:** Add all ingredients to a large slow cooker except vinegar and toppings. Cook on high 4–5 hours or on low 8–10 hours. The longer the cooking time, the better the flavor.
4. **Pressure cooker method:** Using sauté setting on electric pressure cooker add oil, onion, carrots, and garlic (wait to add chipotle peppers). Sauté until onion becomes translucent and carrots begins to soften, 8–10 minutes. Add salt and spices (chili powder, cumin, paprika, oregano, and cilantro) for the last 1–2 minutes of cooking to allow spices to "bloom" and become fragrant and flavorful. Add all remaining ingredients except vinegar and toppings. Cook at high pressure for 10 minutes, then do a quick release of pressure.
5. Stir in vinegar at the end of cooking time and serve with optional toppings: sour cream or plain Greek yogurt, sliced avocado, shredded cheese, pickled jalapeños, or fresh chopped cilantro.

Pro Tip: Store extra chipotle peppers in their original sauce in a sealed container in the refrigerator for several weeks or freeze up to several months. These add great flavor (and heat) to many Mexican dishes. If you have too many leftovers from this meal, freeze extra in individual portions for an easy meal in the future.

Picky Eater Tips: Omit chipotle peppers and sub mild diced green chilis for those sensitive to spicy food. Pull out components of the chili to serve separately to your picky eater, such as lentils, tomatoes, and carrots. Serve with crackers or bread as a familiar side, in addition to a protein they like, such as cheese or chickpeas.

Leftovers: This chili is even better the next day; refrigerate in an airtight container for up to 5–7 days. Freeze up to several months.

Winter/Spring Meal Plan: Week 1

Vegetarian Meal

Easy Pasta Primavera

✓ Vegetarian

Whole Meal Total Time: 30 Min | Prep Time: 10–15 Min | Cook Time: 15 Min

Recommended order of prep:
1. Follow recipe to make <u>Easy Pasta Primavera</u>.

Pro Tip: Add cooked shrimp for more protein and zinc. Use canola oil in place of butter in the recipe for more vitamin E and omega-3 fatty acids and omega-6 fatty acids . Sub different types of vegetables for variety; see "Pro Tip" in the recipe for inspiration.

Dietary Adjustments

Gluten-Free: Use gluten-free penne or rotini to make Easy Pasta Primavera.
Dairy-Free / Vegan: Sub vegan butter or canola oil in place of butter and sub nutritional yeast in place of Parmesan cheese in Easy Pasta Primavera.

Easy Pasta Primavera

Prep Time: 15 Min | Cook Time: 15 Min   Serves: 4

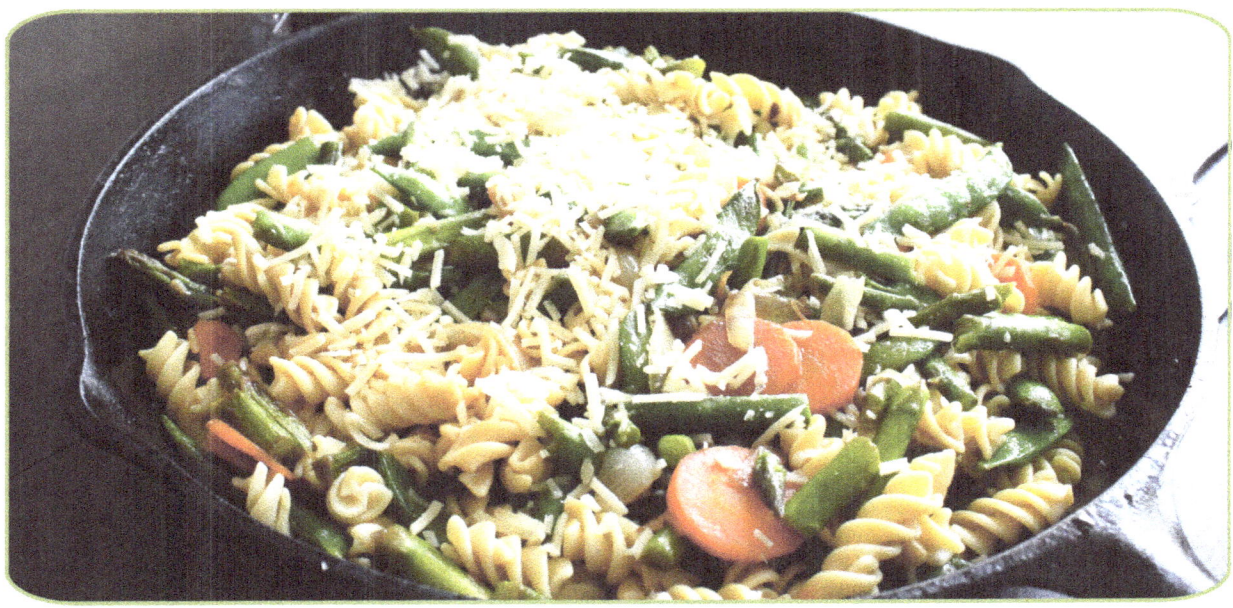

Ingredients
- 2 1/2 cup Whole wheat rotini (8 oz; use gluten-free pasta for gluten-free)

Vegetables
- 1 White onion (sliced)
- 2 clove Garlic (minced)
- 2 tbsp Unsalted butter (sub vegan butter or canola oil for dairy-free and vegan)
- 2 Carrots (cut into 1/4-inch rounds)
- 2 cup Asparagus (cut into 1-inch pieces)
- 2 cup Snap peas
- 1 3/4 cup Chickpeas (drained and rinsed; 14.5 oz can)
- 1/2 tsp Salt

White Wine Sauce
- 2 tbsp Unsalted butter (sub vegan butter or canola oil for dairy-free)
- 1/2 cup White wine
- 2 tbsp Lemon juice (fresh or bottled)
- 1/2 tsp Salt
- 1/8 tsp Red pepper flakes (optional, or to taste)

Serving Suggestion
- 1/2 cup Shredded Parmesan cheese (sub nutritional yeast to taste for dairy-free)

Easy Pasta Primavera (Continued)

Instructions

1. In a large saucepan, cook pasta al dente according to package instructions. Drain and set aside.
2. Slice onion and mince garlic. Add butter for vegetables to a large sauté pan and melt over medium heat. Add onion and garlic and begin to cook, stirring occasionally, about 8–10 minutes while preparing remaining ingredients.
3. Prep vegetables and chickpeas and add to sauté pan with onion and garlic as they are prepared: cut carrots into 1/4-inch rounds, snap asparagus into 1-inch pieces, wash snap peas, and drain and rinse chickpeas. Add salt to vegetables and stir to combine with onion; cook until just starting to soften, for 8–10 minutes.
4. After pasta has finished cooking and is draining in a colander, use the same saucepan as used to cook pasta, and make white wine sauce. Add butter and melt over medium heat, then add wine and simmer to reduce liquid, for about 3–4 minutes. Add lemon juice, salt for sauce, and red pepper flakes to saucepan. Stir to combine and simmer for 2–3 minutes.
5. Add pasta and white wine sauce to sauté pan with vegetables. Stir to evenly coat pasta and vegetables with sauce. Top with Parmesan cheese to serve.

Pro Tip: If cooking this out of season, use frozen asparagus or substitute other seasonal vegetables as desired, such as spinach, kale, radishes, yellow squash, peppers, zucchini, broccoli, or cherry tomatoes. Add cooked chicken, shrimp, or tofu cubes for additional protein.

Picky Eater Tips: Set aside a small amount of vegetables, pasta, and sauce separately to serve individually. Substitute or add veggies you know your picky eater likes. Give the option to try the dish as a whole. Let them sprinkle Parmesan cheese over their dish to give them some autonomy.

Leftovers: Refrigerate in an airtight container up to 5 days. Not recommended to freeze.

Winter/Spring Meal Plan: Week 1

"Challenge" Meal

Oven Baked Pork Chops With Buttery Potatoes & Roasted Brussels Sprouts

√ Gluten-Free

Whole Meal Total Time: 40–50 Min | Prep Time: 30 Min | Cook Time: 15–20 Min

Recommended order of prep:
1. Make recipe for <u>Roasted Brussels Sprouts</u>.
2. Make recipe for <u>Buttery Potatoes</u>.
3. While potatoes and sprouts cook, make recipe for <u>Oven Baked Pork Chops</u>.
4. Serve pork chops with potatoes and Brussels sprouts on the side.

Pro Tip: For easier prep, use frozen Brussels sprouts instead of fresh. Cook at 450° Fahrenheit for 20–25 minutes to make them more crispy.

Dietary Adjustments

Dairy-Free: Use vegan butter or olive oil to make Buttery Potatoes.
Vegetarian: Sub recipe for <u>Rosemary Parmesan Twice-Baked Potato</u> in place of Oven Baked Pork Chops and Buttery Potatoes; top with <u>Crispy Roasted Chickpeas</u> to serve.
Vegan: Sub recipe for <u>Rosemary Parmesan Twice-Baked Potato</u> in place of Oven Baked Pork Chops and Buttery Potatoes and use nutritional yeast instead of Parmesan cheese; top with <u>Crispy Roasted Chickpeas</u> to serve.

Crispy Roasted Brussels Sprouts

Prep Time: 10 Min | Cook Time: 25 Min   Serves: 4

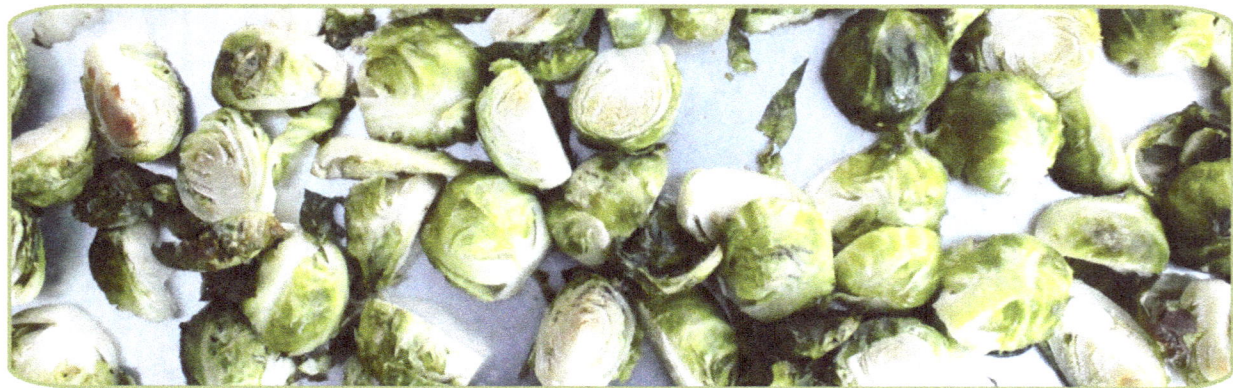

Ingredients
- 4 cup Brussels sprouts (trimmed and cut into halves or quarters)
- 2 tbsp Extra virgin olive oil
- 1/2 tsp Coarsely ground salt

Instructions
1. Preheat the oven to 400° Fahrenheit.
2. Trim Brussels sprouts and cut into approximately the same-sized pieces: in halves, quarters, or leave whole if very small. Spread on a large roasting pan and toss with oil and salt. Arrange sprouts no more than one layer thick on pan.
3. Roast sprouts for 25–30 minutes. Sprouts are done when they are soft enough to pierce with a fork and leaves are starting to char.

Pro Tip: Use this same method of preparation, but grill in a grill basket or sauté in cast iron skillet for variety.

Picky Eater Tips: Offer a small portion of Brussels sprouts roasted until crispy, or try raw shavings if they prefer crunchy textures. Serve with a dip such as ranch or ketchup for familiarity. Add in play to your meal by pretending the sprouts are their favorite type of sports ball or by serving only green food at the meal.

Leftovers: Refrigerate in an airtight container 3–5 days. Reheat in the oven, a skillet, or an air fryer to maintain crispiness. Do not freeze.

Buttery Potatoes

Prep Time: 10 Min | Cook Time: 20 Min   Serves: 4

Ingredients
- 4 Red potatoes (medium, cut into 1-inch cubes)
- 6 cup Water (or more; enough to submerge potatoes)
- 2 tbsp Unsalted butter (use dairy-free spreadable butter for vegan)
- 1/2 tsp Salt

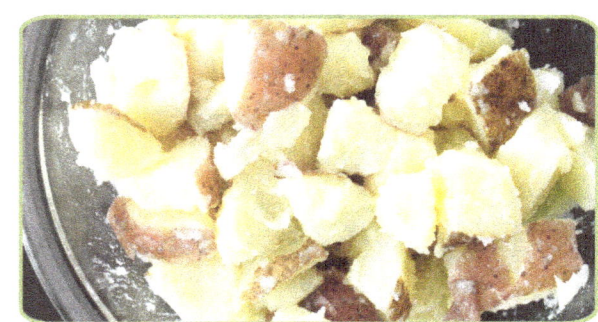

Instructions
1. Scrub potatoes but do not peel. Cut into roughly 1-inch cubes and add to a large saucepan or medium pot.
2. Fill saucepan with water until water just covers potatoes. Cover the pan with a lid and heat on high to bring to a boil, then reduce heat and simmer 20–30 minutes until potatoes are soft enough to insert a fork. Cook longer for a more creamy texture, boiling potatoes until they start to easily fall apart.
3. Drain water from potatoes using a colander or with the lid of the pot. Transfer to serving dish and add butter and salt. Allow butter to melt, then gently stir to evenly coat potatoes with butter.

Pro Tip: For variety, try adding chives, rosemary, or basil to potatoes when adding butter and salt.

Picky Eater Tips: If your picky eater likes potatoes, these can be a good way to introduce other flavors or textures by adding seasonings or mashing them smoother or coarser. Add protein by stirring in a small amount of plain Greek yogurt or topping with cheese. Let your picky eater add salt or butter at the table to give them more autonomy.

Leftovers: Refrigerate in an airtight container up to 5 days. Freeze for 1–2 months. If frozen potatoes are dry, add a small amount of water in dish when reheating.

Oven Baked Pork Chops

Prep Time: 5 Min | Cook Time: 15 Min   Serves: 4

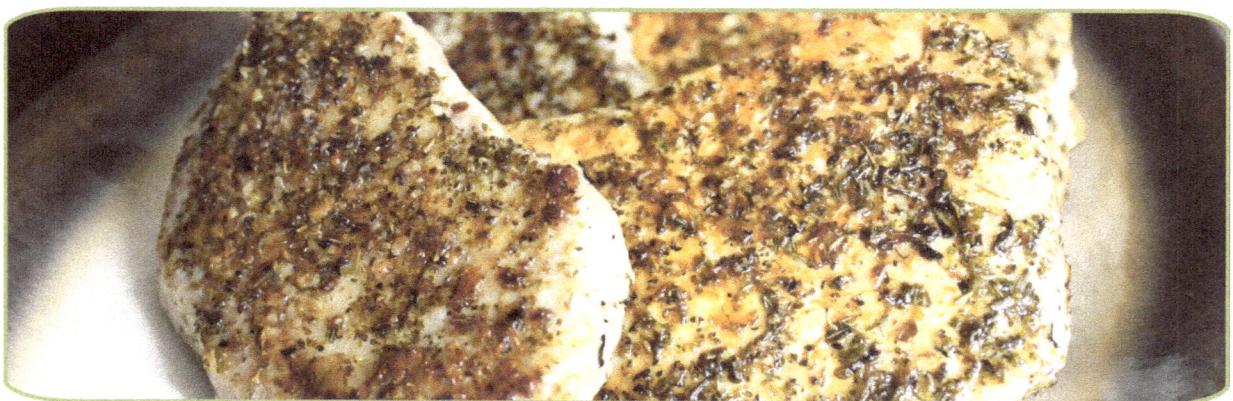

Ingredients
- 1 tbsp Canola oil
- 1 1/2 lb Pork chops (boneless)
- 1 tsp Oregano
- 1 tsp Dried basil
- 1/4 tsp Dried thyme
- 1/2 tsp Salt

Instructions
1. Preheat oven to 400° Fahrenheit. Spread oil on a large baking sheet to coat.
2. Arrange pork chops on the greased baking sheet and evenly coat with oregano, basil, thyme, and salt.
3. Place pork chops in the oven and cook for 15–20 minutes to an internal temperature of 145° Fahrenheit.

Pro Tip: Use a pre-blended pork seasoning or Italian seasoning instead of mixing herbs for an even quicker and easier meal. Instead cooking in the oven, try pan-frying or grilling at 400–450° Fahrenheit for 3–4 minutes per side. Use a food thermometer to make sure not to overcook, or meat will be very tough.

Picky Eater Tips: Set aside a small portion of pork to serve plain, with the option for your picky eater to add the seasoning at the table. Offer a dipping option like barbecue sauce or honey mustard on the side, and include an alternative "safe" protein your picky eater likes, such as string cheese or chicken.

Leftovers: Refrigerate in an airtight container for 3–5 days. Freeze for up to a month.

Rosemary Parmesan Twice-Baked Potato

Prep Time: 5 Min | Cook Time: 45 Min   Serves: 4

Ingredients
- 4 Russet potatoes (large)
- 1/4 cup Extra virgin olive oil (divided)
- 1 tsp Dried rosemary
- 1/2 tsp Coarsely ground salt
- 1/2 tsp Black pepper
- 1 cup Shredded Parmesan cheese (sub nutritional yeast to taste for dairy-free and vegan)

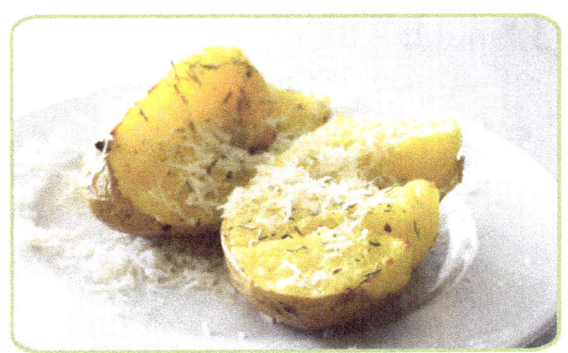

Instructions
1. Preheat oven to 400° Fahrenheit. Scrub potatoes and pierce all over with a fork. Place in a baking dish and bake 30–35 minutes until starting to soften.
2. Remove potatoes from the oven and cut lengthwise in half. Open potatoes and drizzle half of olive oil evenly over each of them. Sprinkle with rosemary, salt, and pepper and return to oven.
3. Return potatoes to oven and roast for another 10–15 minutes until starting to brown and very soft. Remove from oven and drizzle with remaining oil and sprinkle with Parmesan cheese.

Pro Tip: To make this a one-dish meal, additionally top potato with chickpeas before toasting, then add diced tomatoes and chopped spinach before serving. For a quick meal with minimal prep time, bake potatoes ahead of time, then refrigerate until ready to eat. When ready to eat, start at step 2 to finish the potatoes.

Picky Eater Tips: Serve the baked potato plain and allow your picky eaters to sprinkle on rosemary and Parmesan cheese. Offer additional toppings and/or sauces your picky eater likes, such as other types of cheese, salsa, ketchup, or barbecue sauce.

Leftovers: Refrigerate in an airtight container up to 5 days. Do not freeze.

Crispy Roasted Chickpeas

Prep Time: 5 Min | Cook Time: 30 Min   Serves: 4

Ingredients
- 1 3/4 cup Chickpeas (14.5 oz can, drained and rinsed)
- 1 tbsp Extra virgin olive oil
- 1/4 tsp Seasoned salt

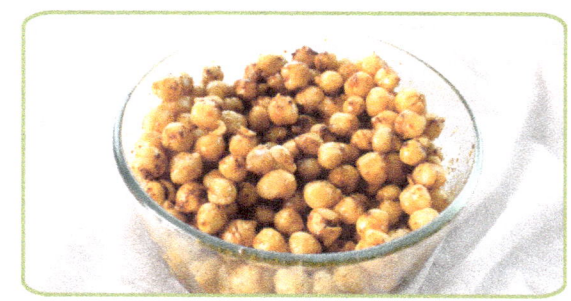

Instructions
1. Preheat oven to 400° Fahrenheit. Drain and rinse chickpeas.
2. Add chickpeas to a baking sheet and toss with oil and salt. Spread evenly across pan, ensuring no overlap.
3. Bake 25–30 minutes, tossing halfway through. For crispier chickpeas, bake longer. Taste one of the chickpeas, and if it's not crispy enough, return chickpeas to the oven for another 5–10 minutes.

Pro Tip: In place of seasoning salt, make your own salt blend: salt + garlic + paprika | salt + oregano + basil | salt + cumin + chili powder. Instead, substitute a different seasoning blend or packet, such as taco seasoning or a ranch seasoning packet.

Picky Eater Tips: Let your picky eater choose their favorite seasoning blend to add to these chickpeas instead of the seasoning mix in the recipe; try taco or ranch to start. Serve a dip with these, like ranch or hummus, for added flavor and familiarity. If your picky eater likes these, they can be a great high-protein alternative to chips or an addition to other recipes.

Leftovers: Allow chickpeas to cool before storing in an airtight container in the refrigerator up to 5 days, or store in airtight container at room temperature 2–3 days. For crispy leftover chickpeas, reheat in oven or toaster oven 5–10 minutes before eating. These are not recommended to freeze.

Winter/Spring Meal Plan: Week 1

Savory Grab & Go

Salmon Stuffed Avocado Boats With Crackers

✓ Dairy-Free

Dietary Adjustments

Gluten-Free: Use gluten-free crackers to serve with Salmon Stuffed Avocado Boats.

Vegetarian / Vegan: Sub recipe for <u>Hummus Stuffed Avocado Boats</u> in place of Salmon Stuffed Avocado Boats.

Sweet Grab & Go

Peanut Butter & Banana Sweet Potato Toast and Flavored Greek Yogurt

✓ Gluten-Free   ✓ Vegetarian

Dietary Adjustments

Dairy-Free / Vegan: Sub soy or coconut yogurt in place of Flavored Greek Yogurt.

Salmon Stuffed Avocado Boats With Crackers

Prep Time: 10 Min | Cook Time: 0 Min   Serves: 1

Ingredients

- 1 Avocado
- 3 oz Canned wild salmon (or salmon in packets)
- 1/2 tsp Lemon juice (use freshly squeezed lemon juice for better flavor)
- 1/8 tsp Salt
- 1/8 tsp Red pepper flakes
- 1 oz Whole wheat crackers (see package for serving size; sub gluten-free crackers for gluten-free)

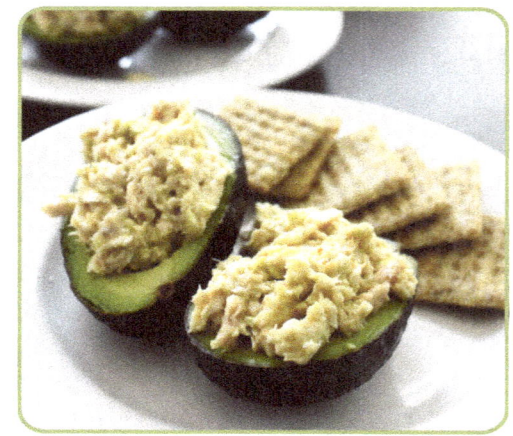

Instructions

1. Slice the avocado in half and remove the pit. Use a spoon to scoop out enough avocado to create a bigger hole that the salmon will fit into. Transfer scooped out avocado to a small bowl.
2. Drain the salmon and add it to the bowl with the scooped out avocado. Add lemon juice, salt, and red pepper flakes and mash until well mixed
3. Fill the hollowed-out avocado halves with the mashed salmon mixture. Scoop out avocado flesh and serve immediately on crackers to prevent avocado from browning.

Pro Tip: Instead of serving in the avocado shell, scoop out all flesh and combine with salmon; serve on crackers or bread as a sandwich. Add a bit of your favorite hot sauce to spice up this recipe. Choose wild-caught salmon instead of farmed for higher vitamin D content.

Picky Eater Tips: Serve salmon, avocado, and crackers separately and let your picky eaters choose what they want. Offer a very small portion of each, especially if foods are new to them. Offer a favorite dressing or sauce to top these, such as ranch dressing. Serve "safe food" options, such as tortilla chips, cheese, or fruit.

Leftovers: Mix up salmon stuffing and refrigerate in airtight container up to 5 days. Leave avocado whole until ready to eat or sprinkle extra lemon juice over avocado half and refrigerate in airtight container up to 2 days.

Hummus Stuffed Avocado Boats With Crackers

Prep Time: 10 Min | Cook Time: 0 Min   Serves: 1

Ingredients

- 1 Avocado
- 1/4 Lemon (juiced; optional)
- 1/4 cup Hummus
- 1 oz Whole wheat crackers (see package for serving size; sub gluten-free crackers for gluten-free)

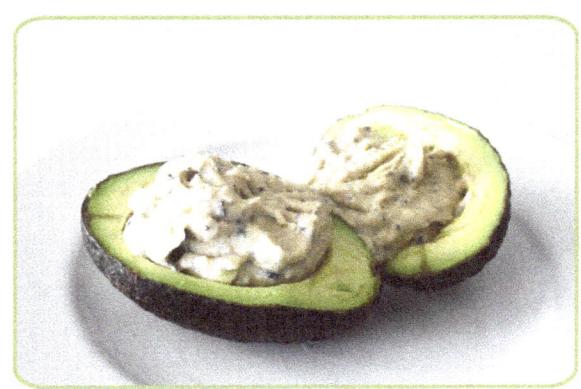

Instructions

1. Slice the avocado in half and remove the pit. Use a spoon to scoop out enough avocado to create a bigger hole that the hummus will fit into. Transfer scooped out avocado to a small bowl.
2. Add hummus to the bowl with the scooped out avocado and mash with a fork until combined.
3. Fill the hollowed-out avocado halves with the hummus mixture. If desired, squeeze lemon juice over top. Scoop out avocado flesh and serve with hummus on top of crackers.

Pro Tip: No time to prep these? Take the ingredients with you and make them when you're ready to eat, such as when you're on your work break at lunch or at the park with your kids. Add a bit of your favorite hot sauce to spice up this recipe.

Picky Eater Tips: Serve hummus, avocado, and crackers separately and let your picky eaters choose what they want. Offer a very small portion of each, especially if foods are new to them. Offer a favorite dressing or sauce to top these, such as ranch dressing. Serve "safe food" options, such as tortilla chips, cheese, or fruit.

Leftovers: Leave avocado whole until ready to eat or sprinkle extra lemon juice over avocado half and refrigerate in airtight container up to 2 days.

Peanut Butter & Banana Sweet Potato Toast

Prep Time: 5 Min | Cook Time: 10 Min   Serves: 2

Ingredients
- 1 Sweet potato (large)
- 2 tbsp All-natural peanut butter
- 2 tbsp Hemp seeds
- 1/4 tsp Cinnamon
- 1 Banana (sliced)

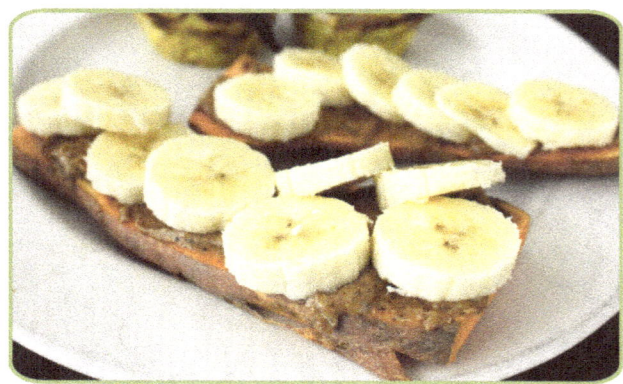

Instructions
1. Trim the ends of sweet potato and discard. Lay potato on its side and cut it lengthwise into 1/4-inch slices.
2. Place sweet potato slices into a toaster or toaster oven and toast for 10–15 minutes until soft and starting to brown. Alternatively, you can broil sweet potato slices in oven 3–6 minutes per side.
3. Use a butter knife to spread peanut butter evenly on toasted sweet potato. Sprinkle hemp seeds and cinnamon evenly over peanut butter, then top with sliced banana. Serve warm.

Pro Tip: Substitute peanut butter for any nut or seed butter. Instead of a banana, try sliced strawberries or mango for variety. Add a drizzle of honey or use cinnamon sugar in place of cinnamon for additional sweetness.

Picky Eater Tips: Offer each component separately and let your picky eater build their own stacked toast: banana slices, sweet potatoes, and peanut butter. Cutting the potatoes or bananas into fun shapes or adding a drizzle of honey or sprinkles on top can help make it more exciting and appealing.

Leftovers: These are best enjoyed fresh. If desired, prep and cook sweet potato in advance and refrigerate in airtight container up to 5 days, then reheat potato and make recipe as instructed to reduce prep time day of eating.

Winter/Spring Meal Plan: Week 1

Savory Breakfast

Eggs in a Butternut Squash Nest

✓ Gluten-Free   ✓ Dairy-Free   ✓ Vegetarian

Dietary Adjustments

Vegan: Sub a slice of medium tofu in place of egg in Eggs in a Butternut Squash Nest.

Sweet Breakfast

Blueberry Breakfast Bars & Glass of Milk

✓ Dairy-Free   ✓ Vegetarian   ✓ Vegan

Dietary Adjustments

Gluten-Free: Use gluten-free oats and all-purpose gluten-free flour blend to make Blueberry Breakfast Bars.

Dairy-Free / Vegan: Choose high protein non-dairy milk to enjoy with Blueberry Breakfast Bars, such as soy or pea.

Eggs in a Butternut Squash Nest

Prep Time: 15 Min | Cook Time: 20 Min   Serves: 4

Ingredients

- 1/2 Medium butternut squash (peeled and seeded, then grated or spiralized; about 4 cups shredded squash)
- 2 tbsp Coconut oil
- 8 Eggs (sub a slice of medium tofu for vegan option)
- 1/4 tsp Salt
- 1/4 tsp Black pepper

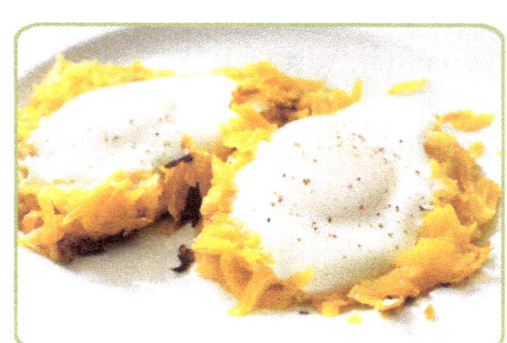

Instructions

1. Peel and seed butternut squash, then use a box grater or spiralizer to grate butternut squash. Set aside.
2. Heat a large skillet over medium heat. Once hot, add half of the coconut oil. Use about 1/2 cup of butternut squash shreds to form a round "nest" with a small well in the center. Crack an egg into the well in the butternut squash nest and season evenly with salt and pepper. Repeat this process to form 4 "nests" with eggs.
3. Place a lid over the skillet and cook 8–10 minutes until eggs are cooked to desired consistency. Once cooked, remove egg nests from skillet and set aside; cover them with a towel to keep them warm. Repeat step 2 to make 4 additional egg "nests."

Pro Tip: For easier prep, use pre-cut butternut squash; sauté squash and serve fried eggs on the side. For a variation on this dish, sub white potatoes, sweet potatoes, beets, or zucchini instead of butternut. With the remaining half of butternut squash, grate the rest and freeze, or cut it into cubes and refrigerate in an airtight container up to 5 days, then roast or grill at 400° Fahrenheit for 15–20 minutes for a side dish.

Picky Eater Tips: Serve the egg and butternut squash separately, especially if these are new foods. Make the egg how your picky eater prefers it – scrambled or hard-boiled instead of fried. Let your picky eater help grate the butternut squash or crack the eggs for more hands-on exposure. Serve a "safe food" alongside this breakfast, such as toast, cottage cheese, or fruit.

Leftovers: Store in an airtight container for 2–3 days in refrigerator. If storing as leftovers, cook egg yolk completely. Do not freeze.

Blueberry Breakfast Bars

Prep Time: 10 Min | Cook Time: 20 Min   Serves: 9

Crumb Crust
- 1/2 cup Flour (sub all-purpose gluten-free flour blend for gluten-free)
- 1/2 cup Slivered almonds
- 1/3 cup Hemp seeds
- 1/3 cup Dark brown sugar
- 2 tsp Cinnamon
- 1/3 cup Coconut oil (softened; sub butter if desired)

Crumb Crust (continued)
- 1 cup Old-fashioned oats

Blueberry Filling
- 2 cup Blueberries (fresh or frozen, thawed)
- 1/3 cup Sugar
- 1/3 cup Chia seeds
- 3 tbsp Lemon juice

Instructions
1. Preheat the oven to 400° Fahrenheit. Prepare an 8x8-inch (or 9x9-inch) baking dish by spraying it with cooking spray.
2. To a medium-sized mixing bowl, add oats, flour, slivered almonds, brown sugar, hemp seeds, and cinnamon; stir to combine. Using a fork or pastry cutter, cut coconut oil into dry ingredients, mixing until small clumps form. Firmly press half of the oat mixture into a thin even layer in prepared baking pan.
3. In a separate small mixing bowl, mix together blueberries, sugar, chia seeds, and lemon juice. Use a potato masher, hand mixer, or food processor to smash blueberries and mix until completely combined. Set aside.
4. Spread the blueberry mixture evenly on top of bottom crust, then crumble remaining oat mixture over top of the blueberry layer. Bake for 18–20 minutes, or until golden brown and bubbly.

Pro Tip: For a variation, substitute all or half the blueberries with another fruit, such as peaches, strawberries, raspberries, or blackberries.

Picky Eater Tips: Let your picky eater help make these bars by measuring ingredients, stirring, or pouring into the baking dish. Let them help decide how to cut the bars and choose additional toppings, such as whipped cream, ice cream, sprinkles, extra blueberries, or nuts. Try their favorite fruit instead of blueberries.

Leftovers: Store in airtight container at room temperature 3–5 days. Refrigerate in an airtight container 5–7 days. Freeze up to 2–3 months.

Winter/Spring Meal Plan: Week 1

Savory Snack

Cauliflower With Buffalo Sauce Dip

✓ Gluten-Free   ✓ Dairy-Free   ✓ Vegetarian   ✓ Vegan

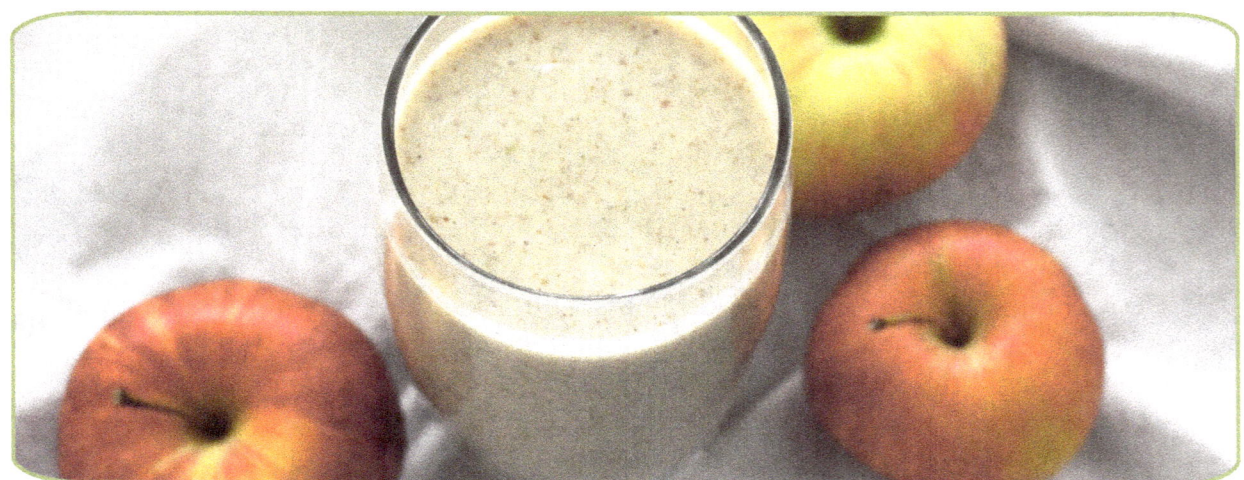

Sweet Snack

Apple Pie Smoothie

✓ Gluten-Free   ✓ Vegetarian

Dietary Adjustments

Dairy-Free: Use soy yogurt to make Apple Pie Smoothie.
Vegan: Use soy yogurt to make Apple Pie Smoothie.

Cauliflower With Buffalo Sauce Dip

Prep Time: 10 Min | Cook Time: 0 Min   Serves: 1

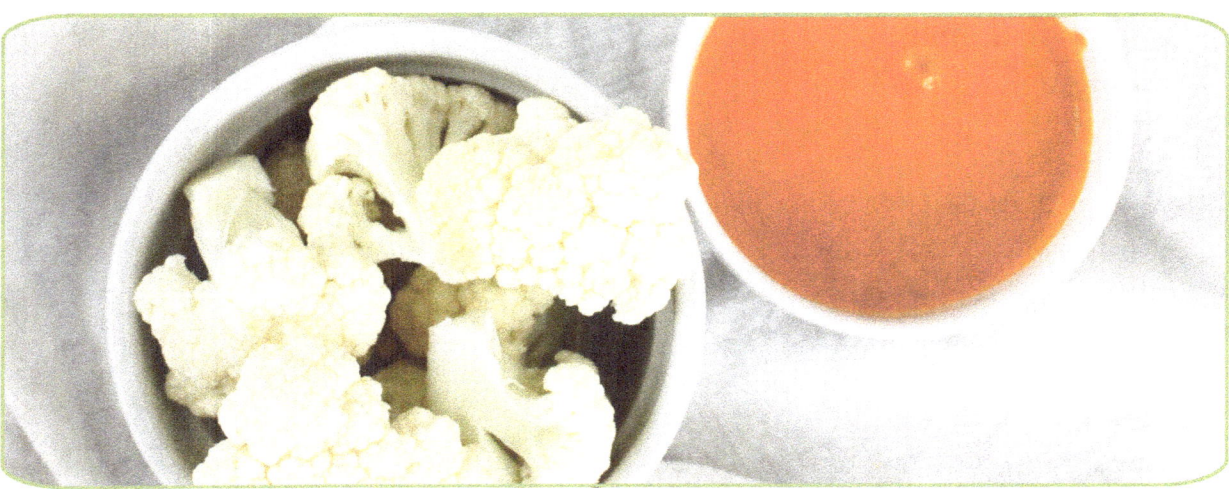

Ingredients
- 1/4 head Cauliflower (cut into florets)
- 2 tbsp Buffalo sauce

Instructions
1. Cut cauliflower into bite-sized florets. Serve with buffalo sauce to dip.

Pro Tip: Substitute your favorite dip for variety: salad dressing, oil & vinegar, or plain Greek yogurt + Ranch seasoning packet.

Picky Eater Tips: Offer a milder dip like ranch or yogurt in addition to buffalo sauce. Roast the cauliflower to bring out a sweeter flavor. Serve other options to dip to let your picky eater choose what they like, such as celery, carrots, crackers, or chips.

Leftovers: Store cut cauliflower in airtight container up to a week. Brown spots can be cut off cauliflower and discarded; the rest of the vegetable is still safe to eat.

Apple Pie Smoothie

Prep Time: 10 Min | Cook Time: 0 Min   Serves: 1

Ingredients
- 1 Granny Smith apple (medium; peel for less chewy texture)
- 1/2 cup Plain Greek yogurt (sub soy or coconut yogurt for dairy-free; sub vanilla Greek yogurt for added sweetness)
- 1 tbsp Ground flaxseed
- 3/4 cup Unsweetened soy milk (can sub other type of milk if desired)
- 1 tsp Vanilla extract
- 1 tsp Cinnamon (ground)
- 1/2 tsp Nutmeg
- 1 tsp Maple syrup

Instructions
1. Dice apple and add to a high-speed blender along with all remaining ingredients in the order listed in recipe. Blend until smooth. Sprinkle smoothie with extra cinnamon to serve, if desired.

Pro Tip: Substitute other types of apples if desired. Use hemp seeds instead of flaxseed or add a scoop of your favorite vanilla protein powder for a higher protein option. If using sweetened protein powder, omit maple syrup. Leaving the peel on the apple will increase the fiber, but the texture of the smoothie will be more chewy, especially if using a lower-quality blender.

Picky Eater Tips: Smoothies are great for picky eaters because they're easy to customize: let your picky eater choose the type of apple, how much cinnamon and nutmeg to add, and add more maple syrup if desired. Set aside some apple slices separately. Let your picky eater help make the smoothie by measuring ingredients and pressing the button on the blender. Offer a small portion to taste in a fun cup or using a silly straw. Alternatively, try serving a smoothie bowl with toppings they can add, like granola, chocolate chips, or cinnamon.

Leftovers: Refrigerate in an airtight container for 2–3 days; add more milk and blend again before serving if too thick. The texture is best if it's blended immediately before drinking. Freeze leftovers in popsicle molds to enjoy, or freeze in an ice cube tray to blend with milk and make another smoothie.

Winter/Spring Meal Plan: Week 2

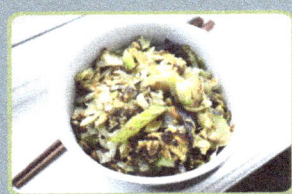
30-Minute Meal 1: Egg Roll Bowls With White Rice

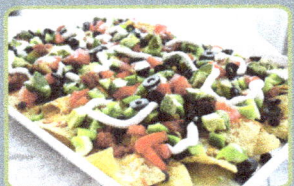
30-Minute Meal 2: Loaded Nachos

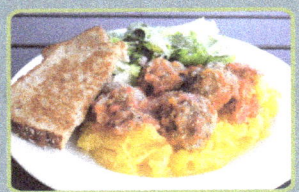
Slow-Cooker: Spaghetti Squash & Meatballs With Garlic Bread

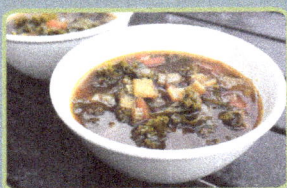
Vegetarian: Spicy Cajun Black Bean Soup and Corn Bread

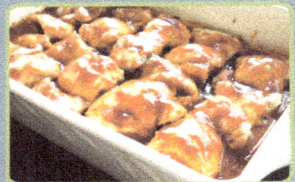
Challenge: Barbecue Chicken Thighs, Baked French Fries, and Garlicky Roasted Green Beans

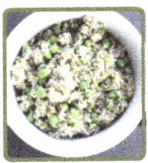
Savory Grab & Go: Pesto Tuna & Green Pea Quinoa Bowls

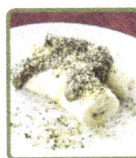
Sweet Grab & Go: Sunflower Banana Boat and Edamame With Salt

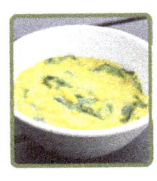
Savory Breakfast: Savory Golden Oats

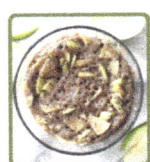
Sweet Breakfast: Microwave Apple Spice Cake

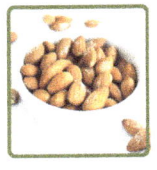
Savory Snack: Salt & Vinegar Almonds

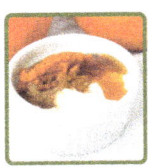
Sweet Snack: Pumpkin Yogurt

Winter/Spring Meal Plan: Week 2

30-Minute Meal 1

Egg Roll Bowls With White Rice

✓ Gluten-Free   ✓ Dairy-Free   ✓ Vegetarian

Whole Meal Total Time: 30 Min | Prep Time: 15–20 Min | Cook Time: 10–15 Min

Recommended order of prep:
1. Make recipe for <u>White Rice</u>.
2. While rice cooks, make recipe for <u>Egg Roll Bowls</u>.

Pro Tip: This recipe is extremely versatile and works great to use up different veggies such as zucchini, peppers, bean sprouts, or spinach. Try various proteins in addition to or as a substitute for eggs, such as shrimp, chicken, pork, steak, or tofu. Instead of rice, serve with pre-made wontons or potstickers for variety and extra protein.

Dietary Adjustments

Gluten-Free: Use gluten-free soy sauce or sub tamari in Egg Roll Bolls.
Vegan: Sub firm tofu in place of eggs for Egg Roll Bowls: drain liquid from tofu and stir with a fork until texture resembles scrambled egg pieces.

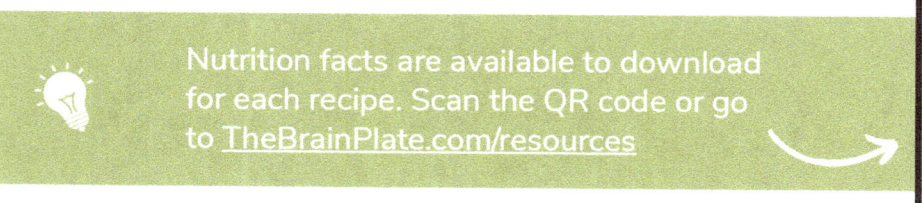

Nutrition facts are available to download for each recipe. Scan the QR code or go to TheBrainPlate.com/resources

White Rice

Prep Time: 5 Min | Cook Time: 20 Min   Serves: 4

Ingredients
- 1 cup Long grain white rice
- 2 cup Water
- 1/2 tsp Salt

Instructions
1. Rinse rice; place white rice in a large bowl and add water to completely submerge rice. Stir the rice around with your hand or a spoon, then drain it through a colander or mesh sieve. Repeat once or twice until water is clear when drained.
2. Add rice, water, and salt to small saucepan. Cover with a lid and turn up heat to bring to a boil, then reduce heat to low and simmer 15–18 minutes until all water has been absorbed.
3. Turn off heat and let rice sit another 10 minutes, then fluff with a fork and serve.

Pro Tip: For more tender rice, add 1/4 cup water for each cup of rice. For chewier rice, reduce water by 1/4 cup for each cup of rice. Don't blend different types of rice because they cook at different rates and will not cook evenly.

Picky Eater Tips: Use a rice variety your picky eater already likes and serve it plain or with a small amount of butter or salt for added flavor. Offer sauces they can choose from, like soy sauce, teriyaki sauce, or orange sauce. Let them scoop their own rice to feel more in control and comfortable.

Leftovers: Refrigerate in an airtight container for up to 5 days, or freeze for up to 3 months.

Egg Roll Bowls

Prep Time: 15 Min | Cook Time: 15 Min   Serves: 4

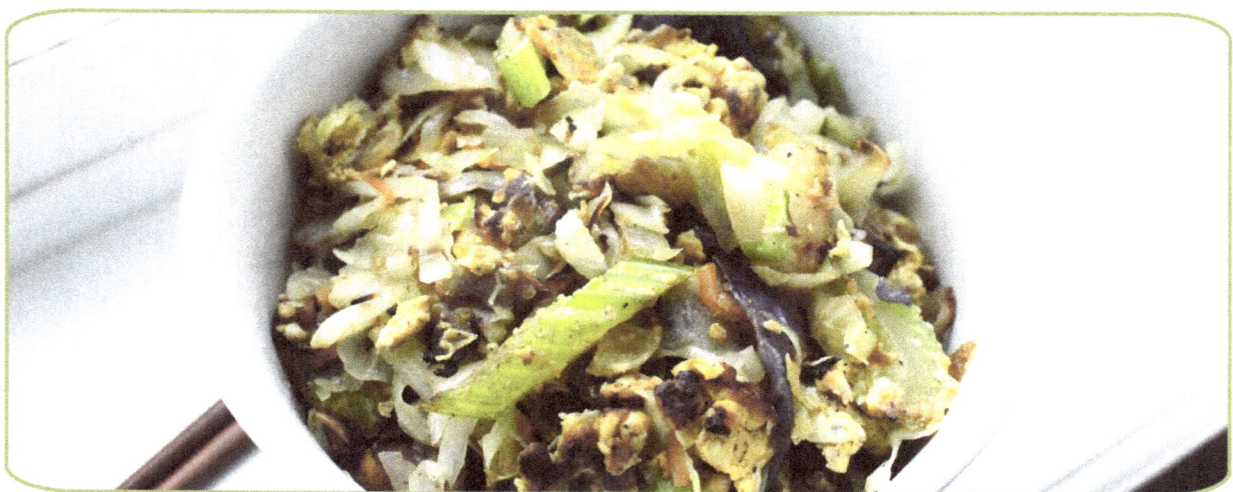

Ingredients

- 3 stalk Celery (sliced on the diagonal; substitute green onion if desired)
- 1 White onion (diced)
- 4 clove Garlic (minced)
- 1 tbsp Fresh ginger (peeled and minced)
- 6 cup Coleslaw mix (12–14 oz package; sub fresh shredded cabbage if desired)
- 2 Carrots (sliced on the diagonal; sub canned or fresh bean sprouts if desired)
- 8 Eggs (sub crumbled extra firm tofu for vegan)
- 1/4 cup Canola oil (divided)
- 3 tbsp Soy sauce (use gluten-free or sub Tamari for gluten-free; sub coconut aminos for soy-free)
- 3 tbsp Rice vinegar
- 1 tbsp Sugar (omit if using coconut aminos)

Instructions

1. Prepare vegetables ahead of starting to cook this recipes. Cut celery into diagonal pieces, dice onion, and mince garlic; set aside together. Peel and mince ginger; set aside separately. If not using pre-made coleslaw mix, shred cabbage. Slice carrots thinly on the diagonal and set aside with cabbage or coleslaw mix.
2. Crack eggs into a separate bowl and set aside; do not mix.

Egg Roll Bowls (Continued)

<u>Instructions (Continued)</u>

3. Heat a large wok or sauté pan over very high heat. Once pan is hot, add half of oil and allow to heat about 30 seconds until oil shimmers and sputters when water is flicked into it. Add celery, onion, and garlic. Cook about 3 minutes, stirring frequently, until onions starts to brown.
4. Move onion and garlic to sides of the pan and add eggs into center of the pan. Break yolks and whites apart with spatula and stir eggs continuously as they cook to break apart. Cook eggs until soft and scrambled.
5. Move eggs to side of pan and add remaining oil and minced ginger to skillet; sauté for about 1 minute until fragrant, being careful not to burn ginger.
6. Add coleslaw mix (or shredded cabbage) and carrots to pan. Continue to cook over high heat, stirring frequently, for about 10 minutes until vegetables are starting to soften and brown.
7. Add soy sauce, vinegar, and sugar to the pan with vegetables, then remove from heat. Stir to evenly distribute sauces.
8. Serve vegetables and eggs in bowls over rice. Top with fish sauce or additional soy sauce to taste.

<u>Vegan Version:</u> Drain liquid from a package of extra firm tofu and press extra water out using a clean towel or paper towel. Once as much liquid as possible has been removed, add tofu to a mixing bowl. Use a fork to mash tofu into small pieces resembling the texture of cooked ground beef crumbles. Add this to recipe in place of egg in step 4.

<u>Pro Tip:</u> Substitute or add various vegetables based on what you have on hand, such as zucchini, cabbage, onion, carrots, peppers, Bok choy, or mushrooms.

<u>Picky Eater Tips:</u> Separate ingredients and serve separately: cabbage, carrots, and scrambled eggs. Let your picky eater add their own sauces, such as soy sauce, fish sauce, or rice vinegar. Serve with "safe food" options such as rice, fruit, or cheese.

<u>Leftovers:</u> Refrigerate in an airtight container for up to 5 days. This dish is not recommended to freeze. Option to wrap leftovers in egg roll wrappers and fry in oil for 3–5 minutes to make egg roll appetizers.

Winter/Spring Meal Plan: Week 2

30-Minute Meal 2

Loaded Nachos

✓ Gluten-Free   ✓ Vegetarian

Whole Meal Total Time: 15–20 Min | Prep Time: 10–12 Min | Cook Time: 20–25 Min

Recommended order of prep:
1. Make recipe for <u>Loaded Nachos</u>. Serve with toppings as desired.

Pro Tip: This meal is very flexible and perfect to serve for picky eaters. Instead of piling all the toppings on, set each on the table and allow your eaters to choose their own dinner.

Dietary Adjustments

Dairy-Free / Vegan: Use plant-based cheese shreds and sour cream, or omit and add avocado cubes instead for Loaded Nachos.

Loaded Nachos

Prep Time: 15 Min | Cook Time: 10 Min   Serves: 6

Ingredients

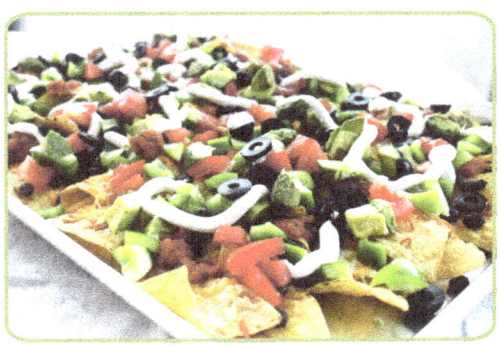

- 12 oz Corn tortilla chips
- 1 cup Shredded cheddar cheese (use dairy-free shreds for vegan option)
- 1 Green bell pepper (diced)
- 2 Tomatoes (diced)
- 1 Avocado (diced)
- 1 cup Black olives (sliced)
- 1 3/4 cup Black beans (14.5 oz can)
- 1 cup Salsa
- 1/2 cup Sour cream (sub plant-based sour cream for dairy-free and vegan)
- Additional nacho toppings as desired: ground beef or turkey cooked with taco seasoning, chopped lettuce, fried egg, cooked corn, or diced green onion

Instructions

1. Preheat oven to 350° Fahrenheit. Spray a large baking sheet with cooking spray.
2. Arrange chips on prepared baking sheet and spread shredded cheese evenly over chips. Place in the oven and bake 10–12 minutes until cheese has melted and is starting to brown. Note: you can place nachos in the oven while it preheats.
3. While cheese melts on chips, dice bell pepper, tomato, and avocado. Slice olives; drain and rinse black beans.
4. Once cheese has melted, remove chips from oven. Top nachos evenly with prepared peppers, tomatoes, avocados, olives, black beans, salsa, sour cream, and any additional toppings as desired.

Pro Tip: For more veggies, serve toppings over a bed of shredded lettuce and top with tortilla chip crumbles instead of serving over chips. Top with cottage cheese or plain Greek yogurt instead of sour cream for extra protein.

Picky Eater Tips: Serve toppings separately and allow picky eaters to build their own nachos. For more food exposures, let them help prep the toppings, including simple steps like pouring the salsa into a bowl to serve.

Leftovers: Nachos are best if eaten immediately. If storing leftovers, store toppings separately from chips. Reheat chips in oven or toaster oven to serve.

Winter/Spring Meal Plan: Week 2

Slow-Cooker Meal

Slow-Cooker Spaghetti Squash & Meatballs With Garlic Bread

✓ Dairy-Free

Whole Meal Total Time: 4 1/2–8 Hrs | Prep Time: 30 Min | Cook Time: 4–8 Hrs

Recommended order of prep:

1. Starting 4–8 hours before planning to eat, make recipe for <u>Slow-Cooker Spaghetti Squash & Meatballs</u>.
2. About 15 minutes before ready to eat, make recipe for <u>Garlic Bread</u>.
3. While garlic bread cooks, use tongs and a fork to scrape out flesh of spaghetti squash into spaghetti-like strands.
4. Serve spaghetti squash topped with meatballs and sauce with garlic bread on the side.

Pro Tip: For super-fast prep for this meal, use pre-made meatballs instead of making them from scratch.

Dietary Adjustments

Gluten-Free: Use gluten-free breadcrumbs to make Slow-Cooker Spaghetti Squash & Meatballs; use gluten-free bread to make Garlic Bread.
Dairy-Free: Use vegan butter to make Garlic Bread.
Vegetarian: Sub recipe for <u>Slow-Cooker Spaghetti Squash & Lentil Bolognese</u> in place of Slow-Cooker Spaghetti Squash & Meatballs.
Vegan: Sub recipe for <u>Slow-Cooker Spaghetti Squash & Lentil Bolognese</u> in place of Slow-Cooker Spaghetti Squash & Meatballs and use vegan butter to make Garlic Bread.

Slow-Cooker Spaghetti Squash & Meatballs

Prep Time: 30 Min | Cook Time: 4 Hrs   Serves: 4

Ingredients

- 1 Spaghetti squash (medium, washed)

Marinara Sauce

- 3 1/2 cup Crushed tomatoes (28 oz can)
- 6 oz Tomato paste
- 1 cup Water
- 2 tsp Oregano
- 1 tsp Dried basil
- 1/2 tsp Salt
- 1/2 tsp Black pepper

Meatballs

- 1 lb Extra lean ground beef (sub ground turkey if desired)
- 1/4 cup Seasoned breadcrumbs (Italian-style; sub gluten-free breadcrumbs for gluten-free)
- 1 Egg (whisked)
- 1 tbsp Extra virgin olive oil
- 1/2 tsp Salt
- 1/2 tsp Garlic powder

Instructions

1. To a large slow cooker, add all ingredients for marinara sauce: crushed tomatoes, tomato paste, water, oregano, basil, salt, and black pepper. Mix well.
2. In a large mixing bowl, combine all ingredients for meatballs: ground beef, bread crumbs, egg, olive oil, salt, and garlic powder. Mix well, then roll into small meatballs the size of golf balls. Place in slow cooker, submerged in sauce.
3. Wash the outside of the spaghetti squash to remove dirt, then very carefully cut spaghetti squash in half lengthwise, and scoop out the seeds. If the squash is too big to fit in the slow cooker, cut it into quarters. Carefully place prepped spaghetti squash flesh-side up on top of meatballs. (No need to submerge it in the sauce.) Cook on low 6–8 hours or on high 4–5 hours.
4. Just before ready to eat, use tongs to carefully lift the spaghetti squash out of the slow cooker. Use a fork to scrape out the flesh into a sieve, strainer, or onto a layer of paper towel, and let the excess liquid drain off. Serve spaghetti squash topped with meatballs and sauce.

Pro Tip: If desired, top with shredded cheddar or Parmesan cheese to serve. Try this with chicken breast instead of meatballs for a variation.

Picky Eater Tips: If your picky eater has a favorite type of frozen meatball, use these instead of making from scratch to help introduce other new flavors using something they already like. Serve with a side of regular spaghetti as a "safe" food.

Leftovers: Refrigerate in airtight container up to 5 days. Not recommended to freeze.

Garlic Bread

Prep Time: 5 Min | Cook Time: 5 Min   Serves: 4

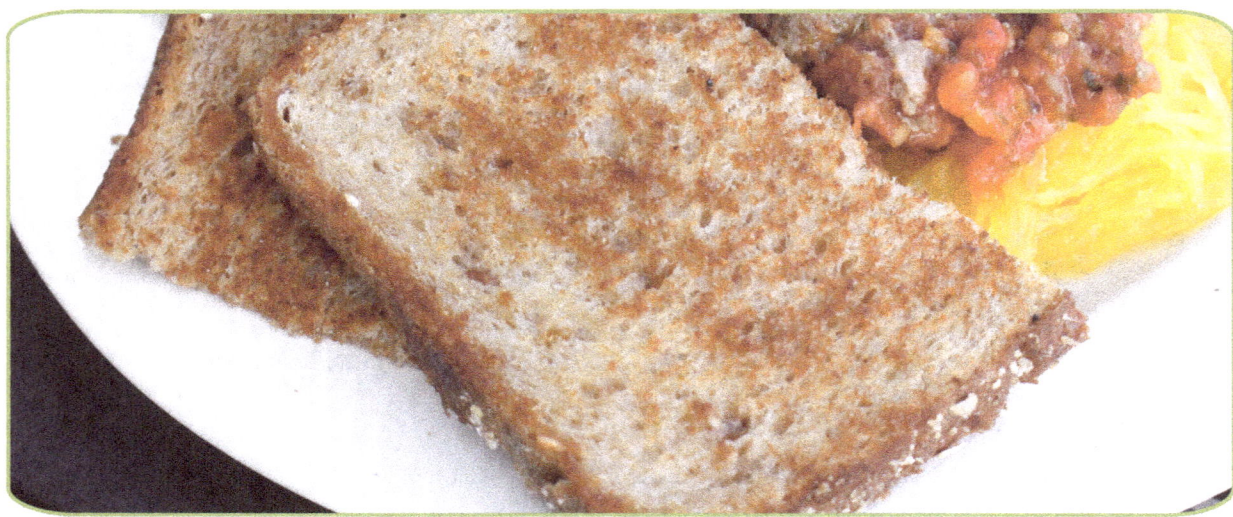

Ingredients
- 4 slice Whole wheat bread (sub gluten-free for gluten-free option)
- 4 tsp Butter (sub dairy-free butter spread for dairy-free and vegan version)
- 1/2 tsp Garlic salt

Instructions
1. Spread 1 tsp butter over each slice of bread and sprinkle with 1/8 tsp garlic salt.
2. Heat a griddle or skillet over medium heat. Once hot, place bread butter-side down and toast for 3–4 minutes until starting to brown.

Pro Tip: Try different seasonings such as an Italian spice blend or seasoned salt for variation.

Picky Eater Tips: If your picky eater likes this, use garlic bread as a way to introduce new flavors to your picky eater by allowing them to pick different spices to add to the toast, such as oregano, parsley, basil, or cumin.

Leftovers: Not recommended to store as leftovers, but if necessary, leftovers can be refrigerated up to a day in an airtight container. Reheat in toaster oven.

Slow-Cooker Spaghetti Squash & Lentil Bolognese

Prep Time: 30 Min | Cook Time: 4 Hrs   Serves: 6

Ingredients

- 2 stalk Celery (diced)
- 1 Carrot (large, cut into rounds)
- 1 Yellow onion (diced)
- 3 1/2 cup Crushed tomatoes (two 14.5 oz cans)
- 6 oz Tomato paste
- 3 cup Water (add 1 cup water for cooking times longer than 6 hrs; sub vegetable broth for richer flavor)
- 1 cup Dried brown lentils
- 2 tbsp Extra virgin olive oil
- 1 tbsp Oregano
- 2 tsp Dried basil
- 1 tsp Salt
- 1/2 tsp Cinnamon
- 1/2 tsp Black pepper
- 1 Spaghetti squash (medium)

Instructions

1. Dice celery, slice carrot into rounds, and dice onion. Add to a large slow cooker with all remaining ingredients except spaghetti squash, adding crushed tomatoes, tomato paste, water, lentils, olive oil, oregano, basil, salt, cinnamon, and black pepper. Stir to mix well.
2. Wash the outside of the spaghetti squash to remove dirt, then very carefully cut it in half lengthwise, and scoop out the seeds. If the squash is too big to fit into the slow cooker, cut it into quarters. Place prepped spaghetti squash flesh-side up on top of sauce. Cover with lid and cook on low 6–10 hours or on high for 3–4 hours.
3. Just before ready to eat, use tongs to carefully lift the spaghetti squash out of the slow cooker. Use a fork to scrape out the flesh into a sieve/strainer (or onto a layer of paper towel) and let the excess fluid drain off. Serve spaghetti squash topped with lentil Bolognese sauce.

<u>Pro Tip:</u> Roast or sauté vegetables before adding to the slow cooker for a richer flavor. Top with shredded cheddar or Parmesan cheese for more protein and flavor. Use fresh basil and oregano for more robust flavor. Serve over whole grain spaghetti instead of spaghetti squash for a more filling meal.

<u>Picky Eater Tips:</u> Offer spaghetti squash and lentils separately instead of serving lentils on top of squash. Offer a familiar pasta on the side. Let your picky eater help scrape out the squash into noodles for an additional hands-on exposure.

<u>Leftovers:</u> Refrigerate in an airtight container up to 5 days. Not recommended to freeze leftover spaghetti squash, but Bolognese can be frozen in an airtight container for several months.

Winter/Spring **Meal Plan: Week 2**

Vegetarian Meal

Spicy Cajun Black Bean Soup and Corn Bread

✓ Vegetarian

Whole Meal Total Time: 25–30 Min | Prep Time: 20–25 Min | Cook Time: 10 Min

Recommended order of prep:
1. Choose stovetop or slow cooker option and make recipe for <u>Spicy Cajun Black Bean Soup</u>.
2. Make recipe for <u>Corn Bread</u>.
3. Serve soup with corn bread on the side.

Pro Tip: Adjust the amount of cayenne pepper according to desired spice level, as this recipe is fairly spicy. Serve with cheese or add peanut butter to corn bread for added protein in this meal.

Dietary Adjustments

Gluten-Free: Use all-purpose gluten-free flour blend to make Corn Bread.
Dairy-Free: Use soy or pea milk to make Corn Bread.
Vegan: Use soy or pea milk to make Corn Bread and see recipe Pro Tip for egg substitute options.

Spicy Cajun Black Bean Soup

Prep Time: 20 Min | Cook Time: 20 Min   Serves: 6

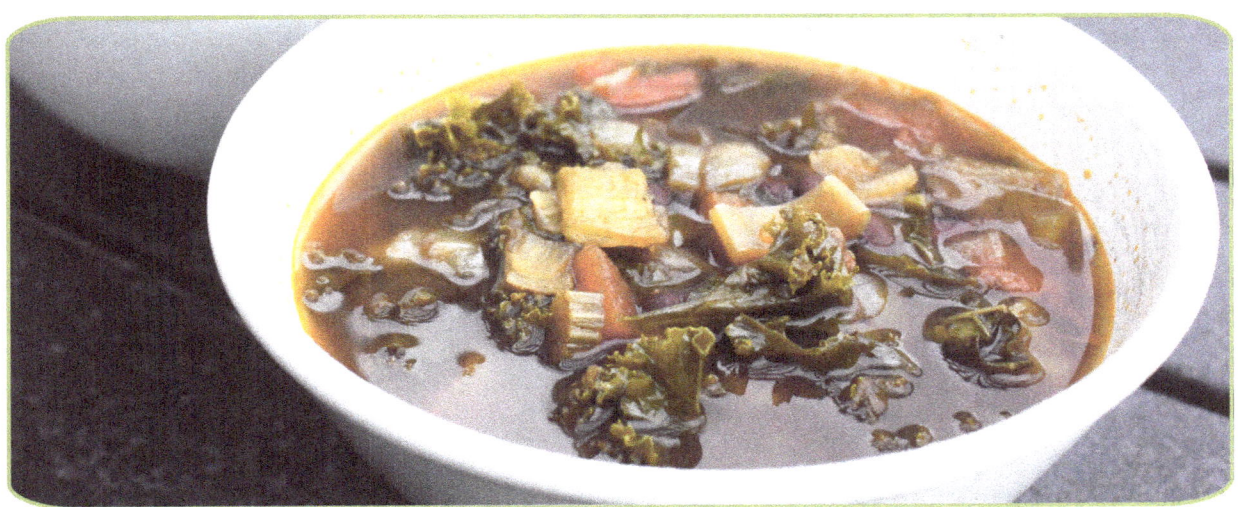

Ingredients

- 2 stalk Celery (diced)
- 1 Yellow onion (diced)
- 1 Yellow bell pepper (diced)
- 2 clove Garlic (minced)
- 2 tbsp Extra virgin olive oil
- 3 cup Kale (roughly chopped, about 3 large leaves)
- 3 1/2 cup Black beans (two 14.5 oz cans, drained and rinsed)

- 2 tsp Salt
- 1 tsp Oregano
- 1 tsp Paprika
- 1/2 tsp Dried thyme
- 1/2 tsp Black pepper
- 1/4 tsp Red pepper flakes
- 6 cup Unsalted vegetable broth
- 1 3/4 cup Diced tomatoes (14.5 oz can)

Instructions

1. Dice celery, onion, bell pepper, and mince garlic; set aside. Heat a medium-sized pot over medium heat. Once hot, add olive oil and prepared vegetables. Sauté for 5–8 minutes until vegetables start to soften.
2. Meanwhile, coarsely chop kale and drain and rinse black beans; set aside.
3. In a small bowl, mix together spices: salt, oregano, paprika, thyme, black pepper, and red pepper flakes. Stir spice mixture into vegetables and cook another minute to allow spices to "bloom" and become fragrant.

Spicy Cajun Black Bean Soup (Continued)

Instructions (Continued)

4. <u>Stovetop method:</u> add all remaining ingredients to pot with vegetables: vegetable broth, chopped kale, drained black beans, and diced tomatoes. Stir to combine and bring to a boil over high heat. Cover and reduce heat, then continue to simmer soup another 30 minutes or more to allow flavors to combine. Add water if the soup becomes too thick.

5. <u>Slow cooker method:</u> transfer vegetables and spices to a large slow cooker and add all remaining ingredients: vegetable broth, chopped kale, drained black beans, and diced tomatoes. Stir to combine and cook on high for 3–4 hours or on low for 6–10 hours.

6. <u>Pressure cooker method:</u> transfer vegetables to pressure cooker (or complete step 1 using the "sauté" option on electric pressure cooker) and add vegetable broth, chopped kale, drained black beans, and diced tomatoes. Stir to combine, put lid on and set to "sealing." Use the manual/pressure cooker and cook for 8 minutes on high pressure. Once finished, let the pressure release naturally for 5 minutes, then do a quick release.

<u>Pro Tip:</u> Substitute canned black eyed peas in place of black beans for a more authentic Cajun flavor. Try fire roasted tomatoes instead of plain diced tomatoes for more flavor. Add additional cayenne pepper to taste for even spicier soup. Use water in place of broth if broth is unavailable. If using salted broth, omit salt and then add salt to taste at the end of cooking.

<u>Picky Eater Tips:</u> Before cooking, set aside some plain black beans and raw chopped vegetables to offer on the side of this cooked soup. Reduce or omit the amount of cayenne pepper for picky eaters sensitive to spicy flavors. Serve with a side of bread, crackers, or cheese as a "safe food" option.

<u>Leftovers:</u> Refrigerate in an airtight container for up to 5 days. Freeze for up to several months.

Corn Bread

Prep Time: 10 Min | Cook Time: 30 Min   Serves: 9

Ingredients

- 1 cup Cornmeal
- 1 cup Flour (sub all-purpose gluten-free flour blend for gluten-free)
- 1 tbsp Baking powder
- 1/2 tsp Salt
- 1 cup Whole milk (sub non-dairy milk for dairy-free or vegan)

- 1/2 cup Brown sugar (packed; sub white granulated sugar if desired)
- 1/3 cup Canola oil (or melted butter, if desired)
- 1 Egg (see Pro Tip for egg substitute for vegan option)
- 1 cup Corn (fresh, frozen, or canned)

Instructions

1. Preheat oven to 350° Fahrenheit and prepare an 8x8-inch square or 9-inch round baking dish by spraying it with cooking spray.
2. In a mixing bowl, combine cornmeal, flour, baking powder, and salt.
3. Create a well in the center of the dry ingredients and add in milk, brown sugar, oil, and egg. Stir until just combined, making sure not to over-mix.
4. Add corn to batter and stir until just combined. Transfer mixture to prepared baking pan.
5. Bake for 30–35 minutes. Check if bread is done by inserting a toothpick; remove from the oven when toothpick comes out clean. Allow corn bread to cool a few minutes before slicing and serving.

Pro Tip: If scaling the recipe up or down, adjust pan size accordingly. You may need to bake corn bread slightly longer for a larger recipe. Add chopped jalapeños when adding corn for a spicy twist. For a vegan version, use an egg substitute or one of these options: 1) 1 tbsp tapioca starch or cornstarch and 2 tbsp water or 2) 1 tbsp ground flaxseed and 2 tbsp water, allowing to sit for 5 minutes to thicken before use.

Picky Eater Tips: Serve with optional toppings and let your picky eater choose which to try: butter, honey, or jelly. Bake these into muffins for an alternative shape. Serve plain bread as a "safe food" alternative in addition to corn bread.

Leftovers: Store in airtight container at room temperature up to 3–5 days. Refrigerate up to a week. Freeze up to a month. It may become slightly dry in the refrigerator or freezer; reheat in microwave topped with damp paper towel.

Winter/Spring Meal Plan: Week 2

Challenge Meal

Barbecue Chicken Thighs, Baked French Fries, and Garlicky Roasted Green Beans

✓ Gluten-Free   ✓ Dairy-Free

Whole Meal Total Time: 75 Min | Prep Time: 40–45 Min | Cook Time: 30 Min

Recommended order of prep:
1. Prep potatoes for <u>Baked French Fries</u> and allow to soak while prepping other meal components. Soak potatoes overnight if desired.
2. Prep <u>Barbecue Chicken Thighs</u> and <u>Garlicky Roasted Green Beans</u>, but wait to start cooking.
3. Finish the recipe for fries, placing them in the oven at the same time as the chicken. When fries and chicken have about 15 minutes left to cook, place green beans in the oven.
4. Serve chicken with fries and green beans on the side.

Pro Tip: If you don't have enough room in your oven for all three recipes, make chicken in the slow cooker instead (cook on high 3–4 hours or on low 5–7 hours), or sauté green beans in a skillet instead of baking in the oven.

Dietary Adjustments

Vegetarian / Vegan: Sub recipe for <u>Barbecue Tofu</u> in place of Barbecue Chicken Thighs.

Baked French Fries

Prep Time: 30 Min | Cook Time: 30 Min   Serves: 4

Ingredients

- 4 Yukon gold potatoes (cut into very thin matchsticks; about 4 cups of fries)
- 1 1/2 tsp Garlic powder
- 1 1/2 tsp Onion powder
- 1 tsp Salt
- 1/2 tsp Black pepper
- 2 tbsp Extra virgin olive oil

Instructions

1. Scrub potatoes, but do not peel. Cut potatoes into thin matchsticks, about 1/4-inch wide and 3-inches long, roughly the same size.
2. Place potatoes in a large bowl and fill it with cold water, enough to submerge potatoes. Soak potatoes for 30–45 minutes to remove some of the starch and make a crispier fry, or prep the night before and soak overnight. Note: you can skip this step if you're running short on time, but this makes for a crispier fry.
3. Preheat the oven to 400° Fahrenheit and line a large baking sheet with parchment paper or silicone baking mat. In a small bowl, mix together seasonings: garlic powder, onion powder, salt, and pepper. Set aside.
4. Drain potatoes and use a clean towel to pat them dry completely before baking.
5. Add oil and half of the seasoning mixture to potatoes and toss until well combined. Transfer to prepared baking sheet one layer thick, being careful to avoid stacking the potatoes on top of each other.
6. Bake for 20 minutes, then remove fries from oven. Sprinkle remaining half of seasoning evenly over fries, then use a spatula to turn fries over. Return to the oven and bake another 10 minutes until fries become crispy. Open the oven several times during baking to release steam, creating a crispier fry.

Pro Tip: Try different seasoning blends, such as steak seasoning, taco seasoning, or try adding your favorite spices such as chipotle powder, cumin, or paprika.

Picky Eater Tips: Let picky eaters choose different seasonings to make these "fries." Let them help by stirring or tossing potatoes with seasoning. Serve with different types of dip, such as ketchup, barbecue sauce, mayonnaise, or honey mustard.

Leftovers: Store in an airtight container for up to 5 days. To freeze, arrange fries in a single layer and freeze solid, then store in an airtight container for up to 3 months. Reheat in toaster oven, oven, or skillet to maintain crispiness; place fries on a baking sheet in a cold oven while it heats, then bake at 400° Fahrenheit for about 5 minutes.

Barbecue Chicken Thighs

Prep Time: 5 Min | Cook Time: 25 Min   Serves: 4

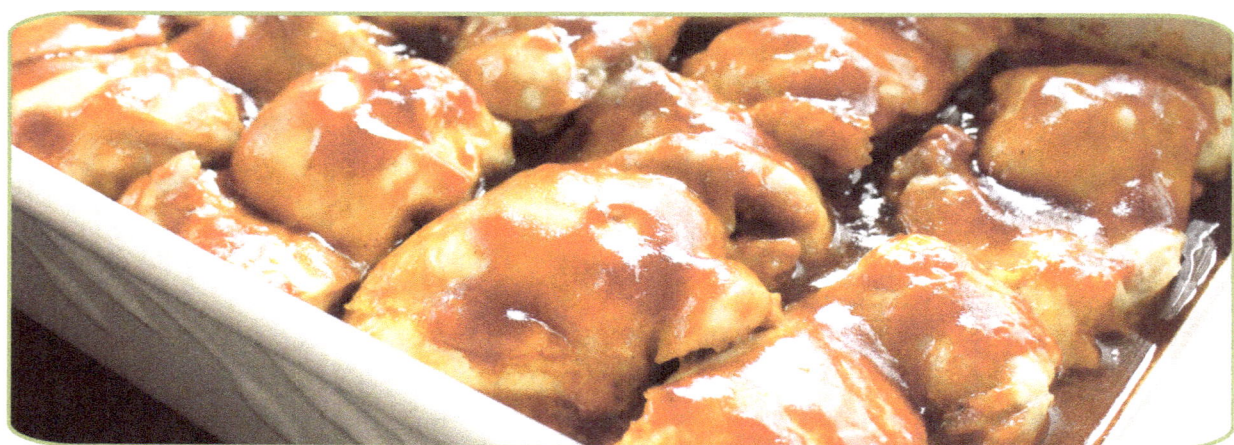

Ingredients
- 1 1/2 lb Boneless, skinless chicken thighs
- 1/2 cup Barbecue sauce (choose gluten-free if desired)

Instructions
1. Preheat the oven to 400° Fahrenheit and prepare a baking dish by spraying with cooking spray.
2. Arrange chicken thighs evenly in baking dish. Spread barbecue sauce evenly over each chicken thigh, turning to coat chicken on all sides.
3. Bake chicken for 20–30 minutes until it reaches an internal temperature of 165° Fahrenheit. Use a food thermometer for best results.

Pro Tip: Choose your favorite barbecue sauce, or sub different variations on barbecue sauce, such as honey mustard or teriyaki sauce, for a variation on this easy dish.

Picky Eater Tips: Swap chicken thighs for chicken breast if preferred. Use your picky eater's favorite barbecue sauce. Leave sauce off of a few pieces of chicken and serve on the side as a dip instead. Offer an alternative "safe food" protein option, such as cheese or chicken nuggets.

Leftovers: Refrigerate in an airtight container for 3–5 days. Freeze for up to 1 month.

Garlicky Roasted Green Beans

Prep Time: 10 Min | Cook Time: 20 Min   Serves: 4

Ingredients
- 4 cup Green beans (fresh, ends trimmed; OR 16 oz package frozen green beans)
- 2 tbsp Extra virgin olive oil
- 1/2 tsp Salt
- 1/2 tsp Garlic powder

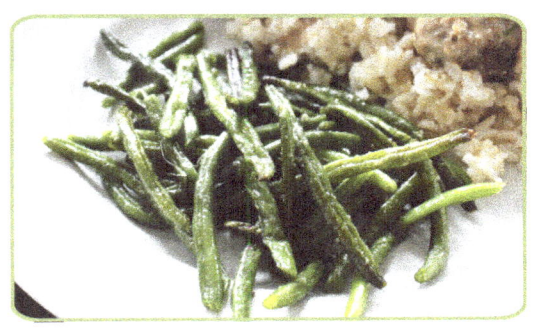

Instructions
1. Preheat oven to 400° Fahrenheit.
2. If using fresh green beans, trim ends and discard.
3. Add green beans to a large baking sheet and toss with oil, salt, and garlic powder. Spread green beans evenly with as little overlap as possible and bake for 20–25 minutes.

Pro Tip: Spice up green beans by sprinkling with chili flakes after roasting. If cooking another food item at a different temperature, use the following guidelines for different cooking times: 350–375° = 25–30 minutes; 425–450° = 14–16 minutes.

Picky Eater Tips: Omit garlic and add only salt. Serve with a dip your picky eater likes. Encourage play at the table and let your picky eater pick up the green beans with their hands. If possible, take your picky eater to a local farmer's market to choose the green beans or pick green beans from the garden. Let them snap the ends off of green beans and help prepare this meal for low-pressure exposures.

Leftovers: Refrigerate in an airtight container up to 5 days. Cooked green beans are not recommended to freeze.

Barbecue Tofu

Prep Time: 20 Min | Cook Time: 15 Min   Serves: 4

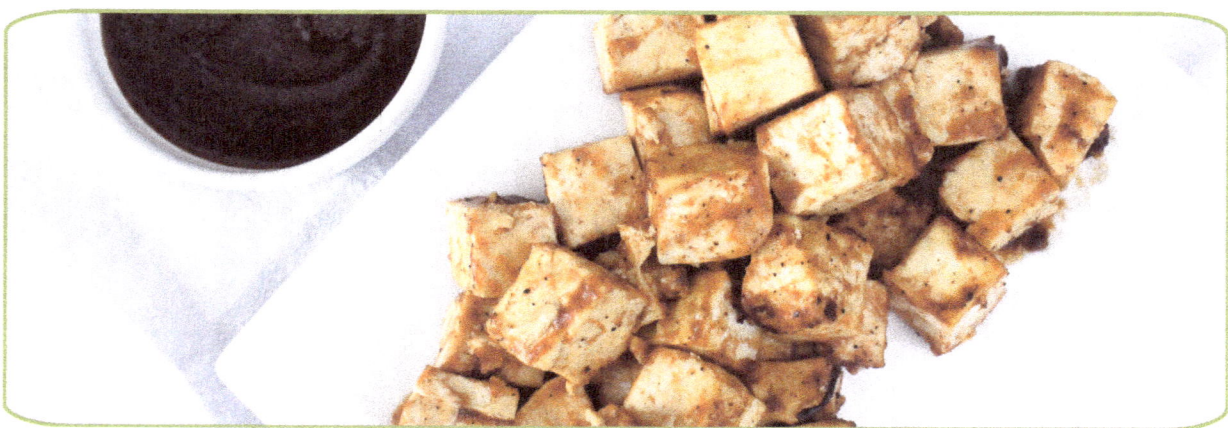

Ingredients
- 28 oz Extra firm tofu (about 2 packages, liquid pressed, cubed)
- 1 cup Barbecue sauce (choose gluten-free if desired)

Instructions
1. Preheat oven to 400° Fahrenheit. Prepare a 9x13-inch baking dish by spraying with cooking spray.
2. Press liquid from tofu: drain liquid from tofu, cut into 1-inch cubes, and place between two clean towels. Using hands, press on tofu to remove as much liquid as possible. Toss tofu cubes with half of the barbecue sauce and allow to marinate for 10–15 minutes while the oven preheats.
3. Place tofu in the oven and bake 15–20 minutes until barbecue sauce starts to become sticky on tofu.

Pro Tip: Marinate tofu overnight in barbecue sauce and serve with extra sauce on the side for more flavor. Try different barbecue sauce flavors for a variation.

Picky Eater Tips: Because tofu is very bland, it can be a good option for picky eaters. Set some plain, uncooked cubes aside and allow to dip in the sauce or choose other sauce to serve, such as teriyaki or soy sauce.

Leftovers: Refrigerate in airtight container up to 5 days. Not recommended to freeze.

Winter/Spring Meal Plan: Week 2

Savory Grab & Go

Pesto Tuna & Green Pea Quinoa Bowls

✓ Gluten-Free

Dietary Adjustments

Dairy-Free: Use dairy-free pesto in Pesto Tuna & Pea Quinoa Bowls.
Vegetarian / Vegan: Sub chickpeas instead of tuna in Pesto Tuna & Pea Quinoa Bowls.

Sweet Grab & Go

Sunflower Banana Boat and Edamame With Salt

✓ Gluten-Free   ✓ Dairy-Free   ✓ Vegetarian   ✓ Vegan

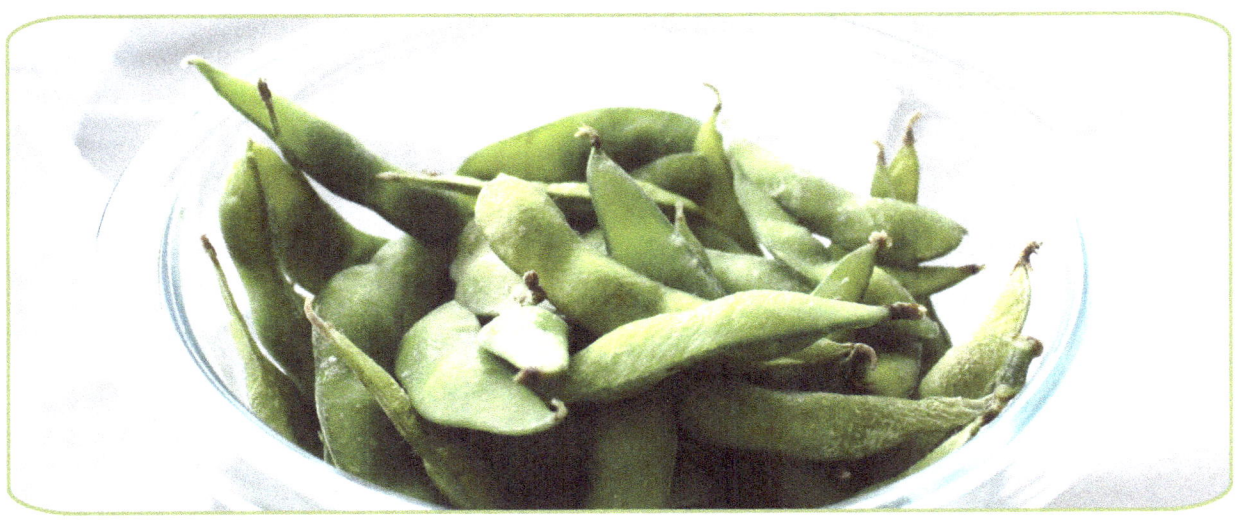

Pesto Tuna & Green Pea Quinoa Bowls

Prep Time: 10 Min | Cook Time: 15 Min

Serves: 4

Ingredients
- 1 cup Quinoa (uncooked)
- 2 cup Water
- 1/4 tsp Salt
- 10 oz Canned tuna (drained, broken into chunks; sub chickpeas for vegan)
- 2 1/2 cup Frozen peas
- 1/4 cup Pesto (choose dairy-free if desired)
- 1/4 cup Nutritional yeast

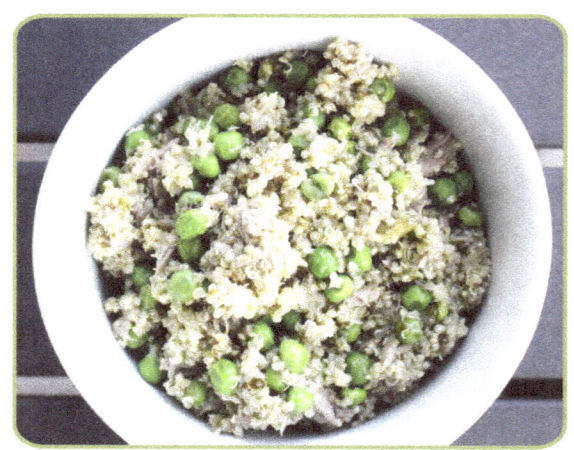

Instructions
1. Combine quinoa, water, and salt together in a medium to large saucepan. Bring to a boil, then reduce heat, cover with a lid, and simmer for 8 minutes.
2. Add tuna and peas to quinoa and stir to combine. Cover with a lid again and continue to cook another 7–8 minutes until quinoa has completely absorbed liquid.
3. Once quinoa is fully cooked, remove from heat and stir in pesto and nutritional yeast to serve.

Pro Tip: Add cherry tomatoes, cucumber, chopped spinach, mushrooms or zucchini for variety and extra veggies. Sub Parmesan cheese in place of nutritional yeast if desired.

Picky Eater Tips: Offer plain tuna, quinoa, and peas separately. Let picky eaters choose to drizzle or dip pesto on their own to adjust the flavor to their liking, or omit entirely. Serve other "safe food" options for protein, starch, and fruit and vegetable if this is completely new.

Leftovers: Refrigerate in airtight container up to 5 days. Not recommended to freeze.

Sunflower Banana Boat

Prep Time: 5 Min | Cook Time: 0 Min   Serves: 1

Ingredients

- 1 Banana (peeled)
- 1 tbsp Sunflower seed butter
- 1 tsp Hemp seeds (sub ground flaxseeds or chia seeds if desired)

Instructions

1. Peel banana and lay on a plate.
2. Spread sunflower seed butter onto banana, then sprinkle hemp seeds over top. Slice and serve immediately.

Pro Tip: Sub peanut or almond butter in place of sunflower seed butter for a variation. Top with sunflower seeds, mini chocolate chips, crushed M&Ms, or chopped nuts.

Picky Eater Tips: Sub other types of nut butters that your picky eater is more familiar with. Let picky eaters build their own "boat" and offer fun toppings such as chocolate chips, granola, dried fruit, or sprinkles.

Leftovers: Refrigerate in airtight container up to a day.

Edamame With Salt

Prep Time: 2 Min | Cook Time: 8 Min   Serves: 1

Ingredients

- 1 cup Frozen edamame in the shell
- 1/8 tsp Salt

Instructions

1. Add edamame to a microwave safe bowl with a few tablespoons of water, just enough to cover the bottom of the dish. Cover with towel or paper towel and microwave on high for 5–8 minutes until heated through.
2. Drain water and season with salt. Shell edamame at the table (shell not edible).

Pro Tip: Toss with soy sauce or sprinkle with chili powder for flavor variation. Instead of microwaving, add edamame to a small saucepan with a small amount of water and steam for 5–8 minutes until heated through.

Picky Eater Tips: Let your picky eaters pop the beans out of the pods themselves for a fun, interactive snack. Offer without salt, or substitute a seasoning packet they choose, such as taco season or ranch packet.

Leftovers: Refrigerate in an airtight container for 3–5 days. Edamame is not recommended to refreeze after cooking.

Winter/Spring Meal Plan: Week 2

Savory Breakfast

Savory Golden Oats

✓ Gluten-Free ✓ Dairy-Free ✓ Vegetarian ✓ Vegan

Dietary Adjustments
Gluten-Free: Use gluten-free oats to make Savory Golden Oats.

Sweet Breakfast

Microwave Apple Spice Cake

✓ Dairy-Free ✓ Vegetarian ✓ Vegan

Dietary Adjustments
Gluten-Free: Use an all-purpose gluten-free flour blend to make Microwave Apple Spice Cake.

Savory Golden Oats

Prep Time: 10 Min | Cook Time: 20 Min   Serves: 4

Ingredients

- 4 cup Water
- 1 cup Old-fashioned oats (use gluten-free if desired)
- 1/2 cup Dry red lentils
- 1 tsp Onion powder
- 1 tsp Turmeric
- 1/2 tsp Garlic powder
- 1/2 tsp Salt
- 2 cup Baby spinach
- 2 tbsp Nutritional yeast

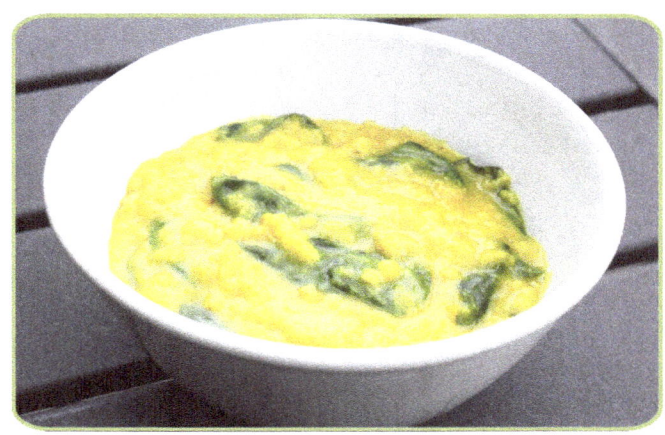

Instructions

1. Add water, oats, lentils, onion powder, turmeric, garlic powder, and salt to a medium-sized saucepan and stir to combine. Cover with a lid and bring to a boil over medium-high heat.
2. Once boiling, reduce heat to medium-low and cook for 15–20 minutes, stirring frequently, until lentils are tender.
3. Stir in baby spinach and nutritional yeast to lentils and oats. Cook another 1–2 minutes, then remove from heat. Serve warm.

Pro Tip: Add red pepper flakes for spice or top with plain yogurt for a tangy twist. For added protein, top with a fried egg, stir in additional nutritional yeast, or sprinkle Parmesan cheese on top.

Picky Eater Tips: Offer a small portion of this savory oatmeal alongside a traditional sweet oatmeal option that your picky eater is more familiar with. Keep some oatmeal separate before adding spinach. Let eaters add their own toppings like cheese, eggs, or season with salt. Have fun with the yellow color of this dish and let them name all the foods that are yellow, invite their favorite yellow toys to the table, or serve as part of a "yellow-themed" menu.

Leftovers: Refrigerate in an airtight container for up to 5 days. Not recommended to freeze.

Microwave Apple Spice Cake

Prep Time: 10 Min | Cook Time: 5 Min   Serves: 4

Ingredients

- 1/2 cup Flour (sub all-purpose gluten-free flour blend for gluten-free)
- 1/4 cup Sugar
- 1 tsp Baking powder
- 4 tbsp Hemp seeds
- 2 tsp Cinnamon
- 1/2 tsp Nutmeg
- 3/4 cup Soymilk (sub other milk type if desired)
- 1 Apple (diced)

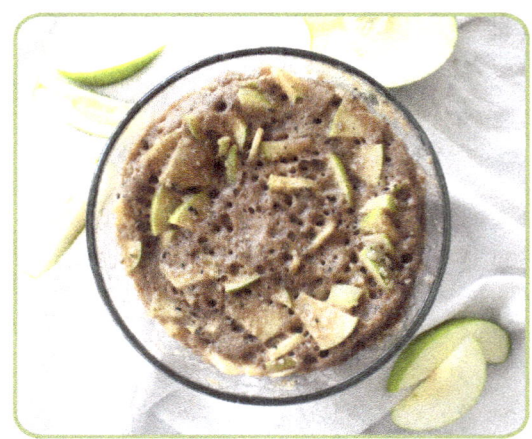

Instructions

1. In a microwave safe bowl, mix together dry ingredients: flour, sugar, baking powder, hemp seeds, cinnamon, and nutmeg.
2. Add milk to dry ingredients and whisk or stir with a fork until thoroughly combined and no clumps remain.
3. Dice apple finely and stir into batter until evenly distributed.
4. Place bowl in microwave and microwave on high 5–6 minutes. See Pro Tip for instructions to cook in individual servings.

Pro Tip: Top with vanilla Greek yogurt, peanut butter, or additional hemp seeds for extra protein. If desired, divide batter into individual portions in microwave-safe containers such as glass bowls, mason jars, or coffee mugs. Microwave individual portions for 1–2 minutes instead of 5–6 minutes.

Picky Eater Tips: Top this cake with something familiar like vanilla yogurt, whipped cream or their favorite nut butter. Set aside some apple slices to serve alongside the cake. Omit the nutmeg for a milder version. Let your picky eater help stir together the batter or measure ingredients for additional hands-on exposure. The microwave format makes it easy to test small portions with different flavors.

Leftovers: Store at room temperature with airtight lid up to 3 days. Refrigerate batter up to 3 days and then microwave for a fresher option. Freeze up to a month.

Winter/Spring Meal Plan: Week 2

Savory Snack

Salt & Vinegar Almonds

✓ Gluten-Free ✓ Dairy-Free ✓ Vegetarian ✓ Vegan

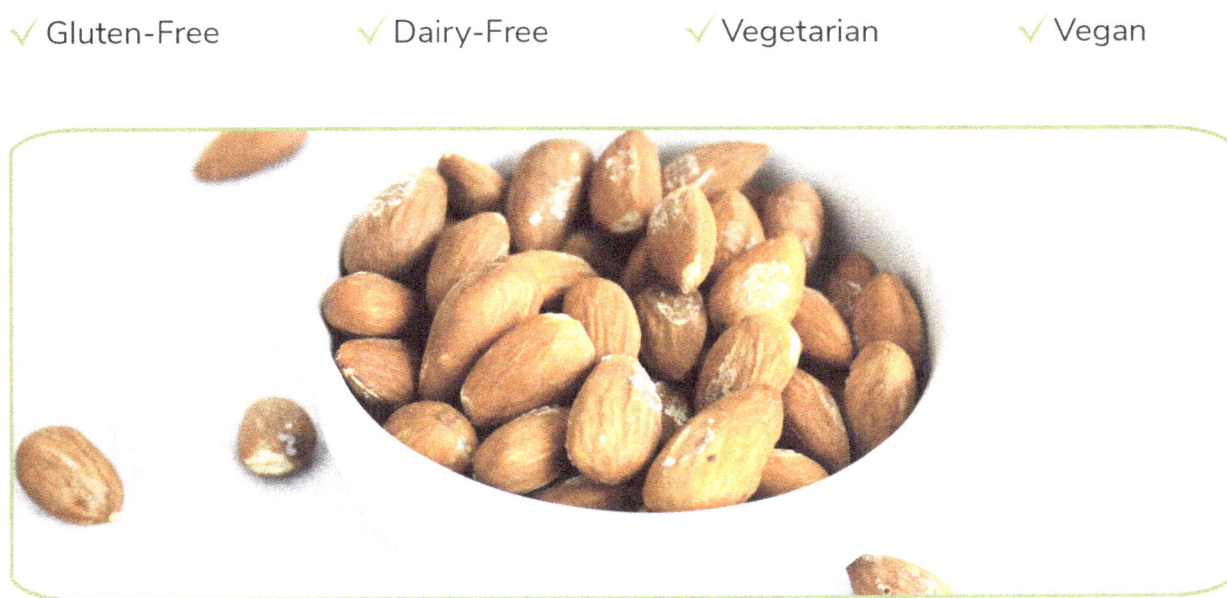

Sweet Snack

Pumpkin Yogurt

✓ Gluten-Free ✓ Vegetarian

Dietary Adjustments

Dairy-Free / Vegan: Use soy or coconut yogurt to make Pumpkin Yogurt.

Salt & Vinegar Almonds

Prep Time: 1 hr | Cook Time: 10 Min   Serves: 4

Ingredients
- 1 cup Almonds (raw, whole)
- 1 cup White vinegar
- 1 tsp Coarse salt

Instructions
1. Add almonds and vinegar to a glass or ceramic bowl (non-metal), submerging almonds completely. Soak 1–2 hours, or longer for a stronger vinegar flavor.
2. Once almonds have completed time to soak, heat oven to 325° Fahrenheit.
3. Drain vinegar from almonds and discard. Add salt and toss to evenly coat.
4. Spread almonds on a baking sheet, no more than one layer deep, and bake for 20 minutes. Remove from oven when almonds are just beginning to brown and allow to cool before serving.

Pro Tip: Spray almonds with vinegar again after baking for a stronger vinegar flavor.

Picky Eater Tips: Serve these almonds alongside plain almonds. Swap different types of nuts and let your picky eater help mix up the batch before putting them in the oven.

Leftovers: Store in an airtight container at room temperature up to several weeks.

Pumpkin Yogurt

Prep Time: 5 Min | Cook Time: 0 Min   Serves: 1

Ingredients
- 1/2 cup Plain yogurt (sub coconut or soy yogurt for dairy-free)
- 1/4 cup Canned pumpkin
- 1 tsp Honey
- 1/8 tsp Ground cinnamon
- 1/8 tsp Nutmeg

Instructions
1. Mix together all ingredients and serve.

Pro Tip: This recipe is a great way to use leftover canned pumpkin to prevent it from going to waste. Adjust the ingredient amounts to taste.

Picky Eater Tips: Serve yogurt, pumpkin, honey, and spices separately and let your picky eater build their own yogurt bowl. Offer additional toppings such as pumpkin seeds, granola, sprinkles, or chocolate chips for more fun.

Leftovers: Refrigerate in an airtight container up to 3–5 days. Do not freeze.

Summer/Fall Meal Plan: Week 3

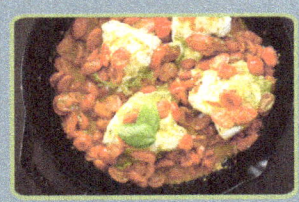

30-Minute Meal 1: Margherita Chicken Over Couscous

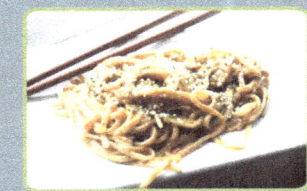

30-Minute Meal 2: Sticky Thai Peanut Noodles With Gingery Snap Peas & Peppers

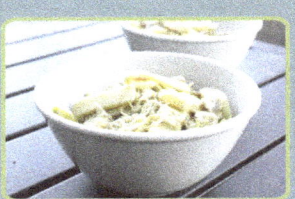

Slow-Cooker: Coconut Lime Curry Slow-Cooker Chicken Over Jasmine Rice

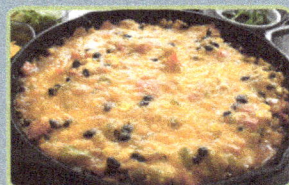

Vegetarian: Black Bean & Quinoa Mexican Skillet With Tortilla Chips

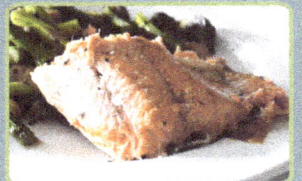

Challenge: Sweet Bourbon Grilled Salmon, Sweet Corn, and Caesar Salad

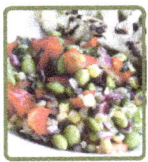

Savory Grab & Go: Edamame Salad With Cilantro Lime Dressing and Cheese Quesadilla

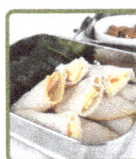

Sweet Grab & Go: Turkey Wraps With Almonds, Cucumbers & Blueberries

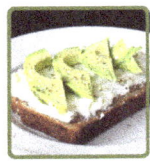

Savory Breakfast: Avocado & Ricotta on Toast

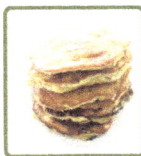

Sweet Breakfast: High Protein Banana Pancakes

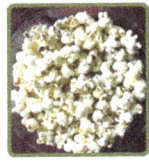

Savory Snack: Parmesan Popcorn

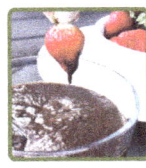

Sweet Snack: Strawberries & Chocolate Fruit Dip

Summer/Fall Meal Plan: Week 3

30-Minute Meal 1

Margherita Chicken Over Couscous

Whole Meal Total Time: 30–35 Min | Prep Time: 15–20 Min | Cook Time: 10–15 Min

Recommended order of prep:
1. Follow recipe to make Margherita Chicken.
2. When chicken has about 5 minutes left to cook, make recipe for Couscous.
3. Serve chicken and sauce over couscous.

Pro Tip: Use fresh basil and garden tomatoes for best flavor. If making this recipe out of season, use canned tomatoes instead of fresh whole tomatoes.

Dietary Adjustments

Gluten-Free: Serve Margherita Chicken with gluten-free bread, gluten-free pasta, or rice instead of Couscous.

Dairy-Free: Sub recipe for Skillet Chicken and Basil Bursted Tomatoes in place of Margherita Chicken.

Vegetarian: Sub recipe for Margherita Crostini in place of Margherita Chicken and Couscous and serve with Sautéed Zucchini.

Vegan: Sub recipe for Mediterranean Tofu and Basil Bursted Tomatoes in place of Margherita Chicken.

Margherita Chicken

Prep Time: 15 Min | Cook Time: 15 Min   Serves: 4

Ingredients

- 1 1/2 lb Boneless, skinless chicken breast
- 1 tbsp Extra virgin olive oil
- 1/2 tsp Oregano
- 1/4 tsp Black pepper
- 4 oz Fresh mozzarella (sliced)
- 1 tbsp Basil leaves (minced)

- 2 tbsp Water (sub unsalted vegetable broth, chardonnay, or pinot grigio for better flavor) 2 tbsp Lemon juice (1/2 lemon)
- 1 tbsp Minced garlic (minced)
- 4 cup Cherry tomatoes
- 1/2 tsp Salt
- 2 tbsp Pesto

Instructions

1. Slice chicken into evenly sized pieces, 1-inch thick, each about 6 oz (the size of 2 decks of cards). Season with oregano and pepper.
2. Heat a large skillet (cast iron preferred) over medium-high heat. Once skillet is hot, add olive oil and arrange chicken breast evenly in pan. Cook chicken 6–8 minutes per side until golden brown and internal temperature reaches 165° Fahrenheit. Remove chicken from skillet and set aside.
3. While chicken cooks, gather other ingredients, slice mozzarella, and mince basil.
4. Once chicken has been removed, add water to pan immediately. Use liquid to deglaze pan: use a spoon to scrape bottom of skillet to loosen and incorporate any seasonings stuck to bottom of pan. Add in garlic and lemon juice and bring to a simmer, stirring to combine, then add cherry tomatoes. Cover and cook 3–5 minutes on high heat until tomatoes start to release their liquid, then remove the lid and cook another 3–5 minutes to reduce liquid.
5. Return chicken to the skillet, placing on top of tomatoes. Top each chicken piece evenly with pesto, then with sliced mozzarella. Cover with a lid and cook 2–3 minutes more until cheese has started to melt.
6. Serve chicken over couscous, topped with tomatoes and garnished with freshly minced basil leaves.

Pro Tip: For a pescatarian option, sub fillets of white fish, such as tilapia or sole.

Picky Eater Tips: Serve meal components separately to allow your picky eater to choose what they like. Set aside some plain cooked chicken before adding back with tomatoes. Set aside some tomatoes and cheese uncooked as an alternative option.

Leftovers: Refrigerate in airtight container up to 5 days. Freeze up to several months.

Couscous

Prep Time: 5 Min | Cook Time: 5 Min   Serves: 4

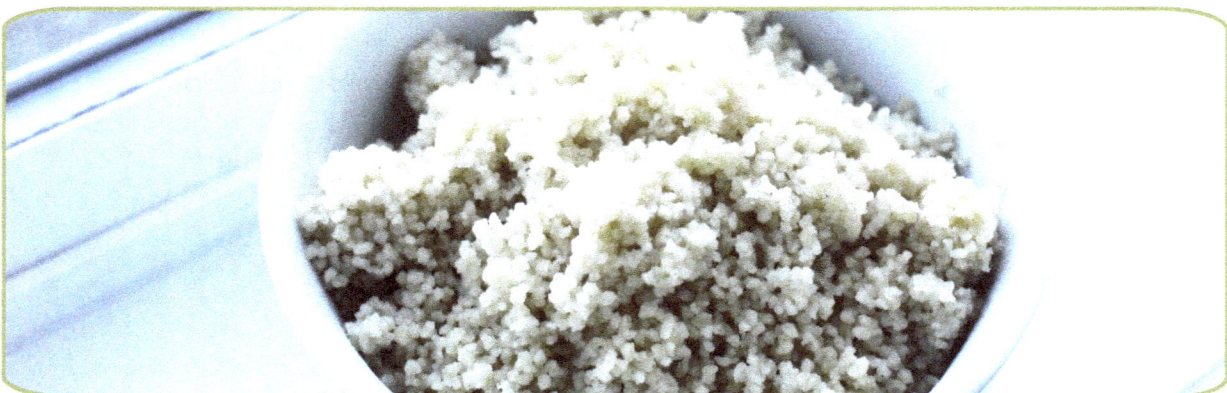

Ingredients
- 1 1/3 cup Water (sub vegetable or chicken broth for more flavor)
- 1 tbsp Extra virgin olive oil
- 1/2 tsp Salt
- 1 cup Dry couscous

Instructions
1. Add water, olive oil, and salt to a medium saucepan. Cover with a lid and bring to a boil over high heat.
2. Once water is boiling, turn off the heat, pour in couscous and stir to combine. Cover the saucepan with a lid and allow to rest for 5 minutes.
3. Remove the lid and fluff couscous with a fork before serving.

Pro Tip: Serve couscous in place of rice in any Mediterranean-inspired dishes for a quick starch option. Use whole grain couscous for higher fiber. Add a squeeze of lemon, fresh parsley or mint for a flavor variation.

Picky Eater Tips: Couscous can be a great option for picky eaters with its naturally mild flavor. Serve other mix-in options for your picky eater to try as a way to expand their palate, such as herbs, lemon juice, chickpeas, or diced vegetables. If this is a new food, rice is a good "safe food" alternative to this dish.

Leftovers: Refrigerate in airtight container up to 5 days. Freeze up to several months.

Easy Skillet Chicken

Prep Time: 5 Min | Cook Time: 8 Min   Serves: 4

Ingredients

- 1 1/2 lb Boneless, skinless chicken breast
- 1 tbsp Extra virgin olive oil
- 2 tsp Dried basil
- 1 tsp Dried parsley
- 1 tsp Dried oregano
- 1/2 tsp Salt
- 1/2 tsp Black pepper

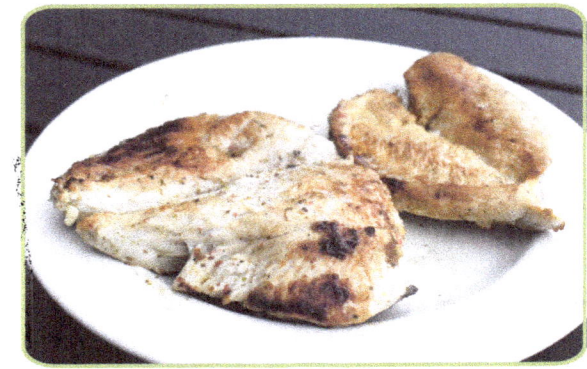

Instructions

1. Slice chicken into evenly sized pieces, each about 6 oz (the size of 2 decks of cards). Make sure pieces are no more than 1-inch thick; slice in half if necessary.
2. Heat a large skillet over medium heat. Once hot, add oil and use a spatula to spread oil evenly over pan. Add chicken to skillet, making sure no pieces overlap.
3. While chicken begins to cook, in a small bowl, mix together spices: basil, parsley, oregano, salt, and pepper. Sprinkle seasoning blend evenly over chicken as it cooks.
4. Cook chicken 3–4 minutes, then flip chicken over and cook another 3–4 minutes until fully cooked through. Chicken should reach an internal temperature of 165° Fahrenheit and be slightly browned.

Pro Tip: Use this same basic recipe with different spices or sauces for an easy variation; try taco seasoning, lemon pepper, oregano and lemon zest, or curry powder. Drizzle with barbecue sauce or serve over salad or quinoa with roasted vegetables.

Picky Eater Tips: Use only salt to season chicken for a very plain version. Serve a very small amount on the plate of your picky eater. Serve chicken with a variety of dipping sauces to add fun, such as ketchup, barbecue sauce, teriyaki sauce, or honey mustard.

Leftovers: Refrigerate in airtight container 3–5 days. Freeze up to a month; if frozen longer, quality will decline.

Basil Bursted Tomatoes

Prep Time: 10 Min | Cook Time: 15 Min   Serves: 4

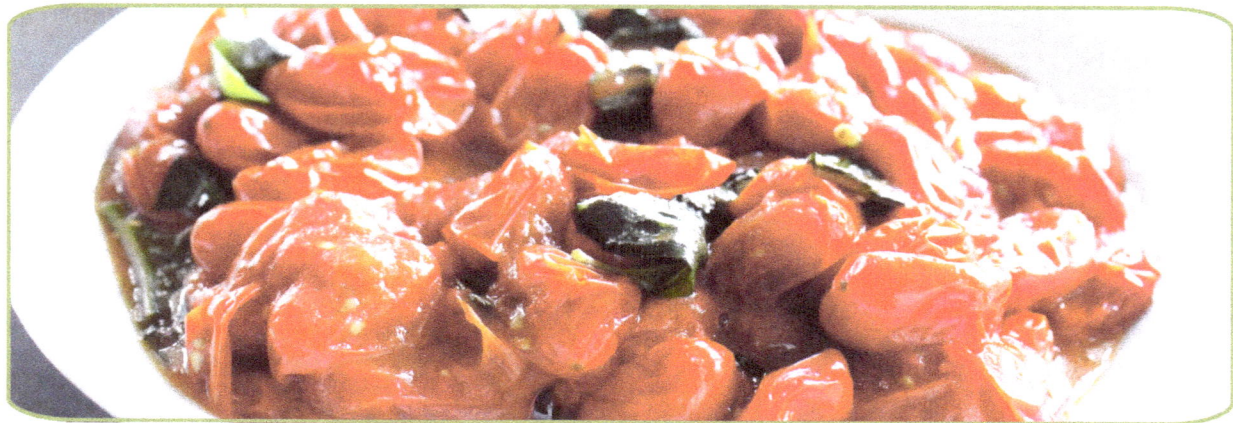

Ingredients
- 1 tbsp Extra virgin olive oil
- 4 cup Cherry tomatoes
- 1/4 cup Basil leaves
- 1/2 tsp Coarsely ground salt

Instructions
1. **Stovetop method:** Heat a large sauté pan over medium-high heat. Once hot, add oil to the pan, then add whole cherry tomatoes. Cook tomatoes until they start to burst, about 15–20 minutes, stirring occasionally.
2. **Oven method:** Preheat oven to 400° Fahrenheit. Place tomatoes on a large baking sheet and toss with oil. Place in oven and cook until tomatoes start to burst, about 15–20 minutes.
3. While tomatoes cook, roughly chop basil and set aside.
4. Once tomatoes have begun to burst, stir in basil and salt and cook just until basil starts to wilt.

Pro Tip: For extra flavor, add shredded Parmesan cheese to cooked tomatoes. You can substitute dried basil instead of fresh, but the flavor won't be as vibrant.

Picky Eater Tips: Set aside some raw tomatoes to offer as an alternative to the cooked version. Leave off basil on a small amount and let picky eaters sprinkle it on themselves for more autonomy. Serve a "safe food" option for a fruit or veggie to reduce the pressure at the table.

Leftovers: Refrigerate in airtight container up to 5 days. Do not freeze.

Margherita Crostini

Prep Time: 10 Min | Cook Time: 5 Min   Serves: 4

Ingredients
- 6 oz French bread (sliced crosswise; sub gluten-free bread if desired)
- 8 oz Fresh mozzarella (sliced)
- 4 Tomatoes (sliced)
- 1/4 cup Pesto
- 2 tbsp Basil leaves (optional, minced)

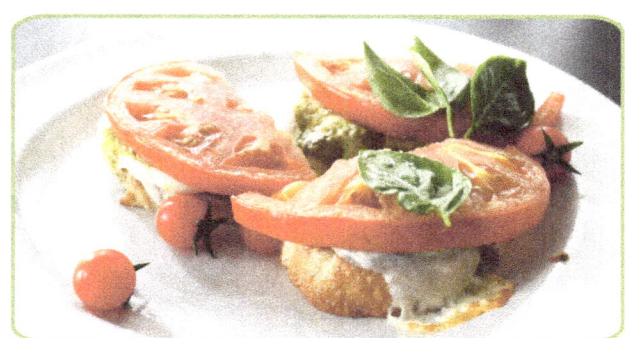

Instructions
1. Set broiler to LOW while preparing ingredients.
2. Slice bread into 1-inch slices and arrange on a baking sheet. Slice mozzarella; slice tomato crosswise and set both aside.
3. Toast bread under the broiler for 2–3 minutes, watching carefully to make sure it doesn't burn.
4. Removed toasted bread from the oven and top with mozzarella cheese slices, pesto, and tomato. Return to the oven and cook for 3–5 minutes more under LOW broiler until cheese is melted and bubbly. Garnish with fresh basil leaves if desired and serve immediately.

Pro Tip: Top crostini with a drizzle of balsamic reduction for a slight twist on this tasty recipe.

Picky Eater Tips: Offer plain toasted bread with cheese on the side. Let picky eaters choose whether to add tomato or basil for a build-your-own approach.

Leftovers: Best if served immediately; refrigerate leftovers in airtight container and reheat in toaster oven, oven, or in skillet. Do not freeze.

Sautéed Zucchini

Prep Time: 10 Min | Cook Time: 15 Min   Serves: 4

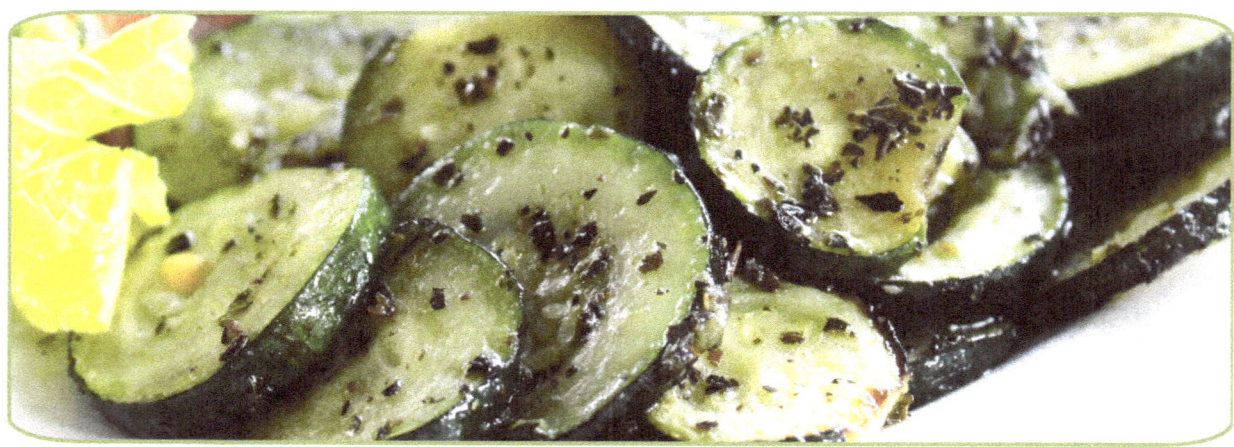

Ingredients

- 3 Zucchini (medium, sliced into rounds)
- 2 tbsp Extra virgin olive oil
- 1 tsp Dried basil
- 1 tsp Oregano
- 1/2 tsp Coarsely ground salt

Instructions

1. Trim ends of zucchini and discard. Cut into 1/4-inch rounds.
2. Heat a large sauté pan over medium-high heat. Once hot, add oil, zucchini, basil, oregano, and salt. Cook 10–15 minutes, stirring occasionally, until squash is tender and starting to brown.

Pro Tip: Zucchini are usually best in summer. Look for firm squash with smooth skin without blemish. Smaller squash are more tender and sweet and usually preferred for roasting; larger squash have bigger seeds and tougher skin. Avoid peeling zucchini to retain nutrients.

Picky Eater Tips: Let your picky eater help pick out a zucchini from the store, slice it, and help stir it while cooking for more hands-on experience. Let them choose different types of seasoning to try, such as an Italian blend or taco seasoning. Serve an alternative fruit or vegetable as a "safe food" to reduce pressure at the table.

Leftovers: Refrigerate in an airtight container up to 5 days. Do not freeze.

Mediterranean Tofu

Prep Time: 15 Min | Cook Time: 10 Min   Serves: 4

Ingredients

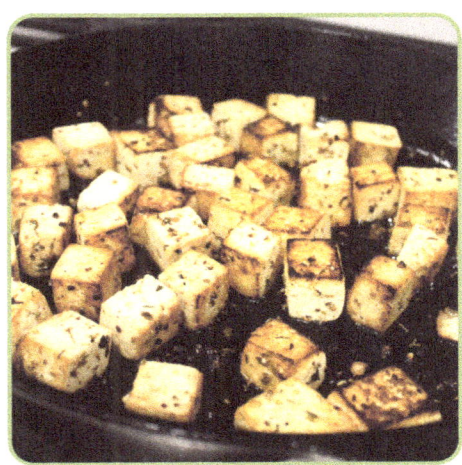

- 14 oz Extra firm tofu (about 1 package, cubed, liquid pressed)
- 1 tbsp Extra virgin olive oil (for marinade)
- 1/4 cup Lemon juice (about 1 large lemon)
- 1 1/2 tsp Garlic (use pre-minced to save time or fresh cloves for better flavor)
- 1 tsp Oregano
- 1/2 tsp Dried thyme
- 1/4 tsp Salt
- 1/4 tsp Black pepper
- 2 tbsp Extra virgin olive oil (for frying)

Instructions

1. Drain water from tofu and cut into 1-inch cubes. Arrange tofu cubes on a clean towel on a plate. Lay a second towel over top of tofu, then set a second plate on top of towel. Set several cans of food or heavy cast iron skillet on top of plate to press liquid from tofu. While liquid presses from tofu, make marinade.
2. Add olive oil (for marinade), lemon juice, garlic, oregano, thyme, salt, and pepper to a shallow dish to make marinade for tofu. Stir to combine well. Add pressed tofu cubes to marinade and stir to coat evenly.
3. Heat a large skillet or sauté pan over medium to medium-high heat. Once hot, add olive oil (for frying), then add tofu. Cook 8–10 minutes, carefully turning tofu several times to ensure even browning on all sides.

Pro Tip: Fresh garlic and lemon juice will provide better flavor, but you can use pre-minced garlic and bottled lemon juice for easier prep. For extra crispy tofu, toss cubes in cornstarch before frying.

Picky Eater Tips: Because tofu is very bland, it can be a good option for picky eaters. Set some plain, uncooked cubes aside and allow to dip in the sauce or choose other sauce to serve, such as teriyaki or soy sauce.

Leftovers: Refrigerate in an airtight container up to 5 days. Not recommended to freeze. To maintain crispiness, reheat in oven, skillet, or toaster oven.

Summer/Fall Meal Plan: Week 3

30-Minute Meal 2

Sticky Thai Peanut Noodles With Gingery Snap Peas & Peppers

✓ Gluten-Free   ✓ Dairy-Free   ✓ Vegetarian   ✓ Vegan

Whole Meal Total Time: 30 Min | Prep Time: 15–20 Min | Cook Time: 10–15 Min

Recommended order of prep:
1. Follow recipe to make <u>Gingery Snap Peas & Peppers</u>.
2. While vegetables cook, make recipe for <u>Sticky Thai Peanut Noodles</u>.
3. Serve noodles with vegetables on the side.

Pro Tip: For a variation on this meal, use peanut sauce over cooked chicken or tofu. Serve alongside or in place of noodles.

Dietary Adjustments

Gluten-Free: Use gluten-free soy sauce or sub Tamari in Sticky Thai Peanut Noodles and Gingery Snap Peas & Peppers.
Vegan: Sub maple syrup instead of honey in Sticky Thai Peanut Noodles.

Gingery Snap Peas & Peppers

Prep Time: 15 Min | Cook Time: 15 Min   Serves: 4

Ingredients

- 2 clove Garlic (minced)
- 2 tbsp Fresh ginger (minced)
- 2 Red bell peppers (sliced into 1/2-inch strips)
- 2 Yellow bell peppers (sliced into 1/2-inch strips)
- 4 cup Snap peas
- 2 tbsp Sesame oil (sub canola oil if desired)
- 2 tbsp Soy sauce (use gluten-free or sub Tamari for gluten-free; sub coconut aminos for soy-free)

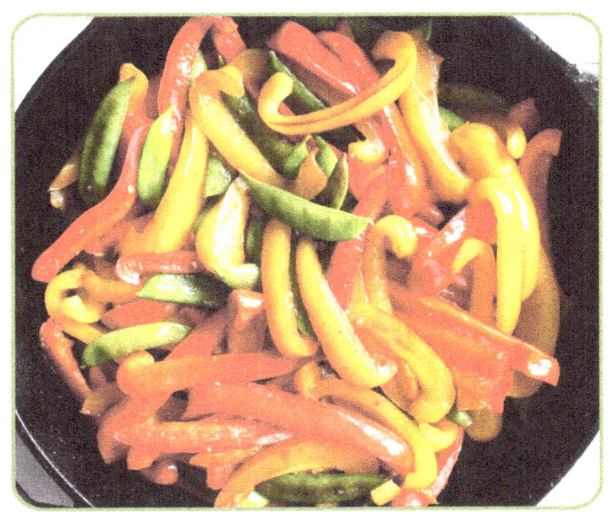

Instructions

1. Mince garlic and ginger and set aside. Cut peppers into 1/2-inch wide strips. Wash snap peas and remove any damaged pieces.
2. Heat a large wok or sauté pan over medium-high heat. Once hot, add oil, garlic, and ginger. Cook 2–3 minutes until fragrant, taking care not to burn.
3. Add bell peppers and snap peas. Cook 8–10 minutes, stirring frequently, until starting to brown and soften.
4. Stir in soy sauce and cook another 1–2 minutes. Remove from heat and serve.

Pro Tip: Substitute or add veggies as desired, such as onion, zucchini, broccoli, water chestnuts, baby corn, carrots, or Bok choy.

Picky Eater Tips: Let your picky eater choose a color of pepper to try. Omit the garlic and ginger for a milder flavor. Set aside some raw peppers and snap peas as an alternative. Let your picky eater add extra soy sauce or teriyaki sauce at the table to give them more autonomy.

Leftovers: Refrigerate in an airtight container up to 5 days. This dish is not recommended to freeze.

Sticky Thai Peanut Noodles

Prep Time: 10 Min | Cook Time: 10 Min   Serves: 4

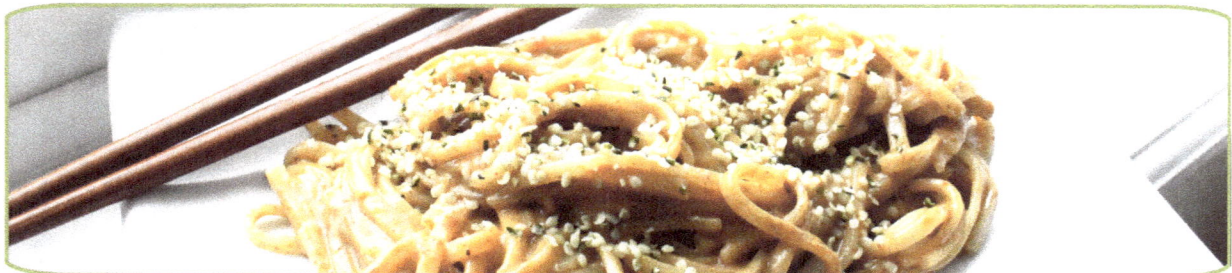

Ingredients

- 8 oz Wide rice noodles
- 1/2 cup All-natural peanut butter (should include only peanuts and salt)
- 5 tbsp Water
- 1/4 cup Soy sauce (use gluten-free or sub Tamari for gluten-free; use coconut aminos for soy-free)
- 1 tbsp Rice vinegar
- 1 tbsp Honey (sub maple syrup for vegan; omit if using coconut aminos)
- 1 tbsp Lime juice (about 1/2 lime)
- 1/4 tsp Red pepper flakes
- 1/4 cup Hemp seeds (to top)

Instructions

1. Cook rice noodles according to package instructions. Drain and add to a large serving bowl.
2. In a separate small bowl, stir together peanut butter, water, soy sauce, rice vinegar, honey, lime juice, and red pepper flakes. Mixture should be the consistency of a thick paste.
3. Once noodles are cooked and drained, stir peanut sauce into rice noodles until well mixed. Sprinkle hemp seeds over noodles to serve.

Pro Tip: Adjust amount of red pepper flakes to desired spice level. You can substitute canola oil in place of sesame oil, but sesame oil will improve the overall flavor. Add cooked chicken breast or fried tofu for extra protein.

Picky Eater Tips: Offer noodles plain with sauce on the side. Serve other toppings for your picky eater to add themselves, such as chopped peanuts or shredded carrots. Try different types of nut butter, such as almond butter or sunflower seed butter, based on what your picky eater is used to. Add more honey to taste.

Leftovers: Refrigerate in airtight container up to 5 days. Not recommended to freeze.

Summer/Fall Meal Plan: Week 3

Slow-Cooker Meal

Coconut Lime Curry Slow Cooker Chicken Over Jasmine Rice

✓ Gluten-Free   ✓ Dairy-Free

Whole Meal Total Time: 2 ½–6 Hrs | Prep Time: 20–25 Min | Cook Time: 2–6 Hrs

Recommended order of prep:
1. Make recipe for <u>Coconut Lime Curry Slow Cooker Chicken</u>.
2. About 20 minutes before ready to eat, make recipe for <u>Jasmine Rice</u>.
3. Serve chicken, vegetables, and curry sauce over rice.

Pro Tip: Save the extra coconut milk from curry chicken recipe and use it in place of some of the water in the jasmine rice recipe, both to prevent food waste and to tie the flavors in the meal together. Sub red bell pepper in place of green bell pepper for more vitamin E.

Dietary Adjustments

Vegetarian / Vegan: Sub chickpeas in place of chicken in Coconut Lime Curry Slow Cooker Chicken.

Coconut Lime Curry Slow Cooker Chicken

Prep Time: 15 Min | Cook Time: 2 Hours   Serves: 4

Ingredients

- 1 Green bell pepper (large, sliced)
- 1 cup Water chestnuts (8 oz can, drained and rinsed
- 1 cup Bamboo shoots (8 oz can, drained and rinsed)
- 1 lb Boneless, skinless chicken thighs (sub 1 3/4 cup chickpeas for vegan)
- 2 tbsp Fresh ginger (minced)

- 2 tbsp Lime juice (1 lime)
- 1 tsp Lime peel (zest)
- 1 cup Coconut milk
- 1/4 cup Sugar
- 2 tbsp Curry powder
- 1 tsp Salt
- 1/4 tsp Red pepper flakes (optional; more for added heat)

Instructions

1. Slice pepper; drain and rinse water chestnuts and bamboo shoots. Place all in a large slow cooker and stir to mix. Push vegetables to edges of slow cooker and place chicken thighs in the center.
2. Mince ginger; juice and zest lime. Add to a separate small bowl along with coconut milk, sugar, curry powder, salt, and red pepper flakes. Stir to mix well and pour mixture over chicken and vegetables in slow cooker, making sure chicken is submerged.
3. Cook on high 2–3 hours or on low 4–6 hours. Serve chicken and sauce over cooked jasmine rice.

Pro Tip: Instead of using a slow cooker, cut chicken into 1-inch pieces and marinate overnight in coconut milk and spices, then cook this on the stove in a large pot for about 20 minutes. If desired, substitute other types of vegetables, such as baby corn, carrot rounds, or broccoli.

Picky Eater Tips: Serve each component of this curry separately: chicken, water chestnuts, bamboo shoots, and curry sauce to let your picky eater build their own dish. Set aside a few plain water chestnuts and bamboo shoots before adding to the slow cooker to let them try these without the curry flavor. Let your picky eater squeeze their own lime wedge at the table for more hands-on experience. Serve a "safe food" option for protein and either a fruit or veggie.

Leftovers: Refrigerate in airtight container up to 5 days. Freeze up to a month.

Jasmine Rice

Prep Time: 5 Min | Cook Time: 20 Min   Serves: 4

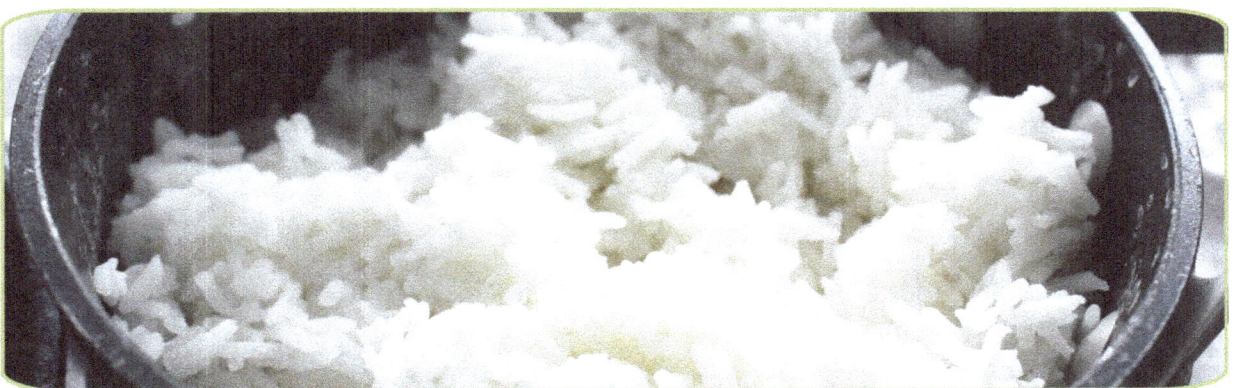

Ingredients
- 1 cup Jasmine rice (rinsed)
- 2 cup Water
- 1/4 tsp Salt

Instructions
1. Rinse rice: place white rice in a large bowl and add water to completely submerge rice. Stir the rice around with your hand or a spoon, then drain it through a colander or mesh sieve. Repeat once or twice until water is clear when drained.
2. Add rinsed rice, water, and salt to small saucepan. Cover with a lid, turn up heat to high and bring to a boil, then reduce heat to low and simmer 10–15 minutes until all water has been absorbed.
3. Turn off heat and let rice sit another 10 minutes, then fluff with a fork and serve.

Pro Tip: For coconut-flavored jasmine rice, sauté rice in coconut oil for 3–4 minutes before adding water. Use coconut milk in place of some or all of the water for additional fat and flavor.

Picky Eater Tips: Serve rice with different types of sauce or dressing, such as butter, teriyaki sauce, or soy sauce. Let your picky eater choose what they want to add. Try a taste test with different types of rice to add exposures to different textures and tastes.

Leftovers: Refrigerate in an airtight container for up to 5 days, or freeze for up to 3 months.

Summer/Fall Meal Plan: Week 3

Vegetarian Meal

Black Bean & Quinoa Mexican Skillet With Tortilla Chips

✓ Gluten-Free   ✓ Vegetarian

Whole Meal Total Time: 40–45 Min | Prep Time: 20–25 Min | Cook Time: 20 Min

Recommended order of prep:
1. Make recipe for <u>Black Bean & Quinoa Mexican Skillet</u>.
2. Serve skillet with tortilla chips on the side.

Pro Tip: Add cooked ground beef, chorizo, soy chorizo, or diced chicken to this dish for additional protein. Try this dish with leftover rice instead of quinoa to use up leftovers and prevent food waste.

Dietary Adjustments

Dairy-Free / Vegan: Omit cheese and top Black Bean & Quinoa Skillet with avocado slices instead.

Black Bean & Quinoa Mexican Skillet

Prep Time: 20 Min | Cook Time: 20 Min   Serves: 4

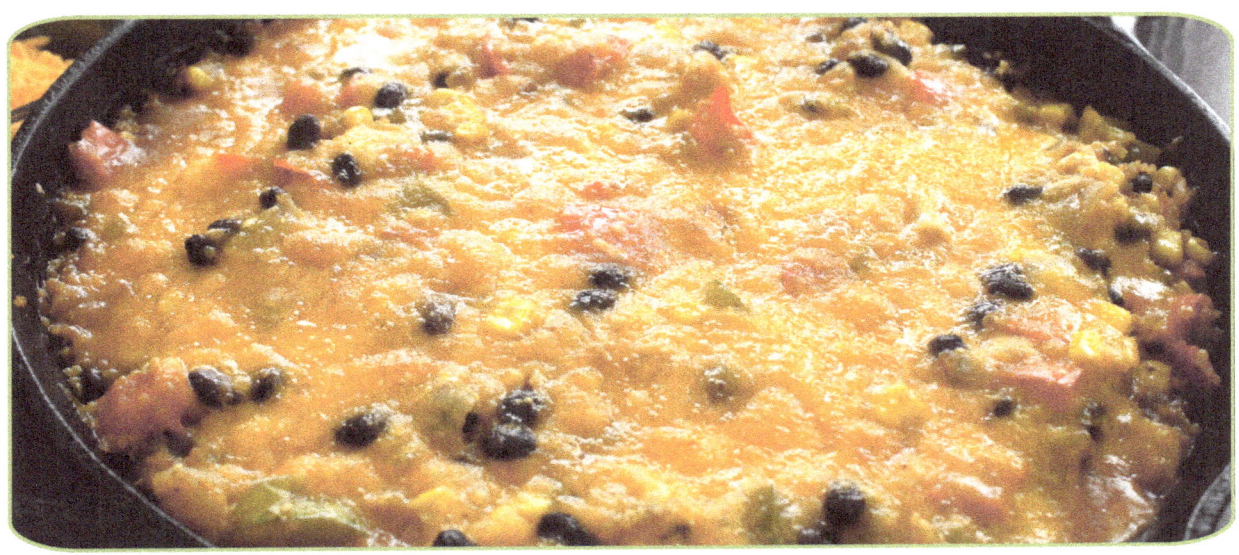

Ingredients

- 1 Yellow onion (diced)
- 2 clove Garlic (minced)
- 2 tbsp Canola oil
- 1 Red bell pepper (diced)
- 1 Green bell pepper (diced)
- 1 jalapeño pepper (minced)
- 2 tsp Cumin
- 1 tsp Chili powder
- 1 tsp Smoked paprika
- 1 tsp Salt
- 1/2 cup Quinoa (uncooked)

- 1 1/4 cup Water
- 1 3/4 cup Black beans (14.5 oz can, drained and rinsed)
- 1/2 cup Frozen corn
- 1 cup Shredded cheddar cheese (sub vegan cheese for dairy-free option OR omit and serve with guacamole or avocado cubes instead)
- Toppings as desired: salsa, shredded cheese, tortilla chips, freshly minced cilantro, sour cream, or avocado cubes

Instructions

1. Dice onion and mince garlic. Heat a large oven-safe sauté pan or cast-iron skillet over medium heat. Once hot, add oil, onion, and garlic. Cook 8–10 minutes until onion is beginning to become translucent.

Black Bean & Quinoa Mexican Skillet (Continued)

Instructions (Continued)

2. While onion and garlic cook, dice bell peppers and mince jalapeño. Once prepared, add to pan with onion along with cumin, chili powder, smoked paprika, and salt. Sauté 2–3 minutes until spices become fragrant.
3. Add quinoa and water to pan with vegetables. Cover with a lid and bring to a boil, then reduce heat and simmer about 15 minutes until liquid has been absorbed.
4. While quinoa cooks, drain and rinse black beans and set aside. Prepare additional toppings as desired and set aside.
5. Once quinoa is fully cooked, stir in black beans and corn until well-combined. If dish still has a significant amount of liquid, leave lid off and continue to simmer until liquid has evaporated, then top dish evenly with shredded cheese.
6. Optional: set oven to high broil. Place the oven-safe sauté pan in oven under broiler for 1–2 minutes until the cheese is bubbly and just starting to brown, watching carefully to avoid burning. Skip this step if you are not using an oven-safe sauté pan.
7. Serve this dish over greens, with tortilla chips, or with corn tortillas and desired toppings.

Pro Tip: Substitute or add other vegetables as desired, such as zucchini, yellow squash, other types of peppers, or tomatoes. Add cooked ground beef, chorizo, soy chorizo, or diced chicken for additional protein.

Picky Eater Tips: Set aside some raw pepper slices, plain black beans, and shredded cheese to serve separately alongside the mixed dish. Offer an additional "safe food" if needed to round out the healthy plate, depending on what your picky eater might need, including options for a protein, starch, and fruit or veggie.

Leftovers: Refrigerate in airtight container up to 5 days. Freeze up to several months.

Summer/Fall Meal Plan: Week 3

Challenge Meal

Sweet Bourbon Grilled Salmon, Sweet Corn, and Caesar Salad

Whole Meal Total Time: 50 Min | Prep Time: 20–30 Min | Cook Time: 12–16 Min

Recommended order of prep:
1. Start marinating salmon for <u>Sweet Bourbon Grilled Salmon</u>.
2. Make recipe for <u>Caesar Salad</u>.
3. Make recipe for <u>Sweet Corn</u>.
4. While corn cooks, cook salmon per recipe instructions.
5. Serve salmon with sweet corn and salad on the side.

Pro Tip: Use a grill mat for salmon for best results. See pro tip in salmon recipe for instructions to cook without a grill. For non-fish lovers, substitute chicken breast in place of salmon.

Dietary Adjustments

Gluten-Free: Use gluten-free soy sauce or sub tamari to make Sweet Bourbon Grilled Salmon. Use gluten-free croutons to make Caesar Salad.

Dairy-Free: Omit Parmesan cheese and sub nutritional yeast or slivered almonds for Grilled Caesar Salad; use dairy-free Caesar dressing.

Vegetarian: Sub recipe for <u>Sweet Bourbon Grilled Tofu</u> in place of Sweet Bourbon Grilled Salmon. Use vegetarian Caesar dressing.

Vegan: Sub recipe for <u>Sweet Bourbon Grilled Tofu</u> in place of Sweet Bourbon Grilled Salmon. Sub nutritional yeast or slivered almonds for Parmesan cheese in Grilled Caesar Salad; use vegan Ceasar dressing.

Sweet Bourbon Grilled Salmon

Prep Time: 30 Min | Cook Time: 10 Min   Serves: 4

Ingredients

- 1 1/2 lb Salmon fillet (fresh, or thawed from frozen)
- 3 tbsp Canola oil
- 3 tbsp Soy sauce (use gluten-free soy sauce or sub Tamari for gluten-free or coconut aminos for soy-free)
- 1/2 cup Bourbon (low-quality bourbon is fine)
- 1 tbsp Brown sugar
- 1 tsp Minced garlic
- 1/2 tsp Black pepper

Instructions

1. Place salmon in a shallow dish. In a separate bowl, make a marinade by whisking together all remaining ingredients: oil, soy sauce, bourbon, brown sugar, minced garlic, and black pepper. Pour marinade over salmon, turning to coat on all sides. Arrange fish so it is covered by as much of the liquid as possible. Marinate in the refrigerator for 20–30 minutes, turning salmon over half-way through to ensure an even marinade.
2. Heat grill to about 450° Fahrenheit. Grill salmon for 6–8 minutes per side on a grill mat until internal temperature is 130–140° Fahrenheit; salmon should look opaque and easily flake with a fork. Pour remaining marinade over fish as it grills. Allow salmon to rest 5 minutes after cooking and before serving to retain moisture.

Pro Tip: Instead of grilling, heat a cast iron skillet to medium-high temperature, add a tablespoon of canola oil, and then add salmon. Sear at high heat. If fish begins to burn before inside is cooked, reduce heat to medium until cooked through. If using frozen salmon, allow to thaw completely before marinating. Instead of pouring remaining marinade over salmon, make a reduction by adding leftover marinade to a small saucepan and simmering over medium-low heat. Serve the reduction over the salmon.

Picky Eater Tips: Serve a very small amount of salmon to start, or serve in a wrap or with chips, allowing your picky eater to choose how they would like to try this. If your picky eater doesn't like fish, you can use this marinade on chicken to serve in addition to salmon. Offer a dip on the side such as teriyaki, aioli, honey mustard, or even ranch dressing to make this feel more familiar.

Leftovers: Refrigerate in an airtight container 3–5 days. Not recommended to freeze.

Caesar Salad

Prep Time: 15 Min | Cook Time: 0 Min   Serves: 4

Ingredients

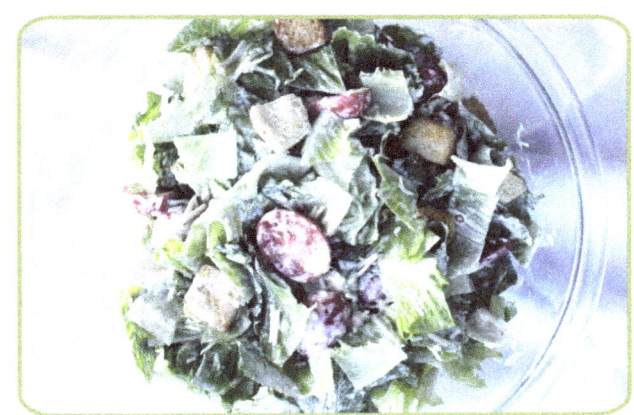

- 6 cup Romaine lettuce (chopped; about 2 Romaine hearts)
- 2 cup Cherry tomatoes (cut in half)
- 1 cup Croutons (sub gluten-free croutons for gluten-free)
- 1/2 cup Grated Parmesan cheese (sub sliced almonds for dairy-free)
- 1/2 cup Caesar salad dressing (use vegan or dairy-free if desired)

Instructions

1. Chop romaine hearts into approximately 1-inch pieces and cut tomatoes in half lengthwise.
2. Add lettuce to a large serving bowl along with croutons, Parmesan cheese, and salad dressing. Toss to combine well and serve immediately.

Pro Tip: Use a pre-made salad mix for an even easier side dish. Substitute roasted chickpeas in place of croutons for a high-protein crunch. Add other ingredients as desired, such as bacon bits, cucumbers, anchovies, or sliced almonds.

Picky Eater Tips: Serve dressing on the side to let your picky eater add on top or use as a dip instead; offer alternative dressing options if they don't like Caesar. Serve salad components separately to let your picky eater build their own bowl. Add other veggies or toppings they like, such as croutons, other types of cheese, or plain cucumber slices. Serve a fruit they like as a "safe food" alternative.

Leftovers: Once dressing has been added, refrigerate for 1–2 days. Do not freeze.

Fresh Sweet Corn

Prep Time: 10 Min | Cook Time: 15 Min   Serves: 4

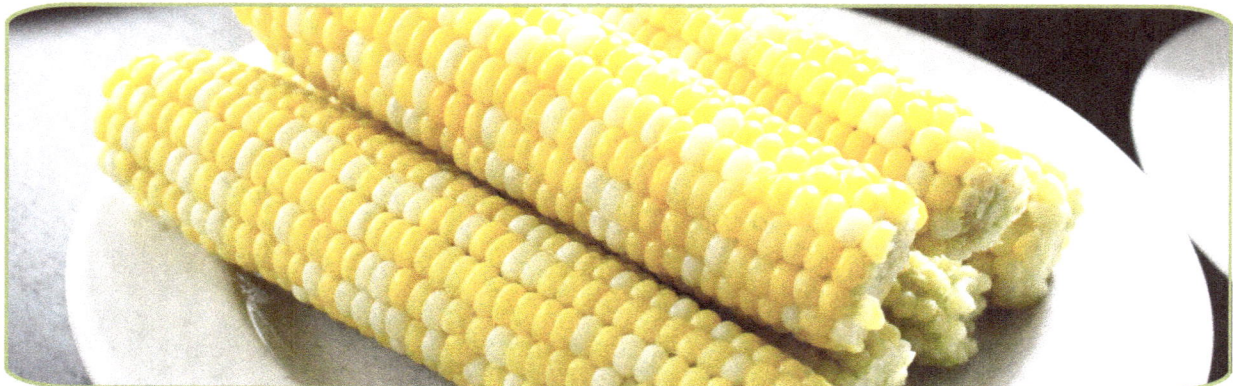

Ingredients
- 4 ear Corn on the cob (6-inch ear, husk removed)

Instructions
1. Shuck corn and remove as many of the silks as possible. Wash and trim any damaged parts of the corn.
2. **Boiled corn option:** Fill a large pot or skillet with a few inches of water and bring to a boil. Place corn in boiling water and cover with lid. Boil 4–5 minutes, then turn corn over and boil another 4–5 minutes. Serve corn with butter and salt, if desired.
3. **Grilled corn option:** Soak corn in the husk 2–3 hours (to prevent husk from burning), then place on preheated grill (about 400–450° Fahrenheit) and cook 4–5 minutes per side until husk is starting to char.

Pro Tip: Fresh sweet corn is in season and in July and August. To choose a good ear of sweet corn, avoid peeling back the husk, as it can dry out the kernels. Instead, choose ears with bright green, tightly wrapped husks, sticky brown silks (not dry or black), and plump kernels you can feel through the husk. If you're not sure, ask your local farmer, as they're experts at spotting the freshest pick.

Picky Eater Tips: Let your picky eater choose whether to eat corn off the cob or to cut it off the cob and eat with a fork. Let them choose and season their own corn. Find fun "corn holders" at the store to poke into the cob to help hold the corn to eat.

Leftovers: Refrigerate in airtight container up to 5 days. To freeze, blanch corn by boiling only 2–3 minutes, then transferring to an ice bath to cool quickly. Freeze on the cob or cut off and freeze in reusable containers, mason jars, or freezer-safe bags.

Sweet Bourbon Grilled Tofu

Prep Time: 30 Min | Cook Time: 15 Min   Serves: 4

Ingredients

- 2 lb Extra firm tofu (about 2 packages, liquid pressed)
- 2 tbsp Canola oil
- 3 tbsp Soy sauce (use gluten-free or sub tamari for gluten-free)
- 1/2 cup Bourbon (low-quality bourbon is fine)
- 1 tbsp Brown sugar
- 1 tsp Minced garlic
- 1/2 tsp Black pepper

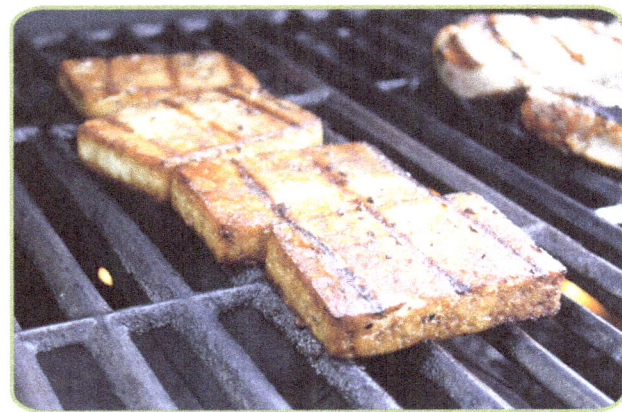

Instructions

1. Drain water from tofu and slice each block into 5 even pieces. Press liquid from tofu by laying slices between two clean towels and pressing down firmly with your hands. Once as much liquid as possible has been removed, arrange tofu slices in a shallow dish with no pieces overlapping.
2. In a separate bowl, make a marinade by whisking together all remaining ingredients: oil, soy sauce, bourbon, brown sugar, minced garlic, and black pepper. Pour marinade over tofu, turning to coat on all sides. Arrange tofu so it is covered by as much of the liquid as possible.
3. Marinate tofu in the refrigerator for 20–30 minutes, turning tofu slices over halfway through to ensure even marinade. If time allows, marinate for several hours.
4. Heat grill to about 450° Fahrenheit. Place tofu either directly on the grill or use a grill mat. Grill for 6–8 minutes per side until starting to char.
5. While tofu grills, pour the remaining marinade into a small saucepan and simmer over medium-low heat. Serve marinade reduction over tofu.

Pro Tip: Marinate tofu for several hours or overnight for better flavor. As an alternative to grilling, cook tofu in a cast-iron skillet for 6–8 minutes per side.

Picky Eater Tips: Because tofu is very bland, it can be a good option for picky eaters. Set some plain, uncooked tofu cubes aside and allow to dip in the sauce or choose other sauce to serve, such as teriyaki or soy sauce.

Leftovers: Refrigerate in airtight container up to 5 days. Not recommended to freeze.

Summer/Fall Meal Plan: Week 3

Savory Grab & Go

Edamame Salad With Cilantro Lime Dressing and Cheese Quesadilla

✓ Vegetarian

Dietary Adjustments

Gluten-Free: Use corn or gluten-free tortilla to make Cheese Quesadilla.
Dairy-Free / Vegan: Sub recipe for <u>Crispy Vegan Baked Black Bean Tacos</u> in place of Cheese Quesadilla.

Sweet Grab & Go

Turkey Wraps With Almonds, Cucumbers & Blueberries

✓ Gluten-Free

Dietary Adjustments

Dairy-Free / Vegan: Sub avocado, extra almonds, or other type of nut or seed in place of turkey and Havarti cheese in Turkey Wraps With Almonds, Cucumbers & Blueberries. See page 38 for more ideas for protein substitutes.
Vegetarian: Sub slices of Swiss or other cheese in place of turkey in Turkey Wraps With Almonds, Cucumbers & Blueberries. See page 38 for more ideas for protein substitutes.

Edamame Salad With Cilantro Lime Dressing

Prep Time: 20 Min | Cook Time: 5 Min   Serves: 4

Salad
- 2 cup Mukimame (shelled Edamame, frozen)
- 1 cup Frozen corn
- 1 Red bell pepper (diced)
- 1/2 cup Red onion (diced)
- 1/4 cup Cilantro (fresh, chopped)

Dressing
- 1/4 cup Lime juice (about 2 limes)
- 1/4 cup Extra virgin olive oil
- 1 tbsp Red wine vinegar
- 2 tsp Honey (sub maple syrup for vegan)
- 1/4 tsp Salt

Instructions
1. Add mukimame (shelled edamame) and corn to a small saucepan with enough water to just cover the bottom of the pan; vegetables will not be fully submerged. Place on the stove, cover with a lid, and cook over medium heat for about 5 minutes until mukimame are bright green, indicating they are fully cooked. Drain water and set aside to cool.
2. Meanwhile, dice bell pepper and onion. Mince cilantro. Add to a medium-sized serving bowl.
3. Make dressing in a separate small bowl, whisking together lime juice, olive oil, red wine vinegar, honey, and salt together until smooth.
4. Add cooked mukimame and corn to the serving bowl with other vegetables. Pour dressing over vegetables and stir to mix well. Serve immediately or chill in refrigerator up to several hours to allow flavors to blend.

Pro Tip: Make this salad ahead of time and refrigerate until ready to serve to save time during meal prep.

Picky Eater Tips: Serve each component of this salad separately to let your picky eater build their own salad, with the dressing on the side. Offer an alternative dressing like plain olive oil or a bit of ranch. Serve the cilantro separately and allow each person to add their own. Serve a familiar veggie or fruit on the plate as a "safe food" they enjoy.

Leftovers: Refrigerate in airtight container up to 5 days. Not recommended to freeze.

Cheese Quesadilla

Prep Time: 5 Min | Cook Time: 5 Min   Serves: 4

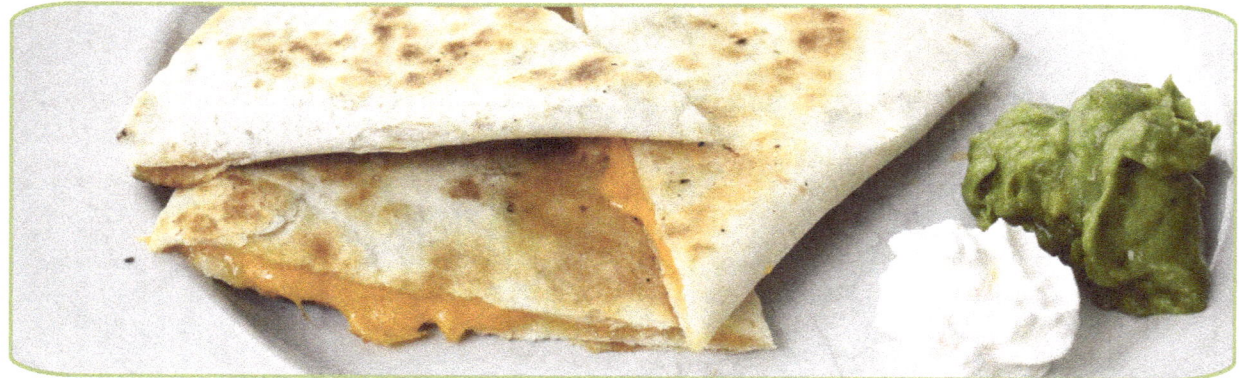

Ingredients
- 4 10-inch tortillas (choose gluten-free or sub 2 corn tortillas in place of 1 flour tortilla for gluten-free option)
- 1 cup Shredded cheddar cheese

Instructions
1. Spread about 1/4 cup shredded cheddar cheese evenly over one half of a tortilla. Fold tortilla in half over cheese.
2. Place in a hot skillet and cook quesadilla for 2–3 minutes, then flip and cook another 2–3 minutes on the other side until cheese is melted and tortilla is starting to brown. Place cooked quesadillas on a plate with a towel over the top to keep warm. Repeat steps 1 and 2 to make remaining quesadillas.

Pro Tip: Add black beans, sliced black olives, sour cream, shredded chicken, pork, beef, or salsa to quesadilla before cooking for variety. Instead of cooking on the stove, cook the quesadilla in the microwave for 1 minute or in the toaster oven for 3–4 minutes.

Picky Eater Tips: Use different types of tortillas and cheese based on what your picky eater likes or to help expand their taste. Let them help assemble the quesadilla, choose the shape (fold in half, make whole, or roll into an enchilada instead), or choose how many triangles to cut it in. Serve plain shredded or sliced cheese and tortilla without cooking or melting the cheese as an alternative.

Leftovers: Refrigerate in an airtight container for up to 5 days. Enjoy leftovers cold (like pizza!) or reheat in microwave, toaster oven, or skillet.

Crispy Vegan Baked Black Bean Tacos

Prep Time: 15 Min | Cook Time: 15 Min   Serves: 4

Ingredients

- 1 3/4 cup Black beans (14.5 oz can, drained and rinsed)
- 2 tbsp Canola oil (to sauté garlic)
- 2 tsp Minced garlic
- 1 tsp Smoked paprika
- 1 tsp Cumin
- 1 tsp Oregano
- 1 tsp Onion powder
- 1 tsp Salt
- 1/4 cup Water
- 8 Corn tortillas (white or yellow)
- 1 tbsp Canola oil (to top tacos)
- Toppings for tacos as desired: lime wedge, shredded lettuce, cubed avocado, salsa, sour cream, or chopped cilantro

Instructions

1. Preheat oven to 450° Fahrenheit. Drain and rinse black beans; set aside.
2. Heat a large sauté pan over medium heat. Once hot, add oil (for sautéing garlic), and minced garlic. Cook, stirring occasionally, 1–2 minutes. Once garlic is fragrant, add in paprika, cumin, oregano, onion powder, and salt. Stir to evenly distribute spices and cook about 60 seconds to "bloom" the spices.
3. Add drained black beans and water to spices. Cook for 3–4 minutes until heated through, then remove from heat. Mash black beans with a potato masher or fork.
4. Stack tortillas on a microwave-safe plate and cover with a wet paper towel. Microwave for 30–60 seconds until soft and pliable. Re-wet paper towel and repeat process if tortillas break while assembling tacos.
5. Place a warm tortilla on a large baking sheet. Spread slightly less than 2 tbsp of bean mixture on half the tortilla. Fold tortilla in half over beans and use a pastry brush to spread oil along the taco, then flip the taco over and brush oil on the other other side. Repeat this process to make tacos with remaining ingredients.
6. Place tacos in oven and bake for 6 minutes, then flip tacos and bake another 6–8 minutes until golden brown. Prep desired toppings while tacos bake.

Pro Tip: Use flour tortillas if desired. Add fresh cilantro for a burst of flavor.

Picky Eater Tips: Let picky eaters help make this dish by smashing black beans or filling tacos. Serve with a variety of toppings to let them try. Set aside a few whole black beans to offer alongside these tacos.

Leftovers: Refrigerate in airtight container up to 5 days. Reheat in air fryer or oven for crispy tacos. Not recommended to freeze.

Turkey Wraps With Almonds, Cucumbers & Blueberries

Prep Time: 10 Min | Cook Time: 0 Min   Serves: 1

Ingredients

- 1/4 Apple (cored, sliced)
- 1 oz Havarti cheese (sliced thinly; sub other cheese type as desired or avocado for dairy-free)
- 3 1/2 oz Deli-sliced turkey breast (choose gluten-free if desired)
- 1/2 cup Blueberries
- 1/4 cup Almonds
- 1/2 Cucumber (large, sliced)

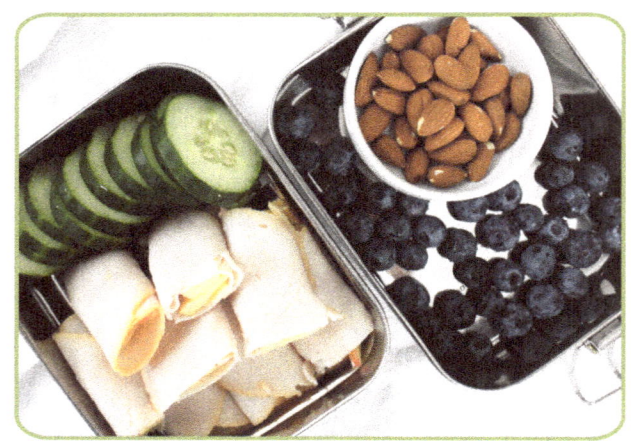

Instructions

1. Cut apple and cheese into thin slices. Layer the apple and Havarti cheese on top of the sliced turkey. Roll into wraps.
2. Serve turkey wraps with the blueberries, almonds and cucumber.

Pro Tip: Sub other type of deli meat or cheese as desired. Use pumpkin seeds or sunflower seeds in place of almonds for a nut-free option.

Picky Eater Tips: Let your picky eater make these rolls to give them more hands-on experience. Let them swap out different carbs, protein, fruit, and veggies using the Quick Options to Build a Healthy Plate on page 38.

Leftovers: Dip apples in a solution of lemon juice and water to prep ahead of time, then refrigerate in airtight container up to 3 days. Do not freeze. Keep almonds in a separate airtight container at room temperature to maintain crispiness.

Summer/Fall Meal Plan: Week 3

Savory Breakfast

Avocado & Ricotta on Toast

✓ Vegetarian

Dietary Adjustments

Gluten-Free: Use gluten-free bread to make Avocado & Ricotta on Toast.
Dairy-Free / Vegan: Use plant-based ricotta OR sub recipe for <u>Avocado Toast</u> in place of Avocado & Ricotta on Toast.

Sweet Breakfast

High Protein Banana Pancakes

✓ Dairy-Free   ✓ Vegetarian

Dietary Adjustments

Gluten-Free: Use an all-purpose gluten-free flour blend to make High Protein Banana Pancakes.
Vegan: Sub recipe for <u>Eggless Crêpes</u> in place of High Protein Banana Pancakes.

Avocado & Ricotta Cheese on Toast

Prep Time: 5 Min | Cook Time: 5 Min   Serves: 1

Ingredients

- 1 slice Whole wheat bread (sub gluten-free bread or rice cakes for gluten-free)
- 1/4 Avocado (sliced)
- 2 tbsp Ricotta cheese (sub plant-based cheese for dairy-free and vegan)
- Salt and pepper (to taste)

Instructions

1. Toast bread to desired crispiness in toaster oven or toaster. While bread toasts, slice avocado into thin slices by cutting the avocado in half around pit, then cut flesh into slices inside shell. Use a spoon to gently scoop out slices and set aside.
2. Spread 2 tbsp ricotta cheese evenly on toast and top with avocado slices. Season with salt and pepper.

Avocado Toast

Prep Time: 10 Min | Cook Time: 0 Min   Serves: 1

Ingredients

- 1 slice Whole wheat bread (sub gluten-free bread or rice cakes for gluten-free)
- 1/4 Avocado
- Salt and pepper (to taste)

Instructions

1. Toast bread in toaster oven or toaster to desired crispiness.
2. Cut avocado in half around pit. Discard pit and cut avocado flesh into squares inside shell (do not cut through peel). Use a fork to mash avocado inside the shell.
3. Spread mashed avocado on toast. Sprinkle with salt and pepper to taste.

Pro Tip (Both Recipes): For more protein, top with a fried egg or chickpeas.

Picky Eater Tips (Both Recipes): Serve toast with spreads on the side. Add a sprinkle of cinnamon or honey to ricotta for a sweeter twist. Serve avocado in different forms: cubed, mashed, or sliced. Let picky eaters build their own toast and choose extra seasonings like Italian seasoning or seasoned salt for more autonomy.

Leftovers (Both Recipes): These are best if prepped and served immediately. Store avocado half in refrigerator with plastic wrap covering all exposed flesh OR mash avocado and drizzle with lime juice to prevent browning. Keep up to 1–2 days.

High Protein Banana Pancakes

Prep Time: 15 Min | Cook Time: 10 Min   Serves: 4

Ingredients

- 3 Bananas (ripe or thawed from frozen)
- 6 Eggs
- 1 tbsp Canola oil (plus more for skillet)
- 1/2 cup Flour (sub all-purpose gluten-free flour blend for gluten-free)
- 2 tbsp Sugar
- 2 tbsp Ground flaxseed (sub additional flour if no flaxseed available)
- 1 tsp Baking powder
- 1/4 tsp Salt

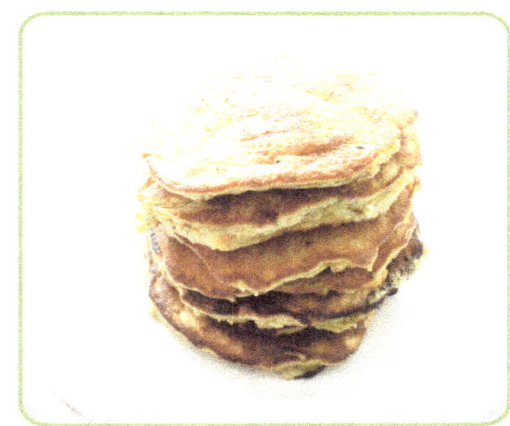

Instructions

1. In a medium-sized mixing bowl, mash bananas with a fork or potato masher until consistency is smooth and almost liquidy. Add eggs and oil and beat gently with a fork for about 30 seconds.
2. Add all remaining ingredients to the egg mixture: flour, sugar, ground flaxseed, baking powder, and salt. Stir until thoroughly combined and batter is smooth.
3. Heat a large griddle or skillet over medium heat. Once hot, add a small amount of oil, using a spatula to spread oil evenly across surface of the griddle.
4. Make pancakes: pour 1/4 cup batter per pancake onto the griddle and cook about 1–3 minutes per side. Cook times vary; flip pancake once starting to see bubbles form in pancake batter. If pancakes burn before bubbles form, lower heat.

Pro Tip: Add fresh blueberries, raspberries, or chocolate chips to pancakes as they cook for variety. Top with peanut butter or almond butter for extra protein and healthy fat.

Picky Eater Tips: Let your picky eater choose what to use to top pancakes: nut butter, yogurt, sprinkles, berries, chocolate chips, or other family favorites. Serve syrup or honey on the side for dipping.

Leftovers: Refrigerate in airtight container up to a week. Freeze up to several months.

Eggless Crêpes

Prep Time: 10 Min | Cook Time: 15 Min   Serves: 4

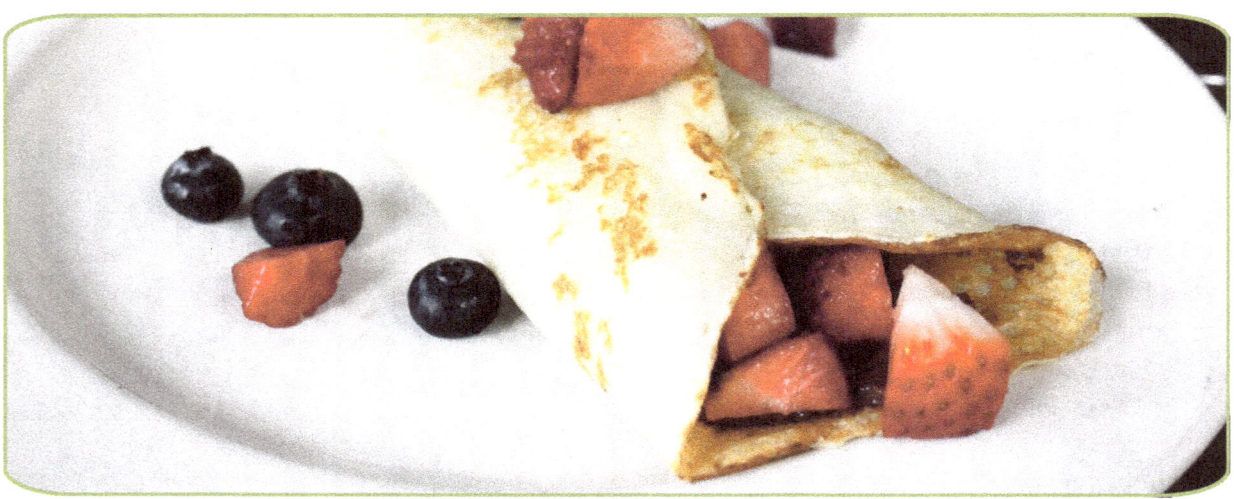

Ingredients

- 1 cup Flour (sub all-purpose gluten-free flour blend for gluten-free)
- 1 tbsp Sugar (omit for savory crêpes)
- 1/4 tsp Salt
- 2 tbsp Canola oil
- 2 cup Soy milk (room temperature; sub dairy or pea milk for soy free)
- Toppings for crêpes as desired (see pro tip for inspiration)

Instructions

1. In a medium-sized mixing bowl, whisk together flour, sugar, and salt.
2. Add oil and soy milk to the dry ingredients and whisk until smooth and well combined with no clumps.
3. Heat a non-stick 10-inch skillet over medium heat. To make sure skillet is hot before cooking, flick a few drops of water in the pan. If they sizzle and evaporate immediately, the skillet is ready.
4. Pour about 1/3 cup of batter into skillet; pick up skillet from stove and tilt it in several directions to allow batter to run and completely cover the bottom of the skillet with a thin layer of batter. Do this quickly before it starts to cook.

Eggless Crêpes (Continued)

Instructions (Continued)

5. Cook crêpe about 2 minutes until it starts to become firm, then flip the crêpe and cook it another 30 seconds, just until starting to brown. To flip, either use a large spatula (flip quickly, in one fell swoop—don't be scared!) or flip with the skillet itself, like a professional chef on a cooking show. Loosen the crêpe from the skillet by shaking the pan back and forth or using a spatula, then flick your wrist, holding the pan to throw the crêpe into the air and catch it in the pan.
6. Repeat steps 5 & 6 to use remaining batter. Stack cooked crêpes on a serving plate, under a towel to keep them warm. Serve with your favorite toppings.

Pro Tip: If you have trouble with the crêpes sticking to the pan, add a drop of canola oil or small amount of butter to the pan before adding batter.
- Sweet crêpe topping inspiration:
    - Chocolate hazelnut spread + sliced strawberries
    - Berries + whipped cream
    - Chocolate or vanilla pudding
    - Cooked apples or pears (simmered over low heat with a little sugar, lemon juice, and cinnamon)
- Savory crêpe topping inspiration:
    - Caramelized onions + sautéed mushrooms
    - Scrambled eggs + fresh basil
    - Sautéed mushrooms + asparagus
    - Eggs + Hollandaise sauce
    - Tomatoes + basil + mozzarella

Picky Eater Tips: These mild crêpes can be a good way to expose picky eaters to new foods. Serve with a variety of fillings like fruit, nut butter, or chocolate spread so picky eaters can create their own combination. Let them build their own crêpe and choose to eat with a fork or pick up with their hands.

Leftovers: Refrigerate in an airtight container up to 5 days. To freeze, fold crêpes into fourths (to save space), then lay crêpes on a silicone baking sheet or wax paper and freeze individually. Once frozen, transfer to a resealable airtight container and freeze up to 2 months. Reheat in the microwave.

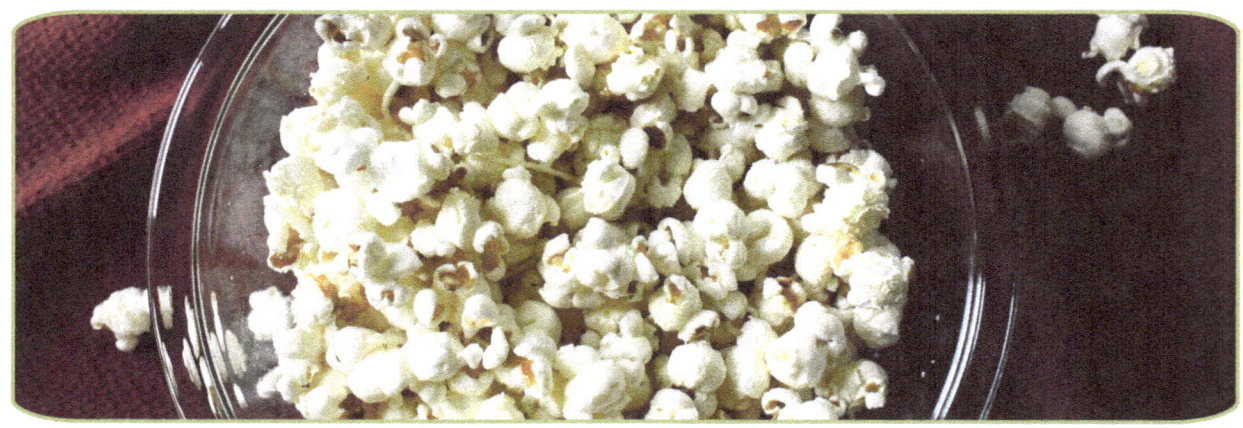

Savory Snack

Parmesan Popcorn

✓ Gluten-Free   ✓ Dairy-Free   ✓ Vegetarian   ✓ Vegan

Dietary Adjustments

Dairy-Free / Vegan: Use vegan butter to make Parmesan Popcorn.

Sweet Snack

Strawberries & Chocolate Fruit Dip

✓ Gluten-Free   ✓ Dairy-Free   ✓ Vegetarian   ✓ Vegan

Parmesan Popcorn

Prep Time: 5 Min | Cook Time: 10 Min   Serves: 4

Ingredients
- 2 tbsp Extra virgin olive oil
- 1/2 cup Popcorn kernels
- 2 tbsp Butter (regular or vegan, melted)
- 1/2 tsp Salt
- 2 tbsp Nutritional yeast
  (sub Parmesan cheese if desired)

Instructions
1. Add oil and one popcorn kernel to a medium saucepan. Cover with a lid and turn heat to medium-high. Once kernel pops, add remaining popcorn, cover with lid again, and cook until popping has slowed to once every few seconds.
2. Meanwhile, melt butter in microwave: place butter in a microwave-safe bowl and heat 30–60 seconds on 50% power, stirring 2–3 times.
3. Remove popcorn from heat and toss with butter, salt and nutritional yeast.

Pro Tip: Make trail mix by adding nuts, dried fruit, chocolate chips, and/or pretzels.

Picky Eater Tips: Let your picky eater help make this popcorn. Allow them to sprinkle nutritional yeast on top, or choose other seasonings to add.

Leftovers: Store in an airtight container at room temperature for several days.

Chocolate Fruit Dip

Prep Time: 15 Min | Cook Time: 0 Min   Serves: 8

Ingredients
- 1 3/4 cup Black beans
  (14.5 oz can, drained and rinsed)
- 1/3 cup Cocoa powder
- 3/4 cup Sugar
- 1/4 cup Almond butter
- 1 tsp Vanilla extract

Instructions
1. Add all ingredients to a food processor and process until very smooth.
2. Transfer into a bowl and serve on toast, as a fruit dip with strawberries or apples, or enjoy a spoonful.

Pro Tip: Refrigerate before serving to allow to thicken.

Picky Eater Tips: This dip can help encourage fruit eating. Let your picky eater help make this dip by measuring ingredients or pressing the button on the food processor. Offer familiar dippers like graham crackers or apple slices for more comfort.

Leftovers: Refrigerate in an airtight container for 5 days, or freeze up to 2 months.

Summer/Fall Meal Plan: Week 4

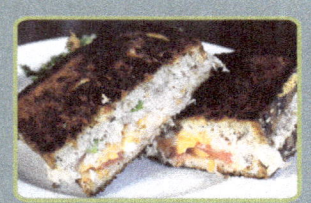

30-Minute Meal 1:
Classic Tuna Melts With
Pan-Fried Cauliflower

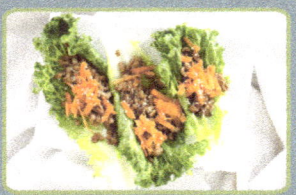

30-Minute Meal 2:
Sesame Pork
Lettuce Wraps

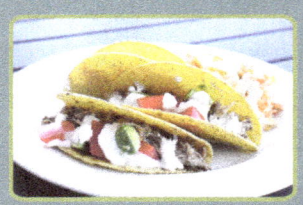

Slow-Cooker: Jerk Chicken
Tacos With Pineapple
Jalapeño Coleslaw

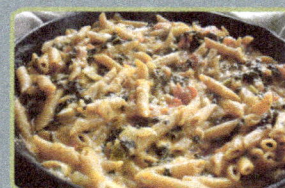

Vegetarian: One Dish
Mac & Cheese With
Tomatoes & Kale

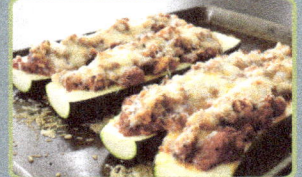

Challenge: Zucchini Pizza
Boats With Garlic Bread and
Watermelon Mint Salad

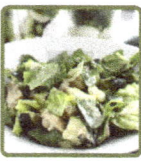

Savory Grab & Go:
Mason Jar Salmon Salad

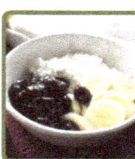

Sweet Grab & Go: Cherries,
Banana, & Cottage Cheese

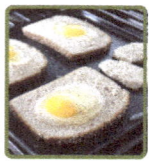

Savory Breakfast:
Egg in a Basket

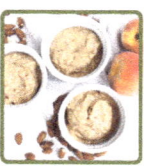

Sweet Breakfast: Peach Almond
Frozen Smoothie Bowls

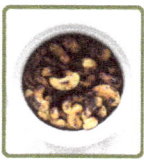

Savory Snack: Spicy
Cashews

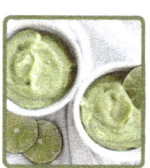

Sweet Snack: Key Lime
Mousse

Summer/Fall Meal Plan: Week 4

30-Minute Meal 1

Classic Tuna Melts With Pan-Fried Cauliflower

Whole Meal Total Time: 30–40 Min | Prep Time: 20–25 Min | Cook Time: 10–15 Min

Recommended order of prep:
1. Make tuna salad for <u>Classic Tuna Melts</u>, but wait to cook.
2. Make recipe for <u>Pan-Fried Cauliflower</u>.
3. While cauliflower cooks, make the Classic Tuna Melts.
4. Serve tuna melts with cauliflower on the side.

Pro Tip: Use pre-cut or frozen cauliflower for an easier recipe, or substitute another vegetable side like a pre-made salad mix. Mix up the tuna salad in advance, then cook these on a busy weekday night for a quick, easy meal.

Dietary Adjustments

Gluten-Free: Use gluten-free bread to make Classic Tuna Melts.
Dairy-Free: Use plant-based cheddar shreds OR sub recipe for <u>Tuna Salad Sandwiches</u> in place of Classic Tuna Melts.
Vegetarian: Sub recipe for <u>Chickpea Melts</u> in place of Classic Tuna Melts.
Vegan: Sub recipe for <u>Chickpea Melts</u> in place of Classic Tuna Melts and use plant-based cheddar shreds.

Classic Tuna Melts

Prep Time: 20 Min | Cook Time: 10 Min   Serves: 4

Tuna Salad Filling

- 12 oz Canned tuna (flaked; packed in water)
- 2 stalk Celery (diced)
- 2 Green onions (sliced)
- 1/3 cup Mayonnaise
- 1 tbsp Lemon juice
- 1 tsp Dijon mustard
- 1/8 tsp Red pepper flakes

Sandwiches

- 1 Tomato (sliced thinly crosswise)
- 8 slice Whole wheat bread (sub gluten-free bread for gluten-free)
- 8 tsp Salted butter (spreadable; sub vegan butter for dairy-free)
- 1 cup Shredded cheddar cheese (sub plant-based cheddar shreds for dairy-free)

Instructions

1. Drain tuna and add to a mixing bowl. Dice celery and slice green onion; add to mixing bowl with tuna along with mayonnaise, lemon juice, Dijon mustard, and red pepper flakes. Stir to mix well and set aside.
2. Thinly slice tomato crosswise into 8 slices and set aside. Spread 1 tsp butter on one side of each slice of bread; set aside.
3. Heat a large griddle or skillet over medium heat. Make sandwiches directly on griddle: lay a piece of bread butter-side down, sprinkle with 1/4 cup of cheese, then top with 1/2 cup of tuna mixture, two slices of tomato, and lay a second slice of bread on top of sandwich, butter side out. Repeat for all sandwiches.
4. Cook sandwiches 3–4 minutes per side, until golden brown and cheese has melted. If bread is browning too quickly before cheese has melted, lower temperature; if cheese is melting before bread has browned, increase temperature. Allow sandwiches to cool slightly, then cut in half to serve.

Pro Tip: For a variation, make "Tuna Melt Nachos" by spreading filling over tortilla chips on a baking sheet, topping with diced tomatoes and shredded cheese. Bake at 350° Fahrenheit for 12–15 minutes until cheese has melted.

Picky Eater Tips: Set aside a small amount of plain tuna for your picky eater to try separately. Let them build their own sandwich and decide how much filling and cheese to add. Ask your picky eater how they would like to cut the sandwich for added autonomy. Offer a grilled cheese sandwich as a "safe food" alternative.

Leftovers: Refrigerate filling separately and make sandwiches fresh for best quality. Refrigerate sandwiches in an airtight container up to 3 days. It's not recommended to freeze sandwiches. Reheat in a toaster oven or on a griddle to maintain crispiness.

Pan-Fried Cauliflower

Prep Time: 15 Min | Cook Time: 15 Min   Serves: 4

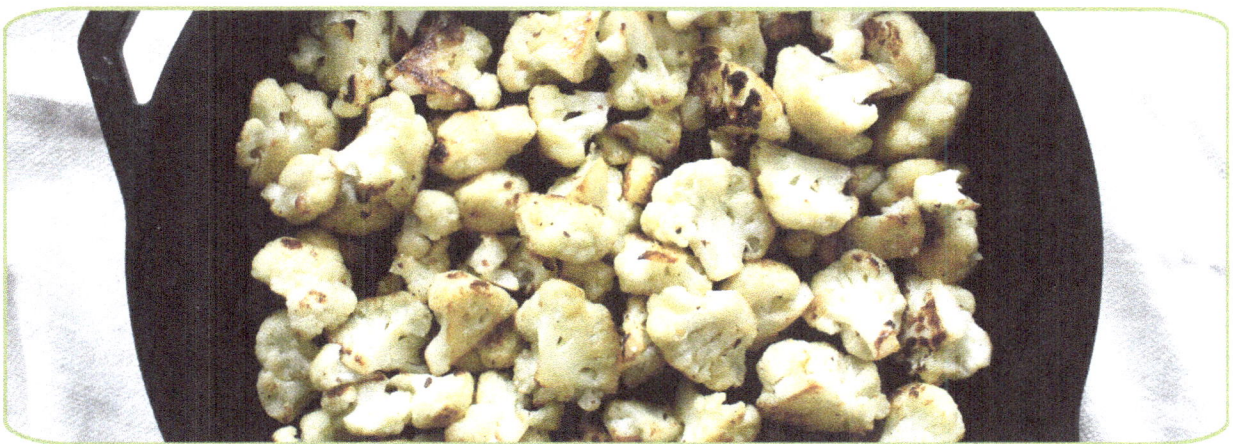

Ingredients
- 1 head Cauliflower (about 2 lbs, cut into florets)
- 2 tbsp Extra virgin olive oil
- 1/4 tsp Coarse salt
- 1/2 Lemon (juiced, optional)

Instructions
1. Cut cauliflower into 1-inch florets.
2. Heat a large sauté pan over medium to medium-high heat. Once hot, add oil and cauliflower to pan; sauté until tender enough to insert a fork and florets are starting to brown, 10–15 minutes. Mix in salt and juice from lemon to serve.

Pro Tip: Use pre-cut or frozen cauliflower for an easier meal. Try these other seasoning ideas for a variation: curry powder | chili powder + cumin + salt + pepper | oregano + Parmesan

Picky Eater Tips: Pan-frying can give more flavor to vegetables and cut the bitterness, so this version of cauliflower may be more appealing to your picky eater. Serve it plain, or let your picky eater choose their favorite dip, like ranch or ketchup, or top with shredded cheese. Set aside a few raw florets to serve alongside the cooked version.

Leftovers: Refrigerate in an airtight container up to 3–5 days. Reheat in the oven or toaster oven for crispier leftovers. Do not freeze.

Tuna Salad Sandwiches

Prep Time: 20 Min | Cook Time: 0 Min

Serves: 4

Ingredients

- 12 oz Canned tuna (flaked; packed in water)
- 2 stalk Celery (diced)
- 1 Carrot (small, finely diced; substitute kohlrabi or cucumber if desired)
- 1/3 cup Mayonnaise
- 1 tbsp Lemon juice (1/2 small lemon)
- 1 tsp Dijon mustard
- 1/8 tsp Red pepper flakes (optional, for spicy flavor)
- 8 slice Whole wheat bread (sub gluten-free bread, tortilla, crackers, or lettuce wrap for gluten-free)

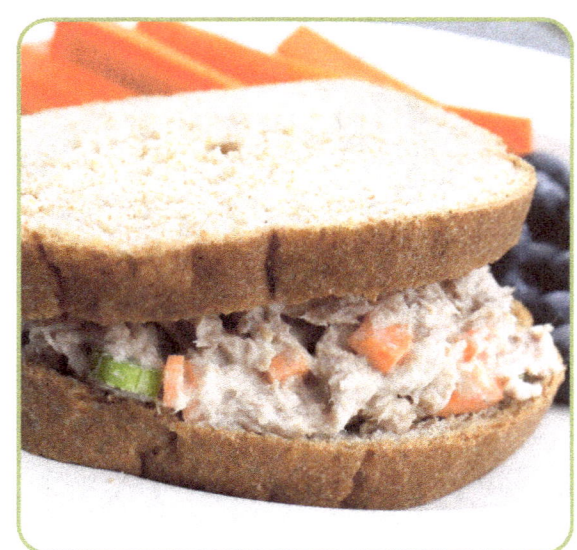

Instructions

1. Drain liquid from tuna and add to a small mixing bowl.
2. Very finely dice celery and carrot. Add to mixing bowl and stir to combine with tuna along with mayonnaise, lemon juice, Dijon mustard, and red pepper flakes. Stir to mix well until tuna becomes creamy.
3. Spread about 1/4 cup tuna salad on a slice of bread and top with a second slice to make each sandwich.

Pro Tip: Toast bread before making sandwiches if desired. Serve tuna salad on crackers or lettuce wraps as an alternative.

Picky Eater Tips: Serve tuna salad on the side with crackers instead of in a sandwich. Try mixing the tuna with less mayo or using plain tuna to keep the texture simpler. Add cheese slices or fruit on the side to round out the meal with familiar options. Let your picky eater help measure ingredients and stir tuna salad together for another hands-on exposure.

Leftovers: Refrigerate tuna salad in an airtight container 2–3 days. Do not freeze.

Week 4 Meal Plan and Recipes

Chickpea Melts

Prep Time: 20 Min | Cook Time: 10 Min   Serves: 4

Tuna Salad Filling

- 1 3/4 cup Chickpeas (14.5 oz can, drained and rinsed)
- 2 stalk Celery (diced)
- 2 Green onions (sliced)
- 1/4 cup Mayonnaise (sub vegan mayo for vegan)
- 1 tbsp Lemon juice (1/2 small lemon)
- 1 tsp Dijon mustard
- 1/8 tsp Red pepper flakes

Sandwiches

- 1 Tomato (sliced thinly crosswise)
- 8 slice Whole wheat bread (sub gluten-free bread for gluten-free)
- 8 tsp Salted butter (spreadable; sub vegan butter for dairy-free)
- 1 cup Shredded cheddar cheese (sub plant-based cheddar shreds for dairy-free)

Instructions

1. Drain and rinse chickpeas and add to a mixing bowl. Smash chickpeas using a potato masher until in small pieces, but mixture is not completely smooth.
2. Dice celery and slice green onion; add to mixing bowl with chickpeas along with mayonnaise, lemon juice, Dijon mustard, and red pepper flakes. Stir to mix well.
3. Thinly slice tomato crosswise into 8 slices and set aside. Spread 1 tsp butter on one side of each slice of bread; set aside.
4. Heat a large griddle or skillet over medium-low heat. Once hot, assemble sandwiches directly on griddle. Lay a piece of bread butter-side down, then spread 1/2 cup of chickpea mixture on bread. Top with 1/4 cup shredded cheese, then layer 2 slices of tomato on top. Lay a second slice of bread on top of sandwich, butter side out. Repeat to make remaining sandwiches.
5. Cook sandwiches 3–4 minutes per side, until golden brown and cheese has melted. If bread is browning too quickly before cheese has melted, turn temperature down; if cheese is melting before bread has browned, increase temperature. Allow sandwiches to cool slightly, then cut in half to serve.

Pro Tip: For a variation, serve this mix in lettuce wrap, on a salad, or with crackers.

Picky Eater Tips: Offer some plain chickpeas or serve some filling next to toast instead of as a sandwich. Let your picky eater choose which type of bread and cheese to use to make the sandwiches. Offer a "safe food" option such as a grilled cheese sandwich.

Leftovers: Refrigerate filling separately and make sandwiches fresh for best quality. Refrigerate sandwiches in an airtight container up to 3 days. It's not recommended to freeze sandwiches. Reheat in a toaster oven or on a griddle to maintain crispiness.

Summer/Fall Meal Plan: Week 4

30-Minute Meal 2

Sesame Pork Lettuce Wraps

✓ Gluten-Free   ✓ Dairy-Free

Whole Meal Total Time: 20–25 Min | Prep Time: 10 Min | Cook Time: 10–15 Min

Recommended order of prep:
  1. Make recipe for <u>Sesame Pork Lettuce Wraps</u>.

Pro Tip: For hungry eaters, serve jasmine or white rice on the side. Serve all components individually and let each person make their own wraps at the table.

Dietary Adjustments

Gluten-Free: Use gluten-free soy sauce or sub tamari in Sesame Pork Lettuce Wraps.
Vegetarian / Vegan: Sub recipe for <u>Sesame Tofu Lettuce Wraps</u> in place of Sesame Pork Lettuce Wraps.

Sesame Pork Lettuce Wraps

Prep Time: 10 Min | Cook Time: 10 Min   Serves: 4

Ingredients

- 2 Carrots (grated)
- 8 leaves Romaine
- 2 tbsp Sesame oil (divided)
- 1 tbsp Minced garlic
- 1 lb Lean ground pork
- 2 tbsp Soy sauce (use gluten-free or sub Tamari for gluten-free; sub coconut aminos for soy-free)
- 1 tsp Honey
- 2 tbsp Sesame seeds

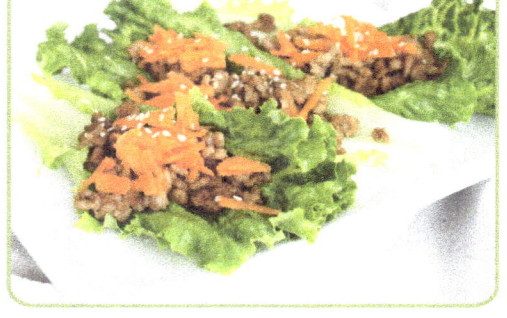

Instructions

1. Peel and grate carrots and set aside. Pull individual leaves off romaine lettuce head, wash, and pat dry; set aside.
2. Heat a skillet over medium heat; once hot, add half of oil and minced garlic. Cook for 1–2 minutes until starting to become fragrant.
3. Add pork to skillet with garlic and use a spatula to break apart as it cooks. Cook for 8–10 minutes, until cooked through and no pink remains.
4. While pork cooks, in a separate small bowl mix together soy sauce, remaining sesame oil, and honey. Once pork is fully cooked, stir in the prepared sauce, then remove from heat.
5. Serve pork mixture in individual lettuce leaves, topped with shredded carrot and a sprinkle of sesame seeds.

Pro Tip: Add additional toppings, like avocado, cucumber slices, or red pepper flakes as desired. Serve with cooked jasmine rice for a more filling meal.

Picky Eater Tips: Offer the pork and toppings separately so picky eaters can build their own wrap. Offer rice or a tortilla instead of lettuce wrap for variety. Serve sauce on the side for more control and autonomy, such as soy sauce or teriyaki sauce. Serve this meal with a familiar "safe food" like fruit or crackers to decrease pressure.

Leftovers: Refrigerate cooked pork separately from lettuce wraps and toppings in an airtight for container up to 5 days. Freeze cooked meat up to several months.

Sesame Tofu Lettuce Wraps

Prep Time: 15 Min | Cook Time: 15 Min   Serves: 4

Tofu Crumbles

- 28 oz Extra firm tofu (drained, mashed into crumbles)
- 2 tbsp Sesame oil (to cook)
- 2 tsp Minced garlic

Serving Suggestion

- 2 Carrots (washed, shredded)
- 16 leaves Romaine

Sauce

- 4 tbsp Soy sauce (use gluten-free or sub Tamari for gluten-free)
- 2 tsp Honey (sub maple syrup for vegan)
- 2 tbsp Sesame oil

- 4 tbsp Sesame seeds (optional)

Instructions

1. Press liquid from tofu: drain liquid from tofu, cut into slices, and place between two clean towels. Using hands, press on tofu to remove as much liquid as possible. Add tofu to a mixing bowl. Use a fork to mash tofu into small pieces resembling the texture of cooked ground beef crumbles; set aside.
2. Make sauce in a small bowl by mixing together soy sauce, honey, and sesame oil for sauce; set aside.
3. Heat a large skillet over medium heat. Once hot, add sesame oil for cooking tofu, then add minced garlic. Cook for 1–2 minutes until starting to become fragrant.
4. Add crumbled tofu and prepared sauce to skillet and cook, stirring occasionally. Spread crumbles evenly in pan between stirring to allow as much liquid to evaporate as possible. Cook about 15 minutes until most of the liquid has evaporated and tofu crumbles are starting to brown.
5. While tofu cooks, peel and grate carrots and set aside. Pull individual leaves off romaine lettuce head, wash, and pat dry.
6. Serve tofu in lettuce leaves, topped with shredded carrot and sesame seeds.

Pro Tip: Top wraps with additional toppings, such as avocado, cucumber slices, or red pepper flakes as desired. Serve with jasmine rice for a more filling meal.

Picky Eater Tips: Offer tofu, toppings, and wraps separately to give picky eaters more choice. Offer a tortilla or rice instead of lettuce. Serve a sauce on the side, such as soy sauce or peanut sauce, for more control and autonomy. Include a "safe food" like fruit or rice at the meal to reduce pressure.

Leftovers: Refrigerate tofu crumbles separately from carrots and lettuce wraps in an airtight container; store up to 5 days. Not recommended to freeze.

Summer/Fall Meal Plan: Week 4

Slow-Cooker Meal

Jerk Chicken Tacos With Pineapple Jalapeño Coleslaw

✓ Gluten-Free   ✓ Dairy-Free

Whole Meal Total Time: 3 ½–6 Hrs | Prep Time: 50–60 Min | Cook Time: 3–6 Hrs

Recommended order of prep:
1. Make recipe for <u>Pineapple Jalapeño Coleslaw</u> and refrigerate until ready to eat.
2. Make recipe for <u>Jerk Chicken Tacos</u>.
3. Prep toppings and set aside until ready to eat.
4. Serve chicken tacos with desired toppings and coleslaw on the side.

Pro Tip: Sub fresh cabbage instead of coleslaw mix if desired. Use a pre-made jerk marinade instead of making from scratch to save prep time.

Dietary Adjustments

Vegetarian: Sub recipe for <u>Slow Cooker Jerk Tofu Tacos</u> in place of Jerk Chicken Tacos.

Vegan: Sub recipe for <u>Slow Cooker Jerk Tofu Tacos</u> in place of Jerk Chicken Tacos. Use vegan mayonnaise to make Pineapple Jalapeño Coleslaw.

Jerk Chicken Tacos

Prep Time: 30 Min | Cook Time: 3 Hrs   Serves: 6

Jerk Marinade

- 1/2 Yellow onion (roughly chopped)
- 2 clove Garlic (peeled)
- 1 Jalapeño pepper (seeded)
- 1 1/2 tsp Extra virgin olive oil
- 1 tbsp Soy sauce (use gluten-free or sub Tamari for gluten-free; sub coconut aminos for soy-free)
- 1 tbsp Lime juice (about 1/2 lime)
- 1 1/2 tsp Apple cider vinegar
- 1 tbsp Brown sugar
- 1 tsp Cinnamon
- 1/2 tsp Dried thyme
- 1/4 tsp Nutmeg
- 1/4 tsp Ground cloves
- 1/8 tsp Cayenne pepper
- 1 tsp Salt

Chicken Tacos

- 1 1/2 lb Boneless, skinless chicken thighs
- 18 Taco shells
- Toppings as desired for tacos: shredded cabbage, diced red onion, diced pineapple, diced avocado, chopped cilantro, sour cream, or lime wedge

Instructions

1. Make jerk marinade. Coarsely chop onion, peel garlic cloves, seed jalapeño, and add them to a food processor along with olive oil, soy sauce, lime juice, vinegar, brown sugar, cinnamon, thyme, nutmeg, cloves, cayenne pepper, and salt. Blend until smooth and set aside.
2. Arrange chicken thighs in a large slow cooker with as little overlap as possible. Pour marinade evenly over chicken. Cook on high 3–4 hours or on low 5–6 hours.
3. Once chicken is fully cooked, shred it by using two forks or by placing chicken in a stand mixer and using the paddle attachment to mix until shredded.
4. Prepare toppings and serve shredded chicken in taco shells with desired toppings.

Pro Tip: Mix up extra marinade and refrigerate it for up to 2 weeks or freeze up to several months. Adjust the amount of cayenne to taste.

Picky Eater Tips: Offer components separately – chicken, taco shells, and toppings – so picky eaters can build their own taco. Omit cayenne for a milder option. Serve with a simple "safe food" alternative, like a cheese quesadilla.

Leftovers: Refrigerate shredded chicken in an airtight container up to 5 days. Freeze meat for up to several months.

Pineapple Jalapeño Coleslaw

Prep Time: 15 Min | Cook Time: 0 Min   Serves: 6

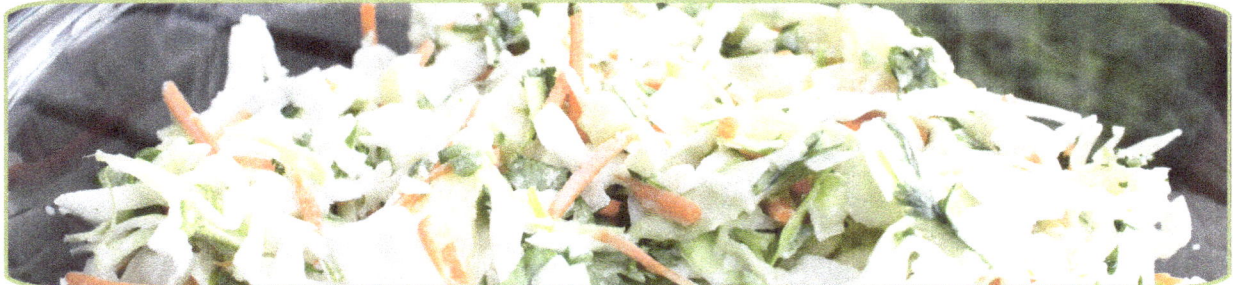

Coleslaw

- 5 cup Coleslaw mix (16 oz package)
- 2 cup Pineapple tidbits (20 oz can; canned in juice; reserve juice for dressing)
- 1 Jalapeño pepper (minced)
- 1/3 cup Cilantro (minced)

Dressing

- 1/2 cup Mayonnaise (sub vegan mayo if desired)
- 1 tbsp Sugar
- 1 tbsp Pineapple juice
- 1 tbsp Lime juice
- 1 tbsp Apple cider vinegar
- 1/2 tsp Salt

Instructions

1. Add coleslaw mix to a large serving bowl. Reserving the juice to use for dressing, drain the pineapple tidbits and add pineapple to bowl with coleslaw mix.
2. Mince jalapeño and cilantro. Add to bowl with coleslaw and stir to combine.
3. In a separate small bowl, whisk together mayonnaise, sugar, pineapple juice, lime juice, apple cider vinegar, and salt. Add dressing to vegetables and toss to mix well. Serve immediately, or refrigerate 2-4 hours or overnight before serving for best flavor.

Pro Tip: Replace the coleslaw mix with fresh shredded vegetables; use mainly cabbage but also add any of the following for color and flavor variation: carrots, kohlrabi, raw beets, or radishes.

Picky Eater Tips: Set aside some plain pineapple and cabbage or slaw mix without dressing for a mild version. Offer an alternative vegetable or fruit as an option for a "safe food."

Leftovers: Refrigerate in airtight container up to 5 days. This recipe is even better the next day. Do not freeze.

Slow Cooker Jerk Tofu Tacos

Prep Time: 20 Min | Cook Time: 2 Hrs   Serves: 4

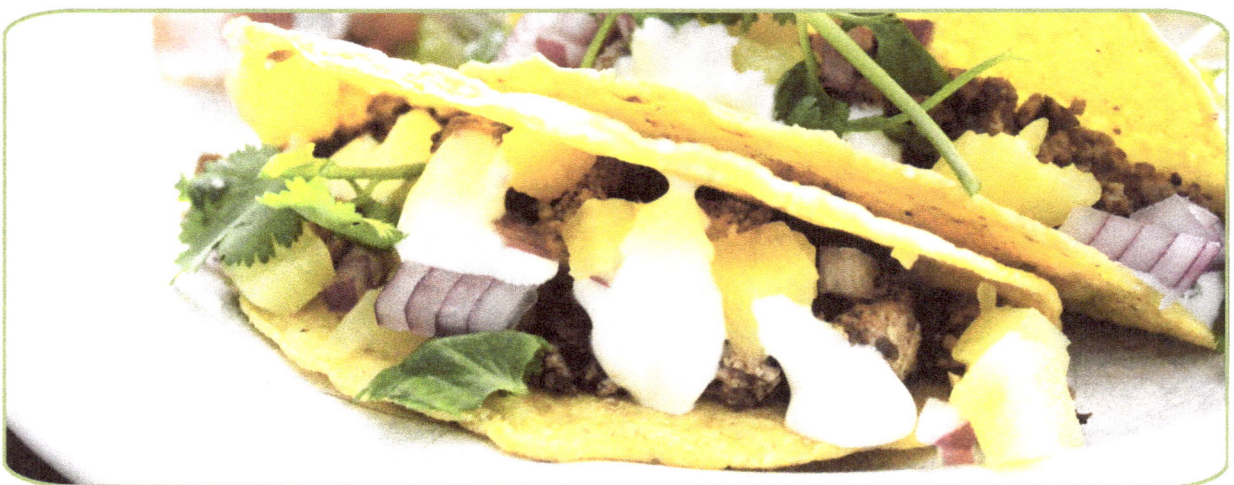

Tofu Tacos

- 14 oz Extra firm tofu (about 1 package)
- Toppings as desired for jerk tofu: diced red onion, diced pineapple, diced avocado, chopped cilantro, sour cream, or a lime wedge
- 12 Taco shells

Jerk Marinade

- 1/2 Yellow onion (roughly chopped)
- 2 clove Garlic (peeled)
- 1 Jalapeño pepper (seeded)
- 1 1/2 tsp Extra virgin olive oil
- 1 tbsp Soy sauce (sub Tamari for gluten-free)
- 1 tbsp Lime juice (1/2 lime)

- 1 1/2 tsp Apple cider vinegar
- 1 tbsp Brown sugar
- 1 tsp Cinnamon
- 1/2 tsp Dried thyme
- 1/4 tsp Nutmeg
- 1/4 tsp Ground cloves
- 1/8 tsp Cayenne pepper
- 1 tsp Salt

Instructions

1. Drain water from tofu and cut each block into 5 slices. Press liquid from tofu: arrange tofu slices on a clean towel on a plate. Lay a second towel over top of tofu, then set a second plate on top of towel. Set several cans of food or heavy cast iron skillet on top of plate to press liquid from tofu. While liquid presses from tofu, make marinade.

Slow Cooker Jerk Tofu Tacos (Continued)

Instructions (Continued)

2. Meanwhile, make jerk marinade. Coarsely chop onion, peel garlic cloves, seed jalapeño, and add them to a food processor along with olive oil, soy sauce, lime juice, vinegar, brown sugar, cinnamon, thyme, nutmeg, cloves, cayenne pepper, and salt. Blend until smooth and set aside.
3. Once liquid has pressed from tofu, use your hands to tear it into small pieces resembling the texture of cooked ground beef. Add the tofu crumbles to a small slow cooker. Pour marinade evenly over tofu and gently stir to evenly distribute throughout. Note: if using a large slow cooker, add about a half cup of water to prevent tofu from drying out.
4. Cook on high 3–4 hours or on low 5–6 hours. Stir once or twice and add more water if becoming too dry and starting to burn.
5. Prep desired toppings and serve tofu in taco shells with toppings as desired.

Pro Tip: Mix up extra marinade and refrigerate it for up to 2 weeks or freeze it for up to several months. Adjust the amount of cayenne to taste.

Picky Eater Tips: Set some tofu cubes aside before cooking to serve plain. Offer the marinade as a dip for the tofu, or serve familiar options to dip such as ketchup or teriyaki sauce. Provide taco elements separately for self-assembly. Include a familiar grain or fruit as a "safe food."

Leftovers: Refrigerate in airtight container up to 5 days. Freeze tofu crumbles for up to several months.

Summer/Fall Meal Plan: Week 4

Vegetarian Meal

One Dish Mac & Cheese With Tomatoes & Kale

✓ Vegetarian

Whole Meal Total Time: 45–50 Min | Prep Time: 30–35 Min | Cook Time: 10–15 Min

Recommended order of prep:
  1. Follow recipe to make <u>One Dish Mac & Cheese with Tomatoes & Kale</u>.

Pro Tip: Sub other types of vegetables in this mac & cheese if desired, such as mushrooms or zucchini, in place of kale or tomatoes. Use canned tomatoes when not in season.

Dietary Adjustments

Gluten-Free: Use gluten-free pasta to make One Dish Mac & Cheese with Tomatoes & Kale.

Dairy-Free / Vegan: Sub recipe for <u>Butternut Squash Mac & Cheese</u> in place of One Dish Mac & Cheese with Tomatoes & Kale.

One Dish Mac & Cheese With Tomatoes & Kale

Prep Time: 30 Min | Cook Time: 15 Min   Serves: 6

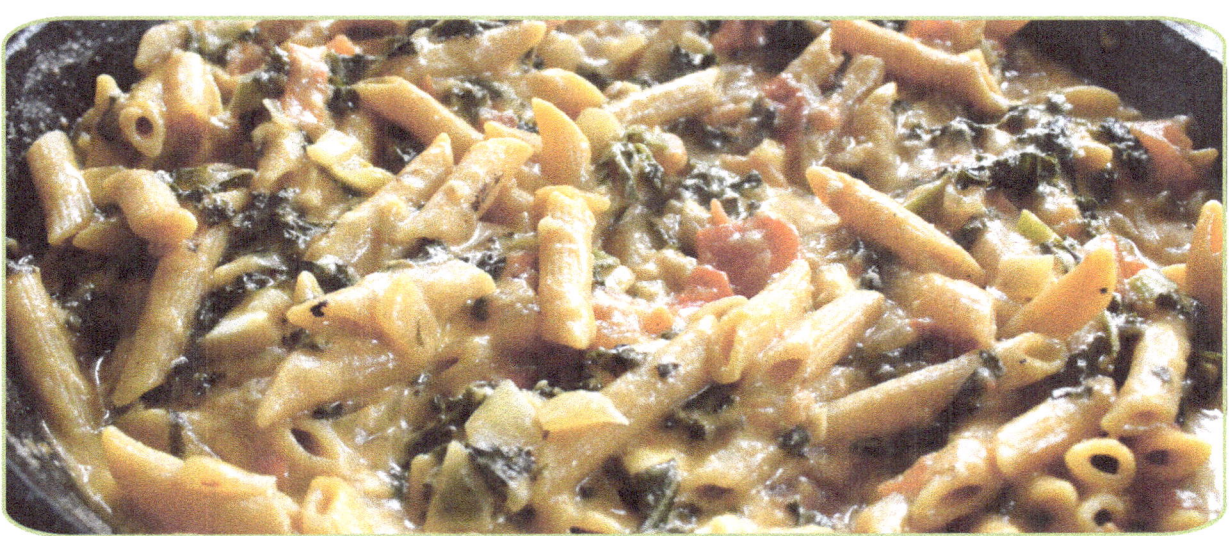

Ingredients

- 1 White or yellow onion (medium, diced)
- 4 clove Garlic (minced)
- 1 tbsp Extra virgin olive oil
- 8 cup Kale (chopped; about 8 large leaves)
- 4 Tomatoes (medium, diced; or sub two 14.5 oz cans diced tomatoes)
- 1 cup Water

- 2 cup Whole milk
- 1/2 tsp Salt
- 4 cup Whole grain penne (uncooked; sub gluten-free pasta for gluten-free)
- 1/4 cup Basil leaves (minced)
- 1/2 cup Plain Greek yogurt
- 2 cup Shredded cheddar cheese
- 1/2 cup Feta cheese

Instructions

1. Dice onions and mince garlic; set aside. Heat a large sauté pan over medium heat. Once hot, add oil, onions, and garlic. Cook until onion is translucent and garlic is fragrant, about 8–10 minutes, stirring every few minutes to ensure even cooking.
2. Meanwhile, strip kale leaves from stems. Roughly chop kale leaves and add to sauté pan with onions. Cook until kale shrinks to about half of its original volume.

One Dish Mac & Cheese With Tomatoes & Kale (Continued)

Instructions (Continued)

3. While kale cooks, dice tomatoes and add to the sauté pan as they are prepared. Note: when tomatoes aren't in season, use canned diced tomatoes; include liquid from can when adding.
4. Add water, milk, and salt to the sauté pan with vegetables. Stir to distribute vegetables and cover with a lid. Turn heat to high and bring to a boil.
5. Once liquid is boiling, add pasta to pan with water and vegetables, stirring to distribute evenly. Make sure pasta is fully submerged in liquid, then reduce heat and cover; simmer until pasta is fully cooked, about 10-13 minutes.
6. While pasta cooks, mince fresh basil leaves and set aside.
7. Once pasta is cooked, remove from heat and add Greek yogurt, shredded cheddar, and feta cheese crumbles to pasta; stir to combine. Stir in chopped basil just before serving.

Pro Tip: Use dried basil and canned tomatoes if fresh aren't available. However, fresh is best and will greatly enhance the flavor of this recipe.

Picky Eater Tips: Set aside some plain pasta, raw tomatoes, plain Greek yogurt, and shredded cheese for your picky eater before mixing them together. Let your picky eater help stir this meal or tear kale for hands-on exposure. Consider renaming this dish so your picky eater doesn't associate it with other types of mac and cheese, which can help increase acceptance. For example, call it "Cheesy Kale and Tomato Pasta."

Leftovers: Refrigerate in an airtight container up to 5 days. Do not freeze.

Butternut Squash Mac & Cheese

Prep Time: 30 Min | Cook Time: 30 Min   Serves: 6

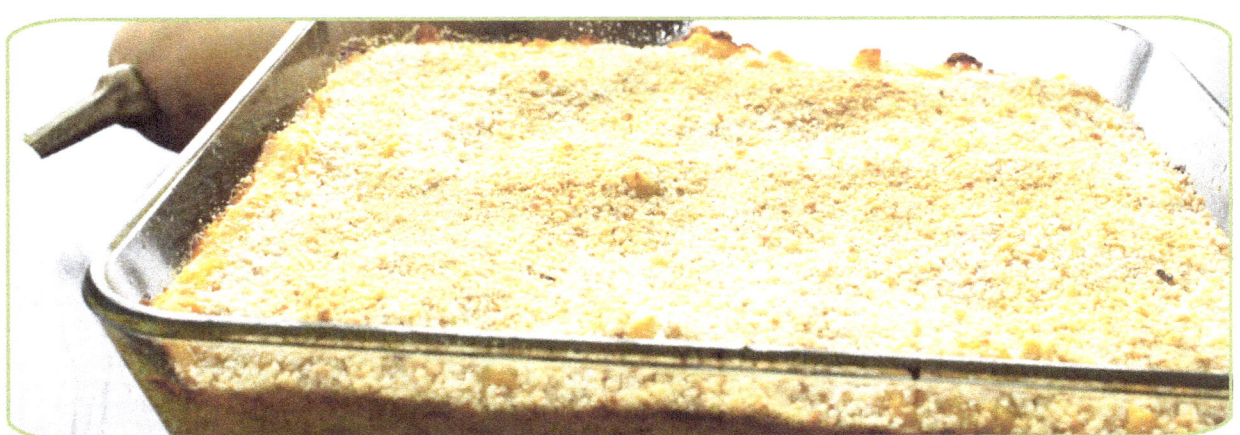

Ingredients

- 2 lb Butternut squash (1 Medium squash; peeled, seeded, and cut into 1/2-inch cubes)
- 3/4 cup Cashews (raw)
- 2 cup Macaroni (dry; sub gluten-free pasta for gluten-free)
- 1 Yellow onion (diced)
- 2 clove Garlic (minced)
- 1 tbsp Extra virgin olive oil
- 1/3 cup Nutritional yeast (sub shredded Parmesan cheese if desired)
- 3/4 tsp Salt
- 1/2 cup Unseasoned breadcrumbs (sub gluten-free breadcrumbs for gluten-free)
- 1/2 tsp Seasoned salt

Instructions

1. Fill a large saucepan or small pot about half full with water and bring to a boil over high heat. While water comes to a boil, peel, seed, and cut butternut squash into small 1/2-inch cubes. Add butternut squash and cashews to water and cook for 15–20 minutes until squash is very soft.
2. While squash cooks, fill a second medium-sized saucepan about 3/4 full with water and bring to a boil. Once boiling, add macaroni and cook al dente according to package instructions. Take care not to overcook. Drain pasta and rinse with water to wash away starch and prevent pasta from sticking together. Set aside.

Butternut Squash Mac & Cheese (Continued)

<u>Instructions (Continued)</u>

3. Preheat oven to 400° Fahrenheit. Prepare a 2.5 quart baking dish by spraying with cooking spray.
4. While squash and pasta cook, dice onion and mince garlic. To reduce the number of dishes, use the same saucepan as used to cook macaroni and heat saucepan over medium heat. Once hot, add oil, onion, and garlic. Sauté for 5–6 minutes until starting to brown and become fragrant.
5. Once butternut squash is cooked to a very soft consistency, reserve 3/4 cup of liquid from the saucepan and drain and discard remaining liquid. To the saucepan used to cook butternut squash, add back in squash, cashews, reserved water, along with cooked onion and garlic, nutritional yeast, and salt. Use an immersion blender to blend until completely smooth. Note: although this looks too thick to blend, it will work! Keep blender below the level of squash and liquid while blending. Alternatively, transfer the mixture to a blender or food processor and blend, taking care to remove lid to release pressure between blending.
6. Add cooked pasta to saucepan with butternut squash sauce and stir to combine. Once mixed well, transfer to prepared baking dish.
7. Bake 15 minutes, uncovered, then remove from oven and top evenly with bread crumbs and seasoned salt. Return to oven and bake another 10–15 minutes until bread crumbs are starting to brown and sauce is bubbly in pasta.

<u>Pro Tip:</u> Stir chili flakes, hot sauce, paprika, cayenne, oregano and/or rosemary into butternut squash sauce for additional flavor. Use pre-cut butternut squash, leftover roasted squash or canned pumpkin puree for an easier meal; make sure to soak or boil cashews so they are soft enough to blend.

<u>Picky Eater Tips:</u> Set aside some of the pasta and sauce separately; serve pasta plain or with a small spoonful of sauce on the side for dipping. Use a fun pasta shape or one your picky eater already likes. Let them help stir the sauce and add toppings at the table, like extra shredded cheese, to give them some control.

<u>Leftovers:</u> Refrigerate in an airtight container up to 5 days. Not recommended to freeze.

Summer/Fall Meal Plan: Week 4

Challenge Meal

Zucchini Pizza Boats With Garlic Bread and Watermelon Mint Salad

Whole Meal Total Time: 50–60 Min | Prep Time: 45–50 Min | Cook Time: 10 Min

Recommended order of prep:
1. Make Watermelon Mint Salad and refrigerate until ready to eat.
2. Make recipe for Zucchini Pizza Boats.
3. When Zucchini Pizza Boats have about 10 minutes left to cook, make recipe for Garlic Bread.
4. Serve pizza boats with watermelon salad and garlic bread on the side.

Pro Tip: For a heartier meal, serve pizza boats over whole grain pasta. This recipe requires very large zucchini – about 10–12 inches long. Find a friend with a garden or ask at your local farmer's market to find these extra large zucchini. Use garden fresh tomatoes instead of canned, if available.

Dietary Adjustments

Gluten-Free: Use gluten-free bread to make Garlic Bread.
Dairy-Free: Use plant-based mozzarella shreds and omit Parmesan cheese for Zucchini Pizza Boats.
Vegetarian: Use plant-based sausage crumbles in Zucchini Pizza Boats.
Vegan: Use plant-based sausage crumbles in Zucchini Pizza Boats; use plant-based mozzarella shreds and omit Parmesan cheese.

Zucchini Pizza Boats

Prep Time: 30 Min | Cook Time: 10 Min   Serves: 6

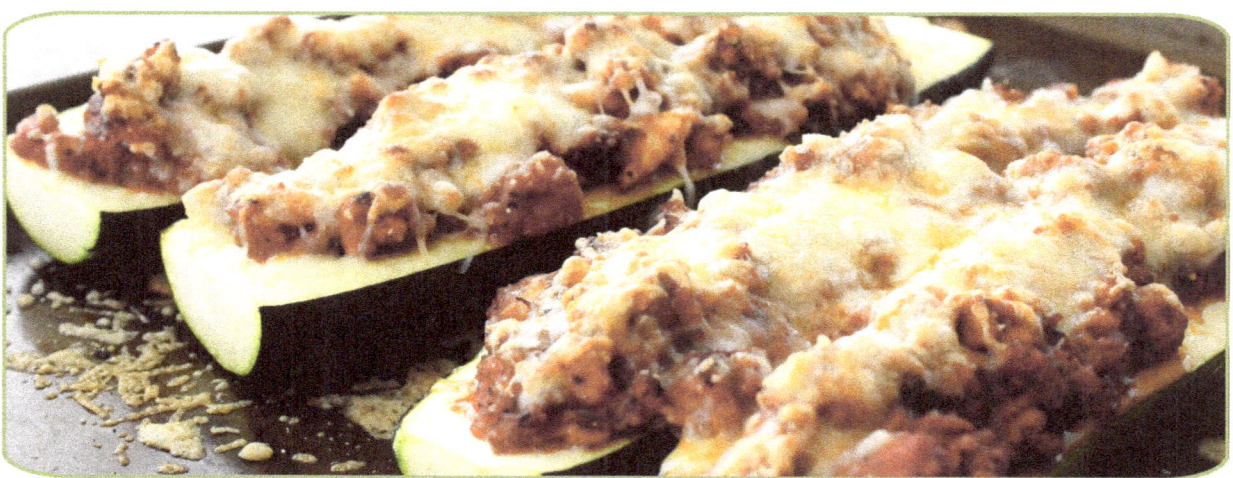

Ingredients

- 3 Very large zucchini (10–12 inches long)
- 1 Yellow onion (diced)
- 2 clove Garlic (minced)
- 2 tbsp Extra virgin olive oil
- 16 oz Ground Italian pork sausage (sub plant-based sausage for vegan)
- 1 tsp Dried basil
- 1/2 tsp Oregano
- 1 3/4 cup Diced tomatoes (14.5 oz can)
- 6 oz Tomato paste
- 1/2 cup Water (more if needed)
- 1 cup Shredded mozzarella (sub plant-based mozzarella shreds or omit for dairy-free)
- 1/2 cup Shredded Parmesan cheese (omit or sub nutritional yeast to taste for dairy-free)

Instructions

1. Heat oven to 400° Fahrenheit.
2. Trim ends of zucchini and discard. Cut zucchini in half lengthwise. Using a knife or a spoon, cut or scoop out middle part of zucchini and discard, leaving about a 1/2-inch of outer part of zucchini to form a "boat." Arrange zucchini on a large baking sheet, cut-side facing up, and bake 25–30 minutes, until soft when pierced with a fork.
3. Meanwhile, dice onion and mince garlic. Heat a large sauté pan over medium heat. Once hot, add olive oil, onion and garlic. Cook 3–4 minutes until fragrant.

Zucchini Pizza Boats (Continued)

Instructions (Continued)

4. Add sausage, basil, and oregano to the pan with onion and garlic. Use a spoon or spatula to break apart sausage into crumbles as it cooks.
5. Add diced tomatoes (do not drain), tomato paste, and water to pan with the sausage. Bring to a boil, then reduce heat and simmer 5–10 minutes while zucchini cooks. If sauce becomes too dry, add another 1/2 cup water.
6. Remove zucchini from the oven and fill zucchini "boats" with prepared sauce. Top evenly with mozzarella and Parmesan cheese, then return zucchini boats to oven and bake another 10 minutes until cheese starts to brown.

Pro Tip: This recipe is designed to use <u>very</u> large zucchini (10–12 inches long). Serve zucchini boats with a side of pasta for hungry eaters. Use fresh tomatoes instead of canned when in season.

Picky Eater Tips: Let picky eaters help build the pizza boats for additional exposure. Let them choose additional toppings like pepperoni or olives to give them autonomy to customize their pizza boats. Offer a "safe food" alternative by topping toast, mini pita, or a tortilla with the sauce and cheese instead of using the zucchini.

Leftovers: Refrigerate in an airtight container for up to 5 days. These are not recommended to freeze.

Watermelon Mint Salad

Prep Time: 15 Min | Cook Time: 0 Min   Serves: 6

<u>Ingredients</u>
- 6 cup Seedless watermelon (about a 5 lb watermelon)
- 2 tbsp Mint leaves (minced)
- 1 tbsp Extra virgin olive oil

<u>Instructions</u>
1. Cut watermelon into 1-inch cubes and add to a large serving bowl.
2. Mince mint leaves finely and add to watermelon along with olive oil. Stir gently to coat watermelon evenly with oil and mint. Chill and serve cold.

<u>Pro Tip:</u> Fresh mint leaves can't be beat in this recipe! Plant mint in a separate pot instead of the ground; it's a perennial plant and takes over the space it's planted.

<u>Picky Eater Tips:</u> Set aside a few pieces of watermelon without mint as a "safe food" option. Cut watermelon into fun shapes to add in play. Let picky eaters tear mint leaves or stir in oil and mint for hands-on experience.

<u>Leftovers:</u> Refrigerate in an airtight container up to 5 days. Do not freeze.

Garlic Bread

Prep Time: 5 Min | Cook Time: 5 Min   Serves: 6

<u>Ingredients</u>
- 6 slice Whole wheat bread (sub gluten-free for gluten-free option)
- 6 tsp Butter (sub dairy-free butter spread for dairy-free and vegan version)
- 3/4 tsp Garlic salt

<u>Instructions</u>
1. Spread 1 tsp butter over each slice of bread and sprinkle with 1/8 tsp garlic salt.
2. Heat a griddle or skillet over medium heat. Once hot, place bread butter-side down and toast for 3–4 minutes until starting to brown.

<u>Pro Tip:</u> Try different seasonings, like Italian herb blend or seasoned salt for variation.

<u>Picky Eater Tips:</u> If your picky eater likes this, use garlic bread as a way to introduce new flavors to your picky eater by allowing them to pick different spices to add to the toast, such as oregano, parsley, basil, or cumin.

<u>Leftovers:</u> Not recommended to store as leftovers, but if necessary, leftovers can be refrigerated up to a day in an airtight container. Reheat in toaster oven.

Summer/Fall Meal Plan: Week 4

Savory Grab & Go

Mason Jar Salmon Salad

✓ Gluten-Free   ✓ Dairy-Free

Dietary Adjustments

Vegetarian: Sub a hard-boiled egg in place of salmon in Mason Jar Salmon Salad.

Vegan: Sub chickpeas or fresh tofu cubes in place of salmon in Mason Jar Salmon Salad.

Sweet Grab & Go

Cherries, Banana, & Cottage Cheese

✓ Gluten-Free   ✓ Vegetarian

Dietary Adjustments

Dairy-Free / Vegan: Sub soy yogurt or plant-based ricotta cheese in place of cottage cheese.

Mason Jar Salmon Salad

Prep Time: 20 Min | Cook Time: 0 Min   Serves: 4

Dressing
- 1/4 cup Extra virgin olive oil
- 1/4 cup Lemon juice (1 large lemon)
- 1/2 tsp Salt
- 2 tsp Dijon mustard

Salad Jars
- 2 Cucumber (diced)
- 14 oz Canned salmon (sub chickpeas or fresh tofu cubes for vegan option)
- 1 head Romaine (chopped)
- 4 Quart mason jar

Instructions
1. In a mason jar, shake or whisk together the extra virgin olive oil, lemon juice, mustard and salt. Divide dressing evenly between 4 quart mason jars.
2. Dice cucumber and add to mason jars on top of dressing. Drain salmon and layer into mason jars, then chop lettuce and add to jars on top of salmon.
3. Store jars in refrigerator up to 3 days. When ready to eat, shake jar well and dump into a bowl or onto a plate to serve.

Vegetarian Version: Sub a hard-boiled egg instead of canned salmon. To make hard-boiled eggs, place eggs in a saucepan and cover with water. Bring to a boil over high heat. Once boiling, turn off the heat but keep the saucepan on the hot burner. Cover and let sit for 10–12 minutes. Drain water from eggs and transfer hot eggs into a bowl filled with ice and water to quickly cool.

Pro Tip: Add different vegetables to salad as desired for a variation, such as carrots, kohlrabi, peppers, or tomatoes. Add chickpeas or a hard-boiled egg for more protein. Sub smoked salmon for more robust flavor.

Picky Eater Tips: Serve ingredients separately and let picky eaters assemble their own version. Offer plain salmon without dressing, or substitute a familiar protein like chicken. Include a "safe" side like crackers or fruit. Serve dressing on the side or let your picky eater choose their favorite dressing for more autonomy.

Leftovers: Store jars in refrigerator up to 3 days. Do not freeze.

Cherries, Banana & Cottage Cheese Bowl

Prep Time: 5 Min | Cook Time: 0 Min   Serves: 1

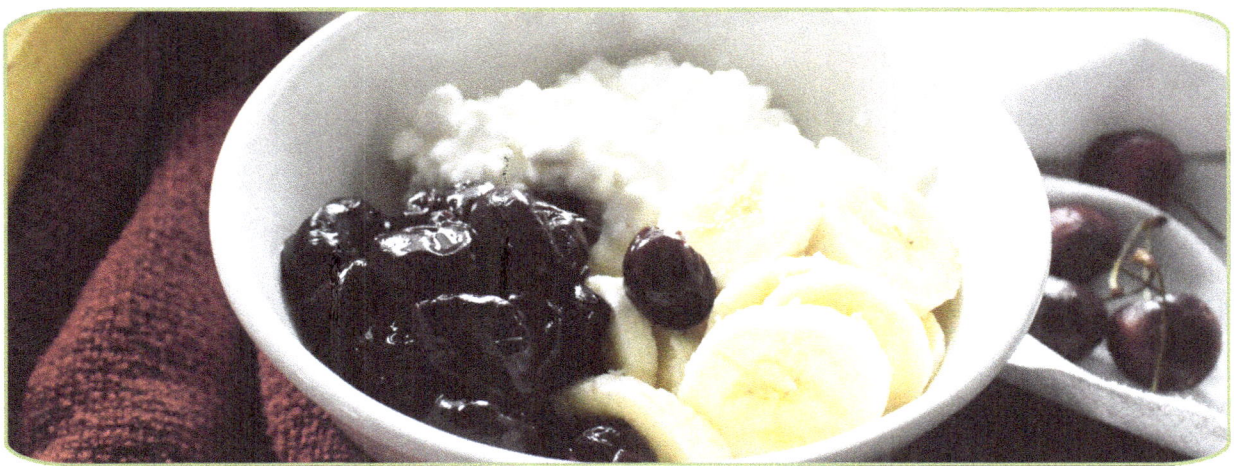

Ingredients

- 1 cup Frozen cherries (thawed)
- 1 cup Cottage cheese (sub plant-based ricotta or soy yogurt for vegan)
- 1 Banana (medium, sliced)

Instructions

1. Thaw frozen cherries by placing in a microwave-safe bowl and microwaving for 30-60 seconds, stirring half-way through cook time.
2. Add cottage cheese to bowl with thawed cherries and slice banana over the top to serve.

Pro Tip: For a sweeter version, use vanilla yogurt or add a sprinkle of sugar over the bowl. Top with chia seeds, ground flaxseeds, sunflower seeds, or nuts for additional protein and a different texture.

Picky Eater Tips: Offer fruit and cottage cheese separately so picky eaters can try each component on its own. Offer yogurt if this feels more familiar to your picky eater. Serve additional toppings, like honey, granola, slivered almonds, or chocolate chips to give your eater more autonomy and make it more fun.

Leftovers: Refrigerate cottage cheese and cherries in an airtight container for up to 3 days. Slice a fresh banana (do not store) for best quality. Do not freeze.

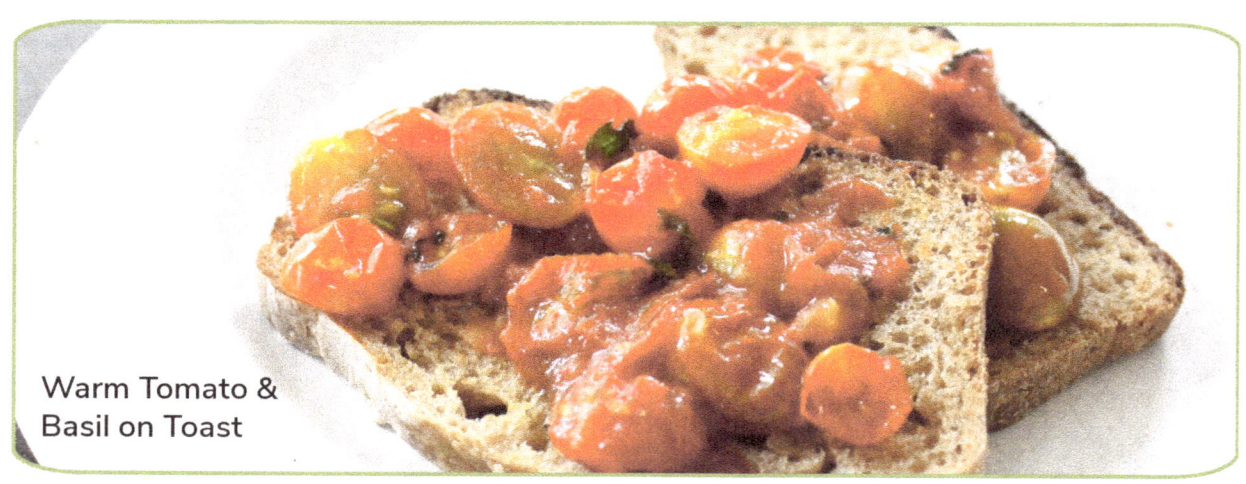

Warm Tomato & Basil on Toast

Savory Breakfast

Egg in a Basket

✓ Dairy-Free   ✓ Vegetarian

Dietary Adjustments

Gluten-Free: Use gluten-free bread to make Egg in a Basket.
Vegan: Sub recipe for <u>Warm Tomato & Basil on Toast</u> in place of Egg in a Basket.

Sweet Breakfast

Peach Almond Frozen Smoothie Bowls

✓ Gluten-Free   ✓ Dairy-Free   ✓ Vegetarian   ✓ Vegan

Egg in a Basket

Prep Time: 5 Min | Cook Time: 5 Min   Serves: 1

Ingredients

- 1 slice Whole wheat bread (sub gluten-free bread if desired)
- 1 tsp Canola oil
- 1 Egg

Instructions

1. Heat a skillet over medium heat. Carefully tear a round piece of bread out of the middle of a slice of bread. Save piece to toast and eat later.
2. Add oil to hot pan. Place bread in skillet and crack egg into hole in the center.
3. Fry egg in bread for 3–5 minutes per side to desired yolk consistency. Toast remaining bread piece in skillet while cooking egg.

Warm Tomato & Basil on Toast

Prep Time: 5 Min | Cook Time: 10 Min   Serves: 2

Ingredients

- 2 Tomatoes (large, cut into quarters)
- 2 tsp Extra virgin olive oil
- 3 tbsp Basil leaves (minced, divided)
- 1/4 tsp Salt
- 4 slice Whole grain bread (toasted; use gluten-free bread or corn tortilla if desired)

Instructions

1. Cut tomatoes into quarters and mince basil leaves.
2. Heat a skillet over medium-high heat. Once hot, add oil, tomatoes, basil, and salt. Cook 4–6 minutes, stirring occasionally, until tomatoes have softened.
3. While tomatoes cook, toast bread in toaster to desired crispiness.
4. Spread the roasted tomatoes and basil evenly over each slice of toast.

Pro Tip (Both Recipes): For additional flavor, add garlic, Parmesan, or sprinkle with Italian or taco seasoning for either of the above recipes. Try balsamic vinegar on Warm Tomato & Basil Toast, or top with an egg or slice of medium-firm tofu for more protein.

Picky Eater Tips (Both Recipes): Let your picky eater help make these recipes by tearing a hole in the bread or topping toast with tomatoes. Offer toppings such as pepperoni, olives, or mozzarella and rename this "Pizza Toast" to make it more fun.

Leftovers (Both Recipes): Refrigerate Egg in a Basket up to a day. Refrigerate the roasted tomatoes separate from toast in an airtight container up to 5 days.

Peach Almond Frozen Smoothie Bowls

Prep Time: 15 Min | Cook Time: 0 Min   Serves: 4

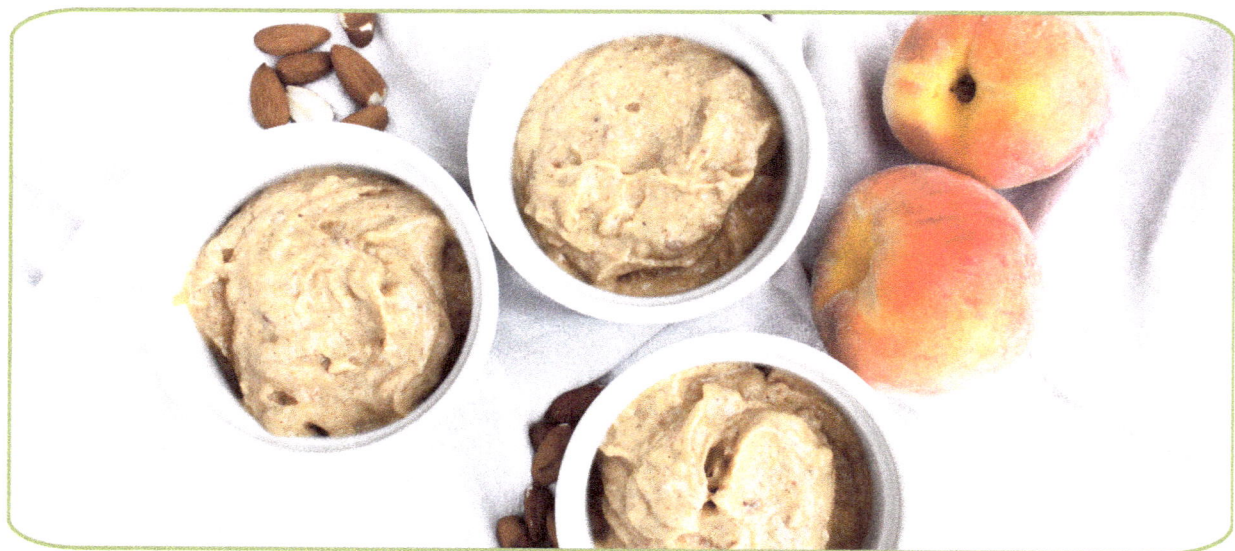

Ingredients
- 2 cup Peaches (sliced and frozen)
- 1/4 cup Almond butter
- 1 tbsp Maple syrup (sub brown sugar if desired)
- 1/2 tsp Vanilla extract

Instructions
1. Add all ingredients to blender or food processor. Blend, stopping occasionally to scrape down the sides. Continue to blend until smooth.

Pro Tip: Sprinkle with cinnamon before serving for a peach cobbler flavor.
Portion leftovers into individual reusable container before freezing to use for a quick breakfast or snack on the go. Adjust amount of maple syrup to taste.

Picky Eater Tips: Let your picky eaters help blend these bowls for hands-on exposure. Offer toppings to go with these, such as chocolate chips, slivered almonds, granola, or sprinkles to add fun. Freeze these in popsicle molds for fun leftovers.

Leftovers: Freeze in an airtight container up to 1 month.

Summer/Fall Meal Plan: Week 4

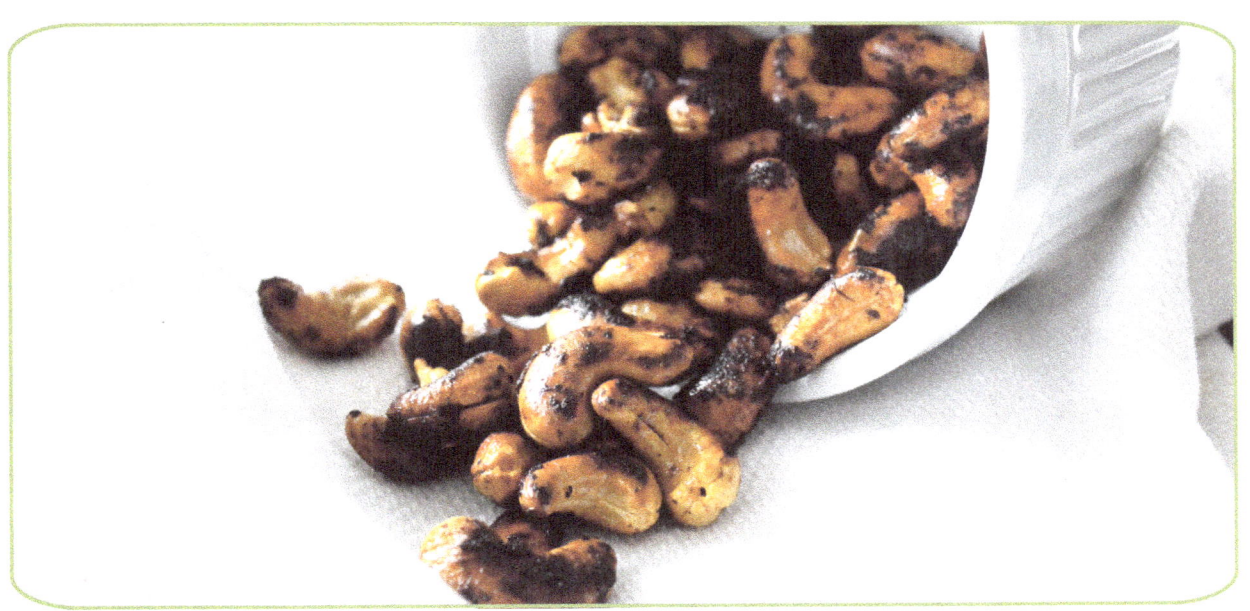

Savory Snack

Spicy Cashews

✓ Gluten-Free   ✓ Dairy-Free   ✓ Vegetarian   ✓ Vegan

Sweet Snack

Key Lime Mousse

✓ Gluten-Free   ✓ Dairy-Free   ✓ Vegetarian   ✓ Vegan

Spicy Cashews

Prep Time: 5 Min | Cook Time: 5 Min   Serves: 4

Ingredients
- 1 cup Cashews (raw)
- 1/2 tsp Smoked paprika
- 1/2 tsp Chili powder
- 1/4 tsp Salt
- 1/4 tsp Red pepper flakes
- 1 tsp Lime juice
- 1 tsp Honey (sub maple syrup for vegan)
- 1/2 tsp Canola oil

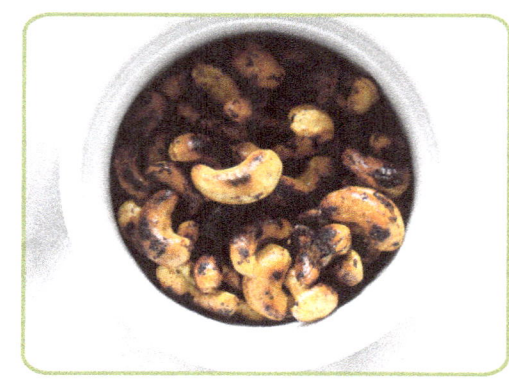

Instructions
1. Add cashews to a medium skillet (dry, without oil) and cook over medium to medium-high heat while assembling remaining ingredients. Cook about 5 minutes, stirring 2–3 times, to begin to toast cashews.
2. Remove cashews from heat and add all remaining ingredients: smoked paprika, chili powder, salt, red pepper flakes, lime juice, honey, and oil. Stir to combine ingredients and evenly coat cashews.
3. Allow to cool, stirring every few minutes to prevent from sticking together.

Pro Tip: This recipe is very spicy; adjust the amount of red pepper flakes to taste. Nuts are a very healthy snack with lots of calories for energy. Portion into individual 1/4 cup containers to help you be mindful of your hunger as you snack; once you're finished with the portion, check in with your body and then decide if you'd like more.

Picky Eater Tips: Offer plain cashews or a mild seasoning as an alternative, with a small side of the spicy version to try. Include a "safe food" or drink like milk to help if the spice is too intense.

Leftovers: Store in an airtight container at room temperature for up to 3–4 weeks.

Key Lime Mousse

Prep Time: 10 Min | Cook Time: 0 Min   Serves: 4

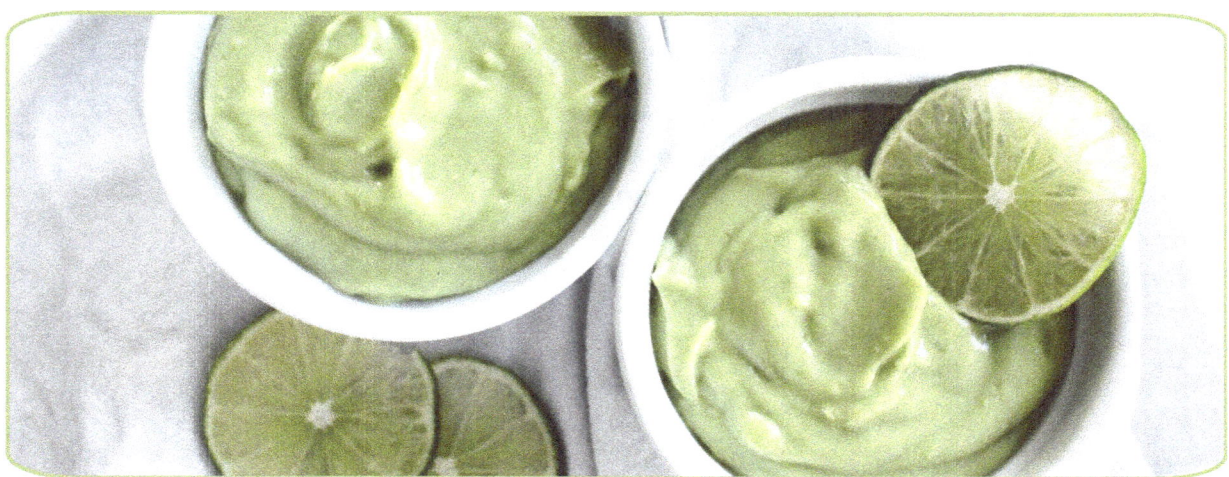

Ingredients

- 2 Avocadoes (large; cubed)
- 1/4 cup Sugar
- 1/3 cup Lime juice (about 3 limes)
- 1 tsp Lime zest
- 2 tbsp Unsweetened soymilk
- 1 tsp Vanilla extract

Instructions

1. In a food processor or blender, combine all ingredients: cubed avocados, sugar, lime juice, lime zest, milk, and vanilla extract.
2. Process or blend until smooth, scraping down sides if necessary. Add more lime juice to taste, if desired.

Pro Tip: Use cream instead of milk for a richer consistency. Easily substitute coconut milk, cashew milk, almond milk, or dairy milk in place of soymilk as desired.

Picky Eater Tips: Serve a small taste alongside a more familiar dessert or safe food. Let picky eaters use the mousse as a dip for grapes or shortbread cookies. Let your picky eater help make the dessert for added exposure. Serve this mousse part of a green-themed menu for fun!

Leftovers: Refrigerate in airtight container up to 3 days. Freeze in popsicle containers for up to several months.

Nutrient and Supplement Guide for Mental Health

Important Considerations *About Dietary Supplements*

The specific ways that nutrients affect the brain and body are incredibly intricate. In this section, we take a closer look at the critical nutrients involved in mental health and how they work. Certain vitamins, minerals, fatty acids, fiber, and amino acids play key roles in mood regulation, the stress response, and cognitive function.

In addition to being found in food, many nutrients are also available as dietary supplements. The term "dietary supplements" refers to a wide range of products intended for ingestion in teas, tinctures, tablets, powders, capsules, or liquid form. All of these can affect mental health – either positively or negatively.

 Interpreting Research Results

When it comes to health claims, it's important to understand the difference between association (aka correlation) and causation. These terms are often confused by the media, but are very different in scientific research. Association describes a relationship where two things change at the same time but may or may not affect each other. For example, ice cream sales and sunburn rates both increase in warmer months, but eating ice cream doesn't cause sunburn. Causation shows a relationship where one variable predictably and directly affects the outcome of another, which requires more rigorous research evidence to confirm. For example, longer periods of sun exposure cause more sunburn.

The quality of research available for dietary supplements varies widely. Some studies include only a small number of people, are done in a specific population, or use cell or animal models. Many have only preliminary findings, use different supplement dosing, or fail to control variables, making it difficult to interpret or generalize the results to a larger population. Translating some study results is possible; for example, most ADHD research is conducted in children, which is often easier to generalize to adults. As registered dietitians and practicing clinicians, we have summarized the available research to give our expert opinion in this section.

Dietary supplements exist to fill in the gaps that might be missing in your diet or for self-treatment of minor conditions. Consult with your mental health team to tailor a supplement regimen based on your specific health needs, lifestyle, and dietary restrictions. For those with multiple dietary restrictions or with limited diet variety, taking a multivitamin instead of, or in addition to, individual supplements may be helpful to ensure you're meeting your basic needs.

Important Considerations *About Dietary Supplements*

Common Types of Dietary Supplements

Vitamins: are naturally-occurring essential nutrients that the body needs in small quantities for various metabolic reactions and cell functions. They are sometimes listed on the label by the name of the vitamin (eg vitamin B2) or by its chemical name (riboflavin). They have different chemical forms, some of which are more bioavailable than others, and thus more easily absorbed and used by the body. Read more on pages 194–206.

Minerals: are naturally-occurring inorganic substances that the body requires in small amounts, such as calcium, iron, and zinc, among others. They also exist in different molecular forms, which affect their bioavailability, such as heme versus nonheme iron. Read more on pages 207–213.

Herbs and botanicals: include different plant parts used for their therapeutic effect, such as leaves, stems, roots, flowers, or seeds. These can be used to make teas, tinctures, extracts, tablets, or capsules. Read more on pages 218–236.

Amino acids: are the building blocks of proteins, found naturally in foods, and sometimes produced by the body. Depending on the type of amino acid, they can be used to build muscle, provide calories, play a part in metabolic reactions to obtain energy from food, work as neurotransmitters, or be made into other important molecules, such as vitamins. Read more on pages 178, 180–182.

Probiotics: are microorganisms including bacteria and yeast. There are hundreds to thousands of different types that make up the microbiota and some of these strains are available in dietary supplements. Additionally, pre- and post-biotics can be found as supplements. Read more on pages 189–192.

Enzymes: are specialized proteins produced by the body that help carry out and increase the efficiency of hundreds of different biological reactions, such as digestion, metabolism, respiration, detoxification, and more. Because these have little direct impact on mental health, these are not discussed in this book.

Important Considerations *About Dietary Supplements*

This guide includes information on a wide variety of nutrients and dietary supplements. It's designed to give you a basic understanding of how these nutrients are connected to mental health and help you ask questions of your mental health team to determine which would best support you. We encourage you to focus on the nutrients you might be missing in your diet, or those important for your specific needs.

For nutrients that can be found in food, you'll find practical guidance in this section on recommended nutrient intake levels, food sources, and when adding dietary supplements might be helpful to fill in nutritional gaps. The Recommended Daily Allowance (RDA) is listed for each nutrient (or Adequate Intake, AI, if the RDA is unavailable) and is based on the amount to meet the needs of up to 97–98% of the adult population. Your needs may differ if you are younger than 20 or older than 50, are pregnant, lactating, or have certain health conditions. Talk with your mental health team to determine your personal needs.

You'll also find information about important safety considerations. While these nutrients are essential, more isn't always better. Some nutrients can cause unpleasant and even dangerous symptoms when taken in toxic doses from either food, supplements, or a combination. Most often, toxicity from nutrients occurs with supplement intake, but some nutrients, such as vitamin A in liver or selenium in Brazil nuts, can build up and cause harmful symptoms. See each nutrient page for more details, including the Tolerable Upper Intake Level (UL), which we'll refer to as the common term, "upper limit." This is the maximum daily intake of a nutrient that can be consumed on an ongoing basis without adverse events for the general population.

 While vitamins and minerals are essential, more isn't always better! Many of these nutrients can be toxic at high levels. Some interact with certain medications, sometimes in significant or dangerous ways. In addition to the RDA, check the information about toxicity in each supplement page to find the Tolerable Upper Intake Level ("upper limit") for each nutrient.

We recommend obtaining nutrients from food whenever possible. Nutrients in food are almost always superior to using supplements because whole foods contain other bioavailable compounds in addition to micronutrients that can work synergistically to have a more potent effect. In other words, nutrients from standalone dietary supplements are not always as effective as the same nutrients found in foods.

How to Choose High-Quality Supplements

In the United States, dietary supplements are considered a category of food rather than a drug, which affects how they are regulated. Under the The Dietary Supplement Health and Education Act of 1994, the Food and Drug Administration (FDA), "is not authorized to approve dietary supplements for safety and effectiveness before they are marketed." Instead, manufacturers are responsible for ensuring safety and potency, but the FDA is not notified before products are on the market.

Once a supplement is on the market, the FDA then has the authority to oversee that manufacturing facilities are complying with current Good Manufacturing Practices (GMPs). GMPs outline a set of manufacturing processes that ensure the identity, strength, quality, and purity of dietary supplements. The FDA periodically inspects manufacturing facilities to ensure compliance, visiting high-risk facilities at least once every three years and other facilities at least once every five years. While the FDA is legally allowed to inspect facilities more frequently than this, resource constraints including staffing and funding shortfalls often impact the agency's ability to meet these targets. In practice, only about 5% of manufacturing facilities are inspected annually, and recent reports show that the FDA has frequently not fulfilled its duty to inspect high-risk facilities within the required timeframe.

 The lack of oversight has led to wide variability in the safety and quality of dietary supplements. Choose a supplement brand with certified third-party testing, as some studies show that many off-the-shelf products do not contain the ingredients in the amounts they were listed on the label.

If a concern is raised about a dietary supplement, the FDA is legally permitted to analyze the supplement for safety and purity, can issue warning letters, require voluntary recalls of products, or pursue mandatory recalls if necessary. The FDA does not routinely analyze supplements before sale.

Several third-party certification programs have been created to fill this gap in oversight. The next page provides an overview of the most common and reputable companies. Each has slightly different standards for certifying products and you should choose a certification based on your needs. For example, if you are a competitive athlete, always choose supplements with third-party testing by a company that tests every batch for banned substances.

Some supplements list on the label that they use "third-party testing," but fail to identify the certifier. You should avoid these and instead choose a supplement with clear labeling, displaying the certification badge directly on the product.

How to Choose High-Quality Supplements

Certification Program	Manufacturing Process	Supplement Quality, Testing for Banned Substances	Post-Market Testing
Banned Substances Control Group	Optional GMP audit program for brands with audits every 2 years	Label accuracy, identity, strength, heavy metals, microbiology, over 500 drugs including testing for 400 substances on the World Anti-Doping Agency Prohibited List, prescription, and over-the-counter drugs. See certification tracks for more details.	Yes – ongoing monitoring and testing programs
Consumer Lab	No facility audits – only tests finished products	Label accuracy, identity, strength, contaminants, how it breaks down in the body. Does not focus on banned substances for sport.	Yes – annual testing using products from store shelves
Informed Choice / Informed Sport	Yes – audits and certifies facilities (Sport audits annually)	Label accuracy, contaminants, ingredient verification, label claims. Tests for over 250 substances on the World Anti-Doping Agency Prohibited List.	Yes – Choice does monthly blind post-market tests; Sport tests every batch
National Sanitation Foundation International	Yes – annual facility audits according to GMP standards	Label accuracy, identity, strength, potency, and contaminants (heavy metals, microbes). NSF Certified for Sport® tests every lot for 280+ banned substances.	Yes – supplements are tested regularly from store shelves
United States Pharmacopeia	Yes – annual facility audits according to CGMP standards	Purity, potency, how well it breaks down in the body, consistency, contaminants. Does not focus on banned substances for sport.	Limited – more focused on pre-market, but periodic checks occur

How to Choose High-Quality Supplements

Choose Supplements With Bioavailable Forms of Nutrients

Vitamins and minerals come in different forms in food and dietary supplements and some are more easily absorbed and used by the body than others. Taking the correct supplement form can enhance its functional use in the body. See the "Dietary supplements" section on each supplement page for more details.

Some dietary supplements claim to be derived from plant or other "natural" sources and purport additional benefits because of this. However, the process of deriving the vitamin from its source often eliminates many of the other benefits of eating the whole foods. Focus instead on increasing plants in your eating pattern and choose the correct form of nutrient.

Check the Ingredients List

Ingredients are mandated to be listed on the supplement bottle, but the FDA does not have the authority to check supplements for safety or purity unless a complaint is made after the supplement is on the market. Always look for third-party verified supplements from one of the certifications on page 171 to ensure that what is listed on the label is actually what is in the product. Here are some tips for what to look for:

- **Fewer ingredients are better:** Quality supplements typically have minimal fillers, artificial colors, or preservatives.
- **Watch for allergens:** For individuals with dietary restrictions (eg, gluten-free, vegan, allergies), ensure the supplement is free from certain ingredients by checking the label for allergen-free or other related certifications.
- **Avoid proprietary blends:** Manufacturers sometimes hide ingredient amounts in proprietary blends. Choose supplements with clearly listed ingredient amounts.

Check the Expiration Date

Some vitamins like vitamin C and vitamin B12 degrade over time, so they become less effective. Check the expiration date on the package and buy supplements from brands and places whose products turnover quickly and don't sit on the shelf too long.

Store Supplements Correctly to Extend Shelf Life

Heat, humidity, and light can degrade supplements, so store supplements in a cool, dry place. Avoid storing them in humid areas such as bathrooms. Instead, a pantry or bedroom drawer may be better for maintaining potency. Keep dietary supplements in a safe place from children and pets to avoid accidental ingestion and overdose.

How to Choose High-Quality Supplements

Check Dosage and Serving Size

Just like you can have too little of a vitamin, you can also get too much. To avoid overdosing vitamins and minerals, always check the RDA (Recommended Daily Allowance) and Tolerable Upper Intake Level (upper limit) listed on each supplement page. Compare the supplement serving size to the recommended daily dosage to ensure you're getting an adequate and safe amount. Consider all sources of foods, dietary supplements, energy drinks, protein shakes, meal replacements, and electrolyte drinks when calculating your nutrient intake.

Take special care to note the unit of measure when comparing nutrient requirements, toxicity, and nutrient amounts in food and dietary supplements. Reference this conversion of common doses.

Measurement Abbreviations and Conversions	
Abbreviation	**Conversions**
Micrograms: mcg or µg	1,000,000 mcg = 1 g 1,000 mcg = 1 mg
Milligrams: mg	1,000 mg = 1 g
Grams: g	1 g = 1,000 mg 1,000 g = 1 kg 28 g = 1 oz
Kilograms: kg	1 kg = 1,000 g 1 kg = 2.2 lbs
International Units: IU	A measurement of the biological effect of a certain amount of the nutrient; the conversion varies for each nutrient. IU are often used for vitamins A, E, and D.

Supplements for Dietary Patterns

Once you have identified a quality supplement, next you need to know if and when you might need one. Some dietary patterns, such as vegetarian or gluten-free, may not include all the necessary nutrients. If you follow one of these eating patterns, talk with your mental health team about adding some of these supplements. Suggested doses are listed per day unless otherwise noted.

Fish-Free

Fish contain a more bioavailable form of omega-3 fatty acids than plants; supplementation may be helpful even if consuming plant sources.

- **Omega-3:** algae oil-based supplement
  - RDA for Alpha-Lipoic Acid (ALA*): 1.1–1.6 g
- **Vitamin D:** 15–20 mcg (600–800 IU) (D3 from lichen or D2)
- **Iodine:** 150 mcg (especially if avoiding seafood entirely)

Dairy-Free

Individuals need to ensure sufficient intake of calcium and other nutrients typically found in dairy.

- **Vitamin B12:** 500–1,000 mcg (if avoiding fortified foods, particularly for vegans or vegetarians)
- **Vitamin D:** 15–20 mcg (600–800 IU)
- **Vitamin K2:** 90–120 mcg
- **Calcium:** 1,000–1,200 mg
- **Magnesium:** 310–420 mg

Gluten-Free

Gluten-free grains are often not fortified. With newly diagnosed celiac disease, initial supplementation may be helpful due to previous malabsorption.

- **B vitamins (B1, B2, B3, B6, B9, B12):** a B-complex supplement can provide sufficient doses; see individual supplement pages for RDA
- **Vitamin D:** 15–20 mcg (600–800 IU)
- **Calcium:** 1,000 mg (if dairy intake is low)
- **Iron (elemental):** 18 mg for women; 8 mg for men
- **Zinc:** 8–11 mg

*ALA stands for Alpha-Lipoic Acid. See pages 184–186 for more information.

Nutrient and Supplement Guide for Mental Health

Supplements for Dietary Patterns

Vegetarian

Vegetarians should consider supplementing nutrients primarily found in meat.

- **Omega-3:** algae oil-based supplement
  - RDA for ALA: 1.1–1.6 g
- **Vitamin B12:** 500–1,000 mcg
- **Vitamin D:** 15–20 mcg (600–800 IU, D3 from lichen)
- **Calcium:** 1,000 mg (if dairy intake is low or non-existent)
- **Iron (elemental):** 18 mg for women; 8 mg for men
- **Zinc:** 8–11 mg

Vegans

Vegan needs are similar to vegetarians, but with a few additional nutrients due to the exclusion of all animal products.

- **Omega-3:** algae oil-based supplement
  - RDA for ALA: 1.1–1.6 g
- **Vitamin B12:** 1,000 mcg daily or 2,500 mcg weekly
- **Choline:** 425–550 mg
- **Vitamin D:** 15–20 mcg (600–800 IU)
- **Calcium:** 1,000 mg
- **Iron (elemental):** 18 mg for women; 8 mg for men
- **Selenium:** 55 mcg
- **Zinc:** 8–11 mg

Standard American Diet / Typical Western Diet

The "Standard American Diet" is defined as an eating pattern high in refined grains, refined sugar, and animal products, while being low in whole fruits, vegetables, grains, and legumes. Although it is best to increase your intake of the latter foods for overall health, supplementation may also be helpful.

- **Omega-3:** algae oil- or fish oil-based supplement
  - RDA for ALA: 1.1–1.6 g
- **Vitamin A:** 700–900 mcg of retinol activity equivalents (RAE)
- **Vitamin C:** 75–90 mg
- **Vitamin D:** 15–20 mcg (600–800 IU)
- **Vitamin E:** 15 mg
- **Calcium:** 1,000 mg (if low dairy intake)
- **Iron (elemental):** 18 mg for menstruating people, 8 mg for non-menstruating people; if eating high amounts of red meat, non-menstruating people may exceed the RDA and should not take a supplement
- **Magnesium:** 310–420 mg
- **Potassium:** 2,600–3,400 mg from food sources

Mindful Choices:

Ingredients, Substances, and Your Mental Health

In addition to what to add to your diet, discussions around mental health often focus on what to leave out. From food additives to sugar, there have been many campaigns to demonize certain foods or ingredients. However, not all research in this area is high quality; many studies have few participants or measure correlation rather than causation. In general, we advocate for a more balanced approach.

 Eating patterns high in ultra-processed foods often lead to imbalances in nutrition, but the emphasis here is on patterns. Including convenience items to reduce stress or enjoying foods with sugar for celebrations are part of a healthy relationship with food. The benefits of engaging in your community almost always outweigh the potential harm of individual ingredients.

There is nothing wrong with removing certain ingredients from your eating pattern, but if doing so causes other harm – such as hyper-fixation on ingredients, avoiding eating when hungry, or limiting participation in social eating – we encourage you to take a step back and look at the bigger picture. As discussed in Section 2, sometimes eliminating foods can lead to feelings of restriction and even disordered eating behaviors. Your overall mental health and well-being are more important than eating a perfect diet.

Instead of putting too much emphasis on eliminating individual ingredients, we encourage you to look at your overall food consumption patterns. Focusing on balancing your plate and cooking at home more often will help you naturally reduce the amounts of additives, preservatives, and sugar, as well as rebalance the types of fats in your eating pattern.

There are other substances apart from additives that are not nutritionally necessary and can have a great impact on mental health. These include depressants, such as alcohol, or stimulants, such as caffeine. Other compounds like tetrahydrocannabinol (THC) sourced from cannabis are psychoactive and can be a hallucinogenic, or act as either a depressant or stimulant. Each of these substances has an initial impact on mental health, and can also affect mental health for hours or days after ingestion. They often interact negatively with mental health medications, so they should be used with caution. The effects of these substances are highly individualized. Be aware of your intake pattern of these substances and how they are likely affecting you and your mental health. Talk with your mental health team regarding their use.

Macronutrients *for Mental Health*

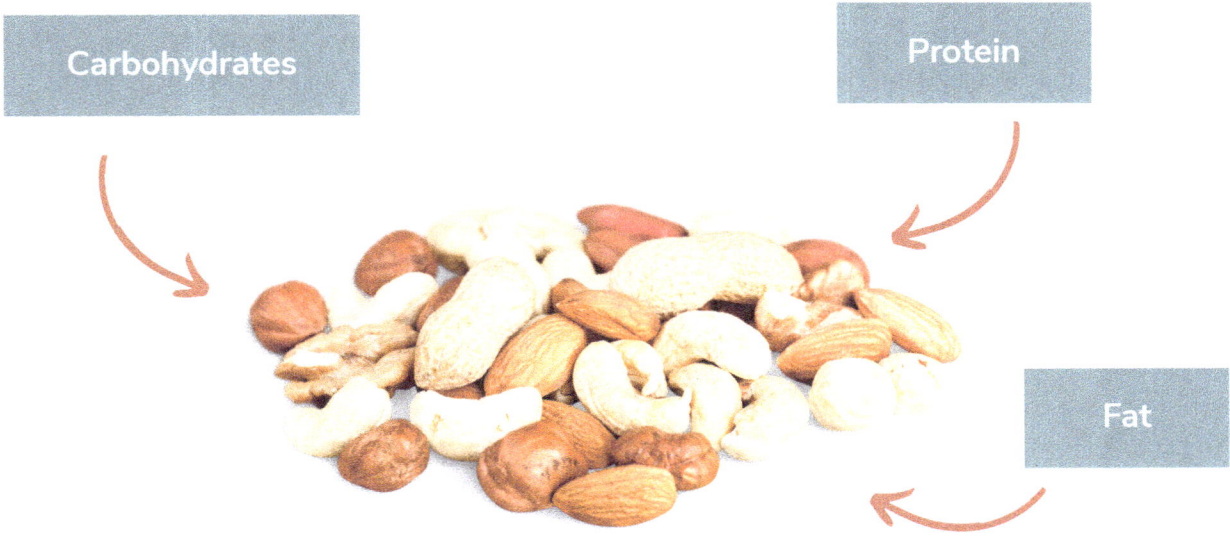

Carbohydrates

Protein

Fat

There are three macronutrients in food: carbohydrates, protein, and fat. "Macro" means "big," as these nutrients are measured in grams (g) rather than milligrams (mg) or micrograms (mcg or µg) like micronutrients. Most foods contain all three of these nutrients in varying amounts but have a primary macronutrient that makes up most of its nutritional content. For example, peanuts contain all three macronutrients but are often categorized as protein because they are a good source of protein. They also contain a significant amount of fat and a small amount of carbohydrates, some of which are fiber.

Each macronutrient plays an important role in the body beyond providing energy – but they do that, too. These are the building blocks of health. If we don't have enough of these nutrients, our physical and mental health will suffer. In this section we explore each nutrient's function in the body, how much we need, and highlight specific components that support mental health.

Macronutrient: Protein

Protein is made up of building blocks called amino acids. There are 20 amino acids used to form protein structures in the body, including muscles, cell membranes, enzymes, and hormones. Amino acids are also the sources to form certain neurotransmitters, such as serotonin, dopamine, and epinephrine (adrenaline).

Nine of these amino acids are defined as "essential," meaning we can't make them in the body, and so we need to eat them. Animal proteins contain the nine essential amino acids in the ratio the body needs them. Plant proteins are best paired as a legume plus grain to meet the correct ratio.

In addition to these 20 amino acids, there are nonprotein amino acids that serve a variety of different functions other than building muscle. Nonprotein amino acids provide energy, work in metabolism, serve as neurotransmitters, and can be made into other important molecules such as vitamins.

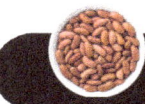
Examples of Protein-Rich Foods

Plant-based proteins: beans, lentils, nuts, seeds, nut butters, spirulina, edamame, tofu, tempeh, seitan, and nutritional yeast
Vegetarian proteins: cheese, cottage cheese, eggs, and Greek yogurt
Meat proteins: chicken, turkey, pork, beef, lamb, ground meat, deli meat, tuna, salmon, tilapia, shrimp, scallops, and other seafood

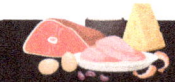
Examples of Amino Acids for Mental Health

Tryptophan: is a building block for serotonin. Tryptophan supplements can increase serotonin levels.
Glutamate: acts as a neurotransmitter and is a precursor to GABA.
Methionine: facilitates the production of neurotransmitters by combining with ATP to produce S-adenosyl-L-methionine (SAMe).
Phenylalanine and tyrosine: are involved in making dopamine, epinephrine, and norepinephrine.
Taurine: elicits a calming effect in the brain by activating GABA receptors.

Macronutrient: Protein

It's important to eat enough protein every day because we can't store protein in our bodies. Eating more than we need isn't necessary. Protein that is consumed beyond the need for building blocks will be broken down for energy. The amount of protein you need depends on your age, activity level, health, stage of life, and other factors. Use these guidelines as a starting point to determine your protein needs.

Protein Intake Guidelines

Minimum protein necessary: The RDA is set at 0.8 grams (g) of protein per kilogram (kg) body weight, or 0.36 g per pound (lb), to prevent protein deficiency. For a 180 lb person, this equals 65 g of protein daily.

Most healthy individuals: Many people benefit from a slightly higher protein goal than the bare minimum, including those in perimenopause, menopause, engaging in light exercise programs, or losing weight. These individuals should aim for 1.0–1.2 g of protein per kg body weight, or 0.45–0.55 g per lb. For a 180 lb person, this equals 82–98 grams of protein daily.

Higher protein needs: Those who are in a growth state such as pregnancy, strength training, or vigorous exercise programs may benefit from a higher protein intake. These individuals should aim for 1.2–1.7 g of protein per kg body weight, or 0.55–0.77 g per lb. Those eating a plant-based diet may also benefit from this higher protein goal to ensure adequacy of all essential amino acids. For a 180 lb person, this equals 98–139 g of protein daily.

Low protein diet: Those with chronic kidney disease may require a lower protein diet, with a goal set between 0.23–0.8 g of protein per kg body weight, or 0.10–0.36 g per lb. The recommendations vary based on disease stage and type of dialysis and you should consult your doctor or dietitian for your needs.

If you eat enough protein each day, you don't need to supplement most amino acids. However, the nonprotein amino acid L-theanine and the nonprotein amino acid derivative creatine have shown promise in impacting certain mental health conditions and brain health. See the following supplement pages for more information.

Amino Acids *for Mental Health*

L-Theanine

<u>Found in</u>: tea leaves; green tea has higher amounts than black tea.

<u>How it works:</u> L-theanine is a nonprotein amino acid that serves other functions in the body besides building muscle. It helps to balance levels of GABA, serotonin, and dopamine, which affect mood, relaxation, and focus. Its chemical structure is similar to glutamate, and because of that L-theanine binds to glutamate receptors and NMDA (N-Methyl-D-Aspartate) receptors. It also may increase levels of BDNF (Brain-Derived Neurotrophic Factor).

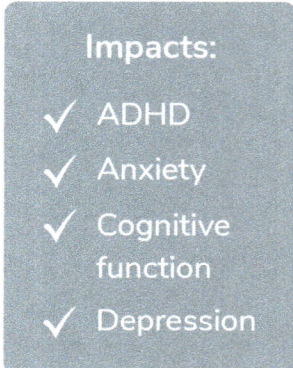

Impacts:

✓ ADHD

✓ Anxiety

✓ Cognitive function

✓ Depression

<u>Dietary supplements:</u> L-theanine supplements are available as capsules, tablets, or in green tea. The dose of L-theanine in tea varies significantly; a serving of 200 ml (6–7 oz) of tea contains between 8–60 mg of L-theanine.

- <u>ADHD:</u> Early-stage research in children shows a possible benefit of taking 2.5 mg of L-theanine per kg body weight; it may be beneficial to combine it with caffeine. A single dose of 200 mg of L-theanine may improve attention similar to a dose of 160 mg of caffeine.
- <u>Anxiety:</u> Early-stage research shows that taking 200 mg daily of L-theanine for 4 weeks may reduce anxiety, but the results of clinical trials are conflicting.
- <u>Cognitive function:</u> Taking a single dose of 100 mg of L-theanine appears to improve attention and reduce error rates on cognitive tests. When combined with caffeine, it may increase alertness. It does not appear to be more beneficial to take it daily and it doesn't seem to improve cognitive function in older adults.
- <u>Depression:</u> Taking 200–250 mg of L-theanine before bedtime for 6–8 weeks may reduce depression symptoms, but these results were from studies with a small sample size, short duration, and one did not have a comparator group.

<u>Side effects:</u> Similar to caffeine, side effects may include headache, jitteriness, dizziness, nausea, or diarrhea. It may cause drowsiness.

<u>Caution:</u> The FDA considers L-theanine to be generally safe at doses less than 500 mg per day. It may interact with blood pressure lowering medication. Choose a brand with third-party certification to avoid potential contamination and ensure purity.

Amino Acids *for Mental Health*

Creatine

<u>Found in:</u> meat, dairy products, and fish. Creatine is also produced in the liver, pancreas, and kidneys. The cumulative amount from an omnivorous diet and synthesis in the body is about 2–4 g daily.

<u>How it works:</u> Creatine is a nonprotein amino acid derivative made from three other amino acids. It serves other functions in the body besides building muscle. Creatine enhances metabolic reactions and energy production in the mitochondria of our bodies' cells. Its role is most important in cells with high energy demands, such as muscle, brain, and heart, where it works by donating a phosphate group to regenerate ATP, which is the primary energy carrier in the body. Its contribution to energy production may be particularly helpful in correcting energy deficits observed in depression and to benefit brain function. It may also have neuroprotective effects from stress and traumatic injury, such as concussion. It appears to also help control inflammation and reduce oxidative stress.

Impacts:

✓ Cognitive function

✓ Depression

✓ Inflammation

✓ Memory

<u>Dietary supplements:</u> Creatine monohydrate is the most cost-effective and best studied form of this dietary supplement. Other types tend to be more expensive and do not appear to be superior. Optimal dosing for mental health remains unclear due to short study duration and variability in underlying dietary intake of creatine in study participants. It appears that the first 5 g of dietary or supplemental creatine is absorbed by muscles, so a higher dose may be needed for cognitive benefits. Many studies use an initial loading dose of creatine to increase the baseline creatine in muscles followed by a lower daily maintenance dose. This is not necessary but may shorten the time to see benefits. Initial loading doses are usually 0.3 g of creatine per kg of body weight for 5–7 days (equal to 0.14 g per lb, or about 25 g of creatine for a 180 lb individual), divided into 4 doses throughout the day.

Creatine is not found in plant proteins, so those following a vegan or vegetarian diet may benefit especially from the addition of supplemental creatine. Vegans can choose a certified vegan creatine monohydrate.

Creatine (continued)

<u>Dietary supplements (continued):</u>

- <u>Alzheimer's disease:</u> Early research shows that taking 20 g of creatine daily for 8 weeks may improve cognition and memory in those with Alzheimer's disease.
- <u>Cognitive function:</u> A single high dose of 20–30 g creatine may enhance energy and cognitive performance after a poor night's sleep; use of this dosing long-term has not been extensively studied so use it with caution. Taking a single dose of 0.35 g per kg body weight (equal to 0.16 g per lb or about 29 g creatine for a 180 lb individual) prior to known sleep deprivation, such as with an early morning wake-up, may help reduce fatigue, brain fog, and improve memory.
- <u>Depression:</u> Early-stage research shows that taking conservative doses of 4–5 g of creatine daily for 2–8 weeks may be beneficial, especially if combined with treatments that include selective serotonin reuptake inhibitor (SSRI) medication. For more impact, a higher dose may be needed, up to 0.14 g per kg body weight (equal to 0.06 g per lb or about 11 g creatine for a 180 lb individual). However, current clinical guidelines* recommend against the use of creatine for depression until more conclusive evidence is available.
- <u>Memory:</u> Taking 2.2–20 g of creatine daily for 5 days–24 weeks may improve performance on certain memory tests.

<u>Side effects:</u> Oral creatine supplements are usually well-tolerated, but high doses may cause gastrointestinal distress, altered bowel habits, muscle cramps, muscle stiffness, dehydration, heat intolerance, and initial weight gain due to water retention. Take supplement doses throughout the day to minimize side effects.

<u>Caution:</u> Supplemental creatine appears to be safe for loading doses of up to 25 g daily or 0.3 g per kg body weight for up to 14 days (equal to 0.14 g per lb). Maintenance doses of up to 10 g daily have been safely used for up to 5 years in some preliminary clinical research. Avoid taking large doses for long durations as there have been case reports of serious adverse effects including kidney damage. If competing in sports, look for a supplement with third-party certification that tests every batch for banned substances to ensure they have not been contaminated. Talk with your medical team before using if you have kidney dysfunction, bipolar disorder, or Parkinson's disease. Avoid using if you are pregnant or breastfeeding.

*Clinical practice guidelines come from the World Federation of Societies of Biological Psychiatry (WFSBP) and the Canadian Network for Mood and Anxiety Treatments (CANMAT).

Macronutrient: Fat

Dietary fat has many jobs in the body. It's a component of cells and hormones, transports nutrients, helps absorb fat-soluble vitamins, and slows digestion to keep us feeling full. There are many different types of fat, which all have different impacts on health. Some types of fat, such as polyunsaturated fats (PUFAs) and monounsaturated fats (MUFAs), promote health while others, such as saturated and trans-fats, cause inflammation when eaten in high amounts.

The nutrition community's understanding of how fat impacts health has evolved as new research has become available. Decades ago, it was found that high-fat diets were associated with poor metabolic health outcomes, such as heart disease and stroke. With new research, it has become clear that the type of fat consumed and what it is replaced by in the diet matters more than the total amount of fat consumed.

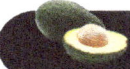 **Monounsaturated Fats**

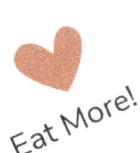 Eat More!

Plant oils: avocado, olive, canola, peanut, safflower, sesame
Nuts: almonds, cashews, hazelnuts, peanuts, pecans, pistachios

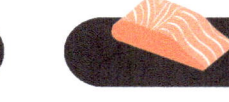 **Omega-3 Fatty Acids**

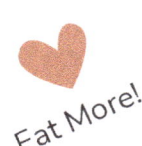 Eat More!

Fatty fish: salmon, mackerel, tuna, cod, herring, sardines
Nuts & seeds: flax, chia, walnuts
Plant oils: flax, soybean, canola

 Omega-6 Fatty Acids

Keep Stable

Nuts & seeds: sunflower, pumpkin, walnuts
Plant oils: corn, soybean, safflower, sunflower

 **Saturated Fatty Acids**

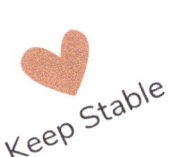 Swap for Plants When Possible

Animal fats: beef, lamb, pork, poultry, butter, cheese
Oils: coconut, palm

Macronutrient: Fat

A higher intake of saturated fat is associated with an increased cardiovascular disease risk, but replacing saturated fat with ultra-processed carbohydrates and simple sugars can make this problem worse. Instead, replacing saturated fats with PUFAs and MUFAs, which primarily come from plant oils, is associated with a decreased risk of cardiovascular disease, better metabolic health outcomes, and improved brain health.

Consuming higher amounts of PUFAs and MUFAs has consistently shown to lower LDL cholesterol levels and improve cardiometabolic health. Omega-3 (alpha-linolenic acid, or ALA) and omega-6 (linoleic acid) fatty acids are defined as essential PUFAs, which means our body cannot produce them from other sources, so we need to eat them. Omega-9 fatty acids, primarily oleic acid, are the main MUFA in our diet. They are also heart-healthy and eating more helps to reduce inflammation.

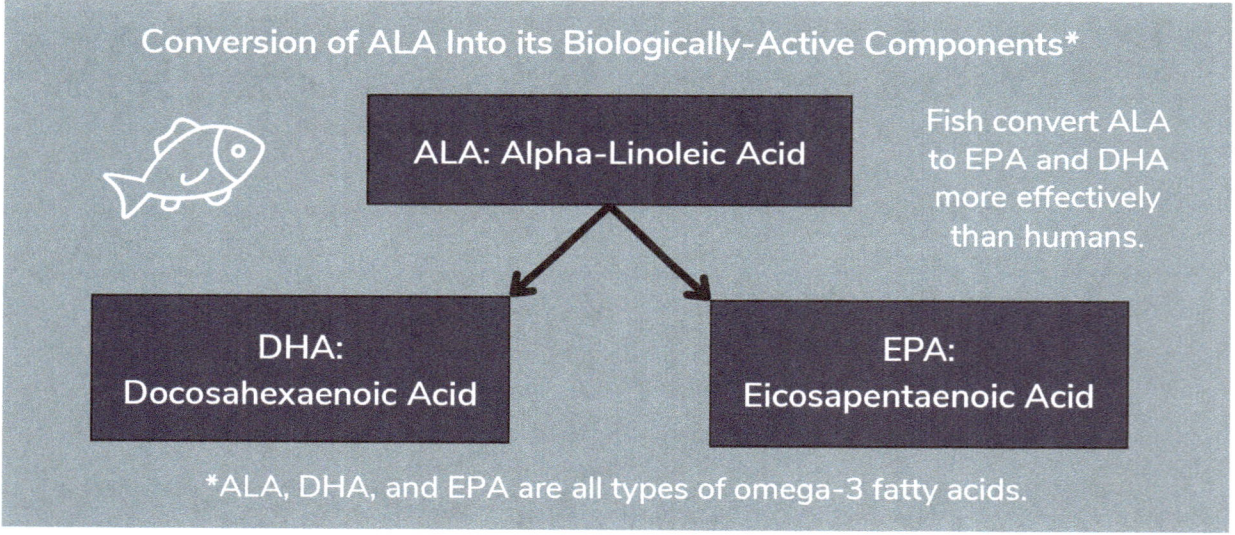

Conversion of ALA Into its Biologically-Active Components*

ALA: Alpha-Linoleic Acid

Fish convert ALA to EPA and DHA more effectively than humans.

DHA: Docosahexaenoic Acid

EPA: Eicosapentaenoic Acid

*ALA, DHA, and EPA are all types of omega-3 fatty acids.

Omega-3 fatty acids have been found to be particularly important for mental health. The plant form of omega-3 fatty acids is ALA, which is converted into DHA and EPA in the body. DHA and EPA are considered biologically active, which means these are the forms of omega-3 fatty acids that provide benefits in the body. Humans have a limited capacity to convert ALA to its active form and so consuming DHA and EPA from food and supplements provides a greater benefit. Each form of omega-3 has a different impact on mental health and is mentioned by its name in the following supplement pages.

Nutrient and Supplement Guide for Mental Health

Fats *for Mental Health*

Omega-3 Fatty Acids: ALA, DHA, and EPA

<u>RDA for ALA:</u> 1.1–1.6 g daily

<u>Found in:</u> ALA is found in plant oils, walnuts, chia, flax, and hemp seeds. DHA and EPA are found in fatty fish such as anchovies, herring, salmon, mackerel, cod, sardines, bluefin tuna, oysters, and mussels.

<u>How they work:</u> DHA and EPA decrease the production of compounds in the body that cause inflammation, including prostaglandins, thromboxanes, and cytokines. They may also contribute to signal transduction in the brain. DHA is found in cell membranes and in high amounts in the brain, indicating its importance in brain structure and development. DHA may help maintain neuronal function and cell membrane integrity in the brain, leading to improved cognitive function and reduced risk of mental health disorders.

Impacts:
- ✓ ADHD
- ✓ Anxiety
- ✓ Cognitive function
- ✓ Depression
- ✓ Inflammation

<u>At risk for deficiency:</u> Groups at risk include those eating low-fish diets. The American Heart Association recommends eating two servings of 3 oz of fatty fish per week. An individual's omega-3 status is difficult to determine and overt deficiency is rare in the United States. Symptoms of severe deficiency include rough, scaly skin and an itchy, swollen, red rash. Insufficient consumption of omega-3 fatty acids is more common than overt deficiency and increases the risk of heart disease, cancer, cognitive decline, Alzheimer's disease, age-related macular degeneration, dry eye, rheumatoid arthritis, and overall inflammation in the body.

<u>Dietary supplements:</u> Fish sources of omega-3 fatty acids that contain DHA and EPA are better used by the body than plant sources that contain ALA. The most common fish sources include fish oil, krill oil, and cod liver oil. A vegetarian source is algal oil, which comes from algae but has lower bioavailability of DHA and EPA compared to fish oils. Look for a supplement with a reputable third-party certification to ensure purity and low mercury levels. Take supplements with meals that include fat for best absorption and to reduce side effects, which can include an unpleasant "fishy" taste in the mouth, bad breath, heartburn, nausea, stomach upset, diarrhea, headache, and smelly sweat.

Fats *for Mental Health*

Omega-3 Fatty Acids: ALA, DHA, and EPA (continued)

<u>Dietary supplements (continued):</u> Individuals with insufficient omega-3 fatty acid intake may benefit more than those consuming high levels of omega-3 fatty acids.

- <u>ADHD:</u> Low blood plasma levels of DHA and EPA are associated with higher rates of ADHD in children. It's unclear if taking ALA, DHA, or EPA supplements can treat or prevent ADHD. Small, early-stage trials show that taking 345–500 mg of DHA daily may improve some social and emotional aspects of ADHD.
- <u>Anxiety:</u> Taking 2.1 g of EPA per day may reduce the severity of anxiety symptoms, but research is limited and more studies are needed.
- <u>Cognitive function:</u> Daily oral intake from food and supplements of 360–800 mg of DHA plus 360–900 mg of EPA may improve cognitive function in healthy adults. It's unclear if taking DHA or EPA alone is beneficial for cognitive function. A higher intake of dietary DHA is associated with a lower risk of Alzheimer's disease, but research about supplementation has had mixed results. It's possible that a higher dose is needed than what has been used in studies to date.
- <u>Depression:</u> Clinical practice guidelines* recommend taking 1–2 g of EPA daily for adjunctive use, but not monotherapy, for patients with major depressive disorder. The guidelines weakly recommend this dose for adjunctive use to treat symptoms of depression in patients with bipolar disorder. Most research shows that DHA supplementation does not improve depression.
- <u>Inflammation:</u> A higher dietary intake of omega-3 fatty acids is associated with a lower risk of heart disease. The American Heart Association recommends eating 6 oz of fatty fish per week, but does not have clinical guidelines for taking supplemental DHA or EPA for healthy adults. Taking 2–4 g of combined DHA and EPA may daily may help with joint inflammation, blood pressure, triglycerides, and cholesterol, which are related to inflammation.

<u>Toxicity:</u> There is no upper limit for ALA, but the FDA recommends limiting intake to less than 3 g daily from DHA and EPA combined from both supplement and food sources. No more than 2 g per day should come from dietary supplements.
High doses can suppress immune function and increase the risk of bleeding. Omega-3 fatty acids may interact with blood thinners or blood pressure medication; discuss with your mental health team before starting supplementation.

*Clinical practice guidelines come from the World Federation of Societies of Biological Psychiatry (WFSBP) and the Canadian Network for Mood and Anxiety Treatments (CANMAT).

Macronutrient: Carbohydrates

Carbohydrates are the body's main energy source and are commonly referred to as "carbs." The body breaks down carbohydrates in foods into three individual monosaccharides (glucose, fructose, and galactose), which are the building blocks of all carbohydrates.

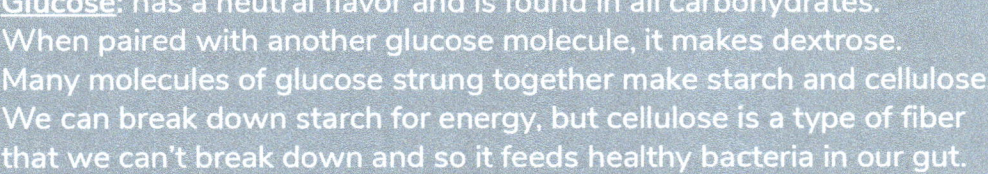
Monosaccharides: Building Blocks of Carbohydrates

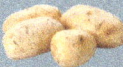

Glucose: has a neutral flavor and is found in all carbohydrates. When paired with another glucose molecule, it makes dextrose. Many molecules of glucose strung together make starch and cellulose. We can break down starch for energy, but cellulose is a type of fiber that we can't break down and so it feeds healthy bacteria in our gut.

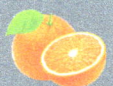

Fructose: gives carbohydrates a sweet flavor. When paired with a glucose molecule, it makes sucrose, commonly known as table sugar. Fructose is converted into glucose in the liver, but in high amounts it's also converted into fat and raises blood triglyceride levels.

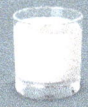
Galactose: is found primarily in dairy and human milk. When paired with a glucose molecule it makes lactose.

Glucose is the primary energy source for the brain and muscles. Balancing glucose levels in the blood is important to make sure enough nutrition is available for the brain and body. The brain uses about 120 g of glucose per day to function optimally. Without enough carbohydrates to break down into glucose, you may feel sluggish, have trouble concentrating, or experience mood swings.

Eating carbohydrates can also allow protein to be used for building blocks rather than being converted into glucose for energy, which means your body will use protein more effectively when you eat enough carbohydrates.

Macronutrient: Carbohydrates

Carbohydrates are found in plant-based foods, which also contain a variety of important nutrients, such as prebiotic fiber, vitamins, minerals, and phytonutrients. For overall health, we encourage you to include whole food sources of carbohydrates when possible and include sweets and refined grains for enjoyment in moderation.

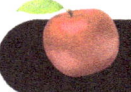

Examples of Fruits

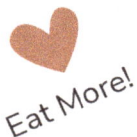
Eat More!

<u>Fresh, frozen, or canned fruit:</u> apples, apricots, bananas, berries, cherries, grapefruits, grapes, kiwis, melons, oranges, pears, peaches, pineapples, pomegranates, nectarines
<u>Dried fruit:</u> raisins, craisins, prunes, dates, apricots, blueberries
<u>Juice:</u> apple, orange, cranberry, pineapple, grapefruit

Eat the whole fruit with the peel intact if possible for more nutrition

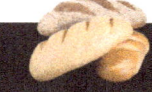

Examples of Minimally-Processed Starches

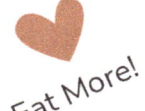
Eat More!

<u>Whole grains:</u> bread, crackers, pasta, brown rice, quinoa, millet, oats, barley, rye, popcorn, corn tortillas
<u>Starchy vegetables:</u> beans, lentils, corn, peas, potatoes, winter squash
<u>Milk products:</u> milk, yogurt (not cheese)

Choose 100% whole grain for more fiber, vitamins, and minerals

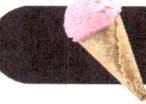

Examples of Refined Sugar & Grains

Be Mindful

<u>Sweets:</u> cookies, ice cream, candy, cake, pastries
<u>Sweeteners:</u> sugar, corn syrup, maple syrup, honey, jelly
<u>Refined grains:</u> white bread, pasta, white rice, flour tortillas, chips, grits
<u>Beverages:</u> soda, juice, drinks sweetened with sugar or high-fructose corn syrup

Nutrient and Supplement Guide for Mental Health

Nutrients for Gut Health

The microorganisms in the intestines, primarily in the colon in the large intestine, make up the gut microbiota. This is an emerging area of research and is greatly impacted by the food we eat. The microbiome includes the microbiota as well as the place in which they live, such as the skin, mouth, or gut. The gut microbiome plays an important role in many areas of health, including mental health by modulating the stress response via the hypothalamic-pituitary-adrenal axis (HPA Axis). The gut microbiota, intestinal cells, and neurons in the enteric nervous system produce some neurotransmitters, including dopamine and up to 90% of serotonin.

The microorganisms included in the gut microbiota vary significantly between people and can change over time. Many factors impact the amount and type of bacteria in the gut, including the environment, genetics, antibiotics, and food we eat.

Microbiome = the microbiota plus the environment in which they live
Microbiota = the microorganisms themselves

The gut microbiome includes the microbiota and the digestive tract, specifically the colon in the large intestine, where they reside. The gut microbiota is made up of microorganisms, primarily bacteria and yeast, but can also include viruses, fungi, parasites, and mold, which normally live in harmony in the intestines. These microorganisms consume prebiotic fiber and produce a number of bioactive substances called postbiotics. A healthy gut microbiome is associated with improved health in a number of areas. There is ongoing research to learn what specific microorganisms may be best for an individual's health.

Prebiotic Fiber

Fiber is a type of carbohydrate that the human body is unable to digest. One of fiber's main roles is to serve as a nutrient for the gut microbiota, which promotes a healthy gut microbiome. Fiber passes through the digestive system and into the large intestine intact, where gut bacteria break it down.

There are two types of fiber: soluble and insoluble. Soluble fiber dissolves in water and helps capture cholesterol for removal. Insoluble fiber provides bulk to food, promotes movement through your digestive tract, and regulates bowel consistency. In general, a high-fiber diet is more beneficial to health than fiber supplements.

Nutrients for Gut Health

Fiber can further be categorized into fermentable and nonfermentable fiber. Fermentable fiber is consumed by bacteria in the gut and is considered a type of prebiotic. Nonfermentable fiber does not directly feed gut bacteria, but can impact the overall gut environment by affecting the bulk and weight of stool and promoting regular bowel movements. Read more about how prebiotic fiber affects mental health on page 192.

Probiotics

Probiotics are live microorganisms, including bacteria and yeast. There are hundreds to thousands of different types that make up the gut microbiota. They are found naturally in fermented foods and are also available in dietary supplements. Eating patterns with a high number of fermented foods are associated with better gut health.

Microorganisms need to be alive to have an impact on gut health. Probiotic supplements that are old or not refrigerated may not contain live specimens and will have little to no impact on gut health. Cooking or freezing probiotic foods may kill the bacteria so they will have less impact on the gut microbiota.

A variety of bacteria and yeast species and doses may have different impacts on types of disease. Using probiotic supplements is an emerging area of research for many health conditions, including mental health. Certain strains of probiotics such as bifidobacterium and lactobacillus may be beneficial for improving symptoms of anxiety and depression. More research is needed to determine the best dose, duration of supplementation, and strains of probiotics to use.

Postbiotics

When the bacteria in the gut consume prebiotic fiber, they produce a wide range of metabolites and byproducts, called postbiotics. Many postbiotics appear to have a positive impact on health. Certain postbiotic compounds, such as short-chain fatty acids, have anti-inflammatory effects. Other gut postbiotics include neurotransmitters themselves, enzymes, or compounds that help to produce and release neurotransmitters and hormones. Additionally, postbiotic supplements may contain inactivated microorganisms and cell components. Because of the limited research available on postbiotic supplements, we recommend focusing on overall gut health rather than individual postbiotics.

Nutrients for Gut Health

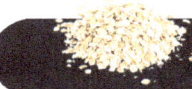 **Examples of Soluble Fiber**

<u>Whole foods:</u> oats, peas, beans, flesh of apples, citrus fruits, carrots, barley; psyllium is often used as an ingredient in high-fiber foods such as tortillas or granola bars

<u>Supplements:</u> psyllium husk; supplements have been shown to help lower LDL cholesterol

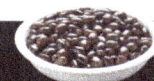 **Examples of Insoluble Fiber**

<u>Whole foods:</u> whole grains, nuts, beans, cauliflower, and the peels of apples and other produce such as zucchini and potatoes

<u>Supplements:</u> cellulose; supplements have not shown the same benefit as fiber included in whole foods

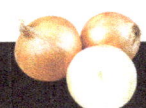 **Examples of Prebiotics**

<u>Whole foods:</u> onions, leeks, asparagus, Jerusalem artichokes, bananas, barley, oats, apples, cocoa, flaxseeds, wheat bran, seaweed, avocado

<u>Supplements:</u> inulin, fructo-oligosaccharides (FOS), galacto-oligosaccharides (GOS), oligofructos (OF), or chicory fiber

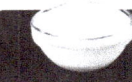 **Examples of Probiotics**

<u>Fermented foods:</u> kefir, kimchi, kombucha, sauerkraut, yogurt, miso, tempeh, natto, some types of pickles, olives, and cheeses

<u>Supplements:</u> refrigerated supplements of probiotics containing bifidobacteria and lactobacillus may be beneficial to support mental health, but more research is needed to determine the appropriate dose and duration of treatment

Nutrients for Gut Health

Prebiotic Fiber

<u>RDA for all fiber:</u> 14 g per 1,000 calories daily

<u>Found in:</u> onions, leeks, asparagus, Jerusalem artichokes, bananas, barley, oats, apples, cocoa, flaxseeds, wheat bran, seaweed, and avocado.

<u>How it works:</u> Most prebiotics are a type of dietary fiber that feed healthy gut bacteria to improve overall microbiome health. The gut microbiome mediates the stress response via the hypothalamic-pituitary-adrenal axis (HPA axis). Intestinal cells, gut bacteria, and neurons in the enteric nervous system produce some types of neurotransmitters, such as dopamine and up to 90% of serotonin, impacting anxiety and depression. This production is impacted by the health of the gut microbiome.

Impacts:
- ✓ Anxiety
- ✓ Depression
- ✓ Inflammation

<u>At risk for deficiency:</u> Most people in the US do not eat enough fiber; at risk groups include those following a low-plant diet, such as a ketogenic or carnivore diet, long-term low-FODMAP diet, or the Standard American Diet with a low intake of vegetables, fruits, whole grains, and/or legumes. People with gastroparesis or other gastrointestinal disorders may not eat enough fiber. Signs of fiber insufficiency include constipation, hemorrhoids, or irritable bowel syndrome. Low fiber consumption is associated with higher cholesterol levels and a higher risk of colorectal cancer, diabetes, and heart disease.

<u>Dietary supplements:</u> Fiber from food is usually best, but prebiotic supplements can promote healthy gut microbiota as well. Look for inulin, fructo-oligosaccharides (FOS), galacto-oligosaccharides (GOS), oligofructos (OF), or chicory fiber in supplements.

- <u>Anxiety, depression, and inflammation</u>: Aim for a total of 3–5 g of prebiotic fiber daily, specifically from FOS and GOS to support gut health. A healthy gut supports neurotransmitter production, the enteric nervous system, and helps manage the HPA stress response. Excess supplementation does not appear to be beneficial.

<u>Toxicity:</u> No upper limit for fiber has been set, but a very high intake of fiber supplements or foods with added fiber may lead to a decreased absorption of nutrients. When introducing fiber, start with a low dose and gradually increase the amount to avoid gas, bloating, and gastrointestinal distress. Drink plenty of water to prevent constipation and bowel obstruction.

Micronutrients *for Mental Health*

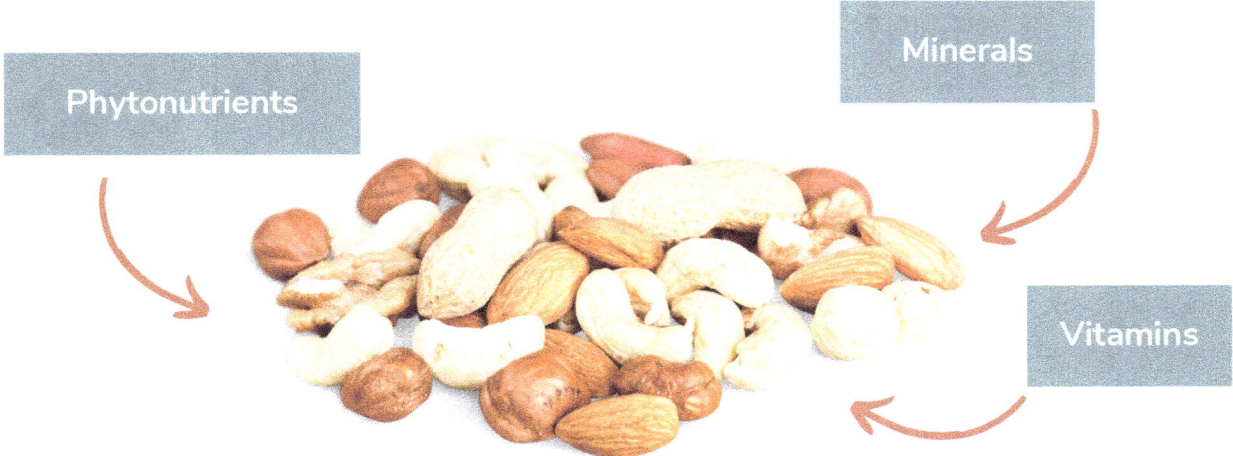

Phytonutrients

Minerals

Vitamins

Micronutrients are naturally-occurring essential nutrients that the body cannot produce, and are needed in very small amounts for a range of physical processes. They include vitamins, minerals, and phytonutrients. Their roles include the production of enzymes that help speed up chemical reactions in the body and hormones for growth and development. Micronutrients help convert food into usable energy for the body by serving as cofactors in metabolic reactions. They also directly impact brain health, regulate mood, and improve cognitive abilities by aiding in brain function, helping the body produce neurotransmitters, and reducing inflammation in the brain.

Overt deficiencies can cause severe health problems, while less-than-optimal intake can often go unnoticed but can lead to reduced energy levels, less mental clarity, and decreased mood. Deficiencies are preventable through eating a diet of diverse foods with supplementation when needed.

 Refer to individual nutrients relevant to you rather than reading this entire section in detail to learn which foods contain different micronutrients, the amount required for health, how they work in mental health, and cautions for toxic levels and possible side effects of supplementation. The "Dietary supplements" section on each page provides evidenced-based information about how much might be helpful for different mental health conditions. Before starting a supplement, talk with your mental health team to determine if, at what dose, and for how long it might be helpful.

Vitamins *for Mental Health*

Vitamin B1 (Thiamine)

<u>RDA:</u> 1.1–1.2 mg daily

<u>Found in:</u> pork, fish, seafood, black beans, acorn squash, fortified or whole grains, beef, yogurt, and sunflower seeds. A significant amount is lost in cooking water as it is leeched from food during boiling.

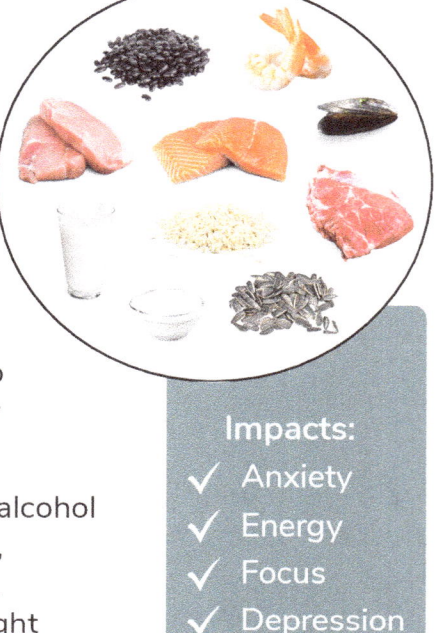

<u>How it works:</u> Thiamine helps make acetylcholine, GABA, and glutamate, which support energy production, mood, focus, and may reduce anxiety. It also helps with the breakdown of food into usable energy by serving as a cofactor in metabolic reactions.

Impacts:
- ✓ Anxiety
- ✓ Energy
- ✓ Focus
- ✓ Depression

<u>At risk for deficiency:</u> Groups at risk include those with alcohol use disorder (especially with low food intake), HIV/AIDs, increased age, diabetes, or a history of bariatric surgery. Signs of early stages of thiamine deficiency include weight loss, low appetite, confusion, short-term memory loss, muscle weakness, and an enlarged heart. Overt deficiency can result in beriberi or Wernicke-Korsakoff syndrome.

<u>Dietary supplements:</u> Thiamine is recommended to take as part of a B-complex vitamin. The most common supplemental forms of thiamine are thiamine mononitrate or thiamine hydrochloride, which are water-soluble and do not require food for absorption. Benfotiamine is converted to thiamine in the body and is fat-soluble, and so it is better absorbed when taken with a meal containing fat. Split large doses of thiamine supplements throughout the day to improve absorption.
- <u>Anxiety, energy, and focus:</u> Sufficient thiamine is needed for neurotransmitter production to manage anxiety, support focus, and to support metabolism for energy production. Taking more than the RDA does not appear beneficial.
- <u>Depression:</u> Taking 300 mg of thiamine daily while starting the SSRI medication fluoxetine may help symptoms improve more quickly in the first 6 weeks of use.

<u>Toxicity:</u> No upper limit has been set. The body reduces absorption of thiamine at high doses. Thiamine is not stored in the body, so if blood levels are high, the body disposes excess in the urine.

Vitamins *for Mental Health*

Vitamin B2 (Riboflavin)

<u>RDA:</u> 1.1–1.3 mg daily

<u>Found in:</u> eggs, organ meats, dairy products, beef, chicken, almonds, mushrooms, salmon, spinach, apples, and fortified grains/cereals. Riboflavin isn't destroyed by heat but can leach into cooking water.

<u>How it works:</u> Riboflavin is used to make flavoproteins, which are found in high amounts in the brain and serve as cofactors in metabolic reactions to produce energy, which is crucial for cognitive function. Riboflavin also helps make serotonin, which may help to reduce anxiety. It may also help maintain the myelin sheath, which can lead to better memory and overall focus. Riboflavin helps reduce inflammation by helping get rid of free radicals, which may reduce the risk of cognitive decline by protecting brain cells from damage.

Impacts:
- ✓ Anxiety
- ✓ Cognitive function
- ✓ Depression
- ✓ Inflammation

<u>At risk for deficiency:</u> Deficiency is rare, but those at risk include pregnant and lactating women, vegan or low-dairy-intake individuals, vegetarian athletes, those with riboflavin transporter deficiency, or those with thyroid insufficiency. Signs of deficiency include skin disorders, edema of the mouth and throat, and hair loss, among other symptoms. Severe, prolonged deficiency can cause anemia and cataracts, which may be irreversible.

<u>Dietary supplements:</u> Riboflavin is recommended to take as part of a B-complex vitamin. It's found in supplements as free riboflavin or riboflavin 5'phosphate, also known as flavin adenine mononucleotide (FMN). FMN is the biologically active form and is slightly better absorbed by the body. However, the difference is not significant and adequate consumption of either form is enough to meet the body's needs.

- <u>Anxiety and depression:</u> Taking 2.1 mg or more of riboflavin daily is associated with reduced risk of anxiety and depression.
- <u>Cognitive function and inflammation:</u> Sufficient riboflavin is necessary to support cognitive function and reduce inflammation, but taking more than the RDA does not appear beneficial.

<u>Toxicity:</u> No upper limit has been set for riboflavin. Riboflavin in amounts of 27 mg or more at one time from food and supplements is poorly absorbed.

Vitamins *for Mental Health*

Vitamin B3 (Niacin)

<u>RDA:</u> 14–16 mg niacin equivalents (NE) daily

<u>Found in:</u> liver, poultry, beef, salmon, tuna, peanuts, potatoes, brown rice, whole grains, and fortified grains. Animal-based sources are more bioavailable than plant-based sources. The amino acid tryptophan can also be converted to niacin in the body.

<u>How it works:</u> Niacin is involved in every aspect of peripheral and brain cell function that are dependent on niacin derived nucleotides, such as nicotinamide adenine dinucleotide (NAD) and NAD phosphate (NADP). These include oxidative reactions, antioxidant protection, DNA metabolism and repair, cellular communication, and converting folate to its active form.

<u>At risk for deficiency:</u> Undernourished groups are most at risk, including those with anorexia, untreated inflammatory bowel disease, alcohol use disorder, AIDS, or liver cirrhosis.
Those deficient in riboflavin, vitamin B6, or iron convert less tryptophan to niacin.

Impacts:
✓ Cognitive function
✓ Inflammation

<u>Dietary supplements:</u> Taking niacin as part of a B-complex vitamin instead of individually can reduce the risk of side effects from high doses. Dietary supplements are available as nicotinic acid and nicotinamide. They are best absorbed when taken on an empty stomach.

- <u>Cognitive function:</u> Taking 17–45 mg* of niacin daily is associated with slowing cognitive decline and a lower risk of developing Alzheimer's disease.
- <u>Inflammation:</u> Consuming adequate niacin at the level of the RDA is necessary to support antioxidant processes in the body. High doses of 500 mg* of niacin or more are used as prescription medication to treat abnormal lipid levels. Take it with a low-fat meal or snack or as directed by your medical team.

<u>Toxicity:</u> The upper limit is set at 35 mg from supplements. Nicotenic acid causes flushing (warm, red skin) on the face, arms, and chest with doses higher than nutritional needs, which is a common side effect when taken as a medication. Niacin is almost completely absorbed by the body even at very high levels of 3,000–4,000 mg. No adverse effects have been found from consuming niacin from food sources.

*Use caution if taking doses higher than the upper limit as this may result in adverse events or side effects. Consult with your medical team when starting or changing a dose of a supplement.

Vitamin B5 (Pantothenic Acid)

<u>RDA:</u> 5 mg daily

<u>Found in:</u> beef, chicken, organ meats, sunflower seeds, tuna, avocado, milk, yogurt, mushrooms, potatoes, egg, peanuts, broccoli, whole grains, and fortified grains. Pantothenic acid is lost during food processing, including boiling, long cooking times, high temperatures, or combining with acidic or alkaline foods.

Impacts:
✓ Anxiety
✓ Cognitive function
✓ Memory
✓ Sleep

<u>How it works:</u> Pantothenic acid is needed for the body to make coenzyme A (CoA) and acyl carrier protein. CoA contributes to the structure and function of brain cells because of its role in making cholesterol, amino acids, phospholipids, and fatty acids. Because of its role in CoA synthesis, pantothenic acid is involved in helping the body make neurotransmitters and steroid hormones, such as cortisol, epinephrine (adrenaline), and testosterone. These are essential to help the body manage stress, necessary for learning, attention, and memory, and can help balance the sleep-wake cycle. Acyl carrier protein plays a role in fatty acid synthesis, which is important for brain structure.

<u>At risk for deficiency:</u> Deficiency is rare except in severe malnutrition.

<u>Dietary supplements:</u> Pantothenic acid is available in supplements as pantethine or calcium pantothenate. Take supplements on an empty stomach. Supplements are often combined with other B-complex vitamins, which are best taken early in the day.

- <u>Anxiety, cognitive function, memory, and sleep:</u> Sufficient pantothenic acid is needed for neurotransmitter and hormone production to manage anxiety, cognitive function, memory, and sleep. It also supports metabolism to provide energy. Taking more than the RDA does not appear beneficial.

<u>Toxicity:</u> No upper limit has been set, as there have been no reports of pantothenic acid toxicity. High doses of 600–900 mg per day of pantothenic acid have been shown to reduce lipid levels.

Vitamins *for Mental Health*

Vitamin B6 (Pyridoxine)

<u>RDA:</u> 1.3–1.7 mg daily

<u>Found in:</u> tuna, salmon, poultry, beef (especially liver), chickpeas, potatoes, banana, fortified grains, winter squash, and nuts. Some losses occur with cooking, mostly in the juices that are released from meat; including these juices retains vitamin B6.

<u>How it works:</u> Vitamin B6 is involved in making neurotransmitters, including dopamine, serotonin, norepinephrine, epinephrine, histamine, and GABA. It also helps maintain normal levels of homocysteine in the blood, which helps promote heart health.

<u>At risk for deficiency:</u> Groups at risk include those with kidney disease, rheumatoid arthritis, untreated celiac or inflammatory bowel disease, or alcohol use disorder. Symptoms of deficiency include dermatitis and a greasy, scaly, red rash, numbness or tingling in hands and feet, sore, red, cracked tongue, and irritability or confusion. Deficiency of vitamin B6 alone is rare; it is often accompanied by deficiency of vitamins B9 and B12.

Impacts:
- ✓ Anxiety
- ✓ Depression
- ✓ Memory
- ✓ Sleep

<u>Dietary supplements:</u> Vitamin B6 is available in oral or sublingual capsules, tablets, or liquid as pyridoxine hydrocholoride or pyridoxal 5' phosphate (PLP). It's recommended to be taken on an empty stomach as part of a B-complex vitamin.

- <u>Anxiety, memory, sleep</u>: Sufficient vitamin B6 is needed for neurotransmitter production to manage anxiety, support memory, and sleep. Taking more than the RDA does not appear beneficial. If restless leg syndrome is affecting sleep, a small study shows that taking 40 mg daily may reduce symptoms to improve sleep.

- <u>Depression</u>: Individuals consuming at least 1.7 mg of vitamin B6 daily seem to have a lower risk of depression than those with a low intake. This association is stronger in females than males. Taking high doses of 25 mg of vitamin B6 daily for 6–12 months may lower the risk of depression in healthy adults who are starting an oral contraceptive containing ethinyl estradiol and levonorgestrel.

<u>Toxicity:</u> The upper limit is set at 100 mg per day. The body absorbs large doses but excretes excess in the urine. Long-term consumption of 1–6 g daily for over 12 months can cause severe sensory nerve damage that can worsen over time.

Vitamins *for Mental Health*

Vitamin B9 (Folate or Folic Acid)

<u>RDA:</u> 400 mcg Dietary Folate Equivalents (DFE) daily

<u>Found in:</u> leafy greens, asparagus, cauliflower, nuts, beans, peanuts, citrus fruit, mushrooms, Brussels sprouts, lentils, okra, broccoli, avocado, fortified/enriched grains, hemp and flax seeds. Cooking with less water helps retain folate.

<u>How it works:</u> Folate helps the body make dopamine, serotonin, norepinephrine, and helps maintain normal homocysteine levels. It's also involved in making DNA and RNA.

<u>At risk for deficiency:</u> Groups at risk include those with low folate intake, alcohol use disorder, or malabsorptive disorders. Pregnant women have increased folate needs. Those with a genetic MTHFR (methylenetetrahydrofolate reductase) polymorphism process folate differently and may have higher folate needs.

Impacts:
✓ Anxiety
✓ Cognitive function
✓ Depression

<u>Dietary supplements:</u> Supplement forms include folic acid and methylfolate (5-MTHF). Those with a genetic MTHFR polymorphism may benefit from taking methylfolate. Folic acid is recommended to be taken on an empty stomach to increase its bioavailability. Folate can be taken alone, as part of a B-complex, prenatal vitamin, or with vitamin B12 to reduce homocysteine levels.

- <u>Anxiety:</u> Sufficient folate is necessary to support neurotransmitter production to manage anxiety, but taking more than the RDA does not appear beneficial.
- <u>Cognitive function:</u> Taking high doses of folic acid supplements alone or with DHA might improve thinking and memory skills in older persons with cognitive impairment. The appropriate dose is unknown; studies have used between 400–15,000 mcg* of folic acid daily, with a duration of 2 months to 2 years.
- <u>Depression:</u> Those with depression who are taking conventional antidepressants may benefit from adding 200–15,000* mcg of folic acid daily for up to 6 months.

<u>Toxicity:</u> The upper limit is set at 1,000 mcg per day from supplements and fortified foods. High folate intake can mask vitamin B12 deficiency, increase the risk of certain cancers, and suppress the immune system. Overdosing folate in pregnancy can cause cognitive delays in children. Doses of 5 mg daily can cause digestive issues and rash; taking 15 mg daily can cause bitter taste, confusion, hyperactivity, impaired judgment, irritability, nausea, and sleep disturbances.

*Use caution if taking doses higher than the upper limit as this may result in adverse events or side effects. Consult with your medical team when starting or changing a dose of a supplement.

Vitamin B12 (Cobalamin)

<u>RDA:</u> 2.4 mcg daily

<u>Found in:</u> foods of animal origin, including meat, dairy products, fish, nutritional yeast, shellfish, poultry, and egg yolks. It's also added to fortified and enriched foods. Heat can destroy up to 50% of vitamin B12 in food.

<u>How it works:</u> Vitamin B12 is required for developing the central nervous system, red blood cell formation, DNA synthesis and function, building new cells, making serotonin, and producing the myelin sheath. It also reduces neuron loss.

<u>At risk for deficiency:</u> Groups at risk include those following a vegan, vegetarian, dairy-free, or gluten-free diet, adults above age 50, those with excessive alcohol consumption, long-term use of metformin or proton pump inhibitor medication, pernicious anemia, history of bariatric surgery, malabsorptive disorders, or pancreatic insufficiency. The symptoms of a deficiency can take several years to appear and may include fatigue, neurological changes, megaloblastic anemia, tongue inflammation and swelling, palpitations, and low counts of red and white blood cells.

Impacts:
- ✓ ADHD
- ✓ Anxiety
- ✓ Depression
- ✓ Memory

<u>Dietary supplements:</u> Groups who are at risk of deficiency due to poor absorption may benefit from high dose supplementation of 100 mcg daily. Vitamin B12 supplements are available as oral or sublingual (under the tongue) cyanocobalamin or methylcobalamin. An intramuscular injection of cyanocobalamin or hydroxycobalamin is best for malabsorptive disorders. Vitamin B12 can be taken as part of a B-complex vitamin or administered individually to correct a deficiency. It's best taken on an empty stomach early in the day; it can be stimulating if taken too late. It has been suggested to impact Alzheimer's disease, but the evidence is unclear as to if there is a benefit.

- <u>ADHD, anxiety, depression, and memory:</u> Sufficient vitamin B12 intake is necessary to support neurotransmitter production for managing anxiety, myelin sheath integrity for reducing ADHD symptoms and improving memory, and producing energy in the body. Sufficient vitamin B12 is associated with lower risk of depression, but high doses above 100 mcg daily do not appear beneficial.

<u>Toxicity:</u> No upper limit has been set. It is not stored in the body and appears to be safe even in very large doses of either oral or intramuscular supplements.

Vitamins *for Mental Health*

Choline

<u>RDA:</u> 425–550 mg daily

<u>Found in:</u> beef, liver, egg yolk, soy, chicken, cod, wheat germ, potatoes, kidney beans, quinoa, milk, yogurt, Brussels sprouts, broccoli, and mushrooms. The liver makes choline, but not enough to meet human needs.

<u>How it works:</u> Choline is a main component of cell membranes, a precursor to acetylcholine, helps with the formation of myelin sheath around nerves, and serves as a source of methyl groups. Choline is not technically a vitamin, but is an essential compound often grouped with vitamin B-complex.

Impacts:
✓ ADHD
✓ Cognitive function
✓ Memory

<u>At risk for deficiency:</u> Overt deficiency is rare; groups at risk include pregnant women or those eating a low animal protein diet. Chronic deficiency can cause nonalcoholic fatty liver disease, muscle, or liver damage. In pregnancy, deficiency is associated with higher risk of neural tube defects. Folate deficiency increases choline needs.

<u>Dietary supplements:</u> The supplement forms choline alfoscerate, aka alpha-GPC or alpha-glycerophosphocholine, and citicoline seem to have the best cognitive outcomes. Alpha-GPC is a precursor to acetylcholine and crosses the blood-brain barrier. Citicoline shows promise in dementia and Alzheimer's disease treatment and may also increase brain dopamine levels.

- <u>ADHD:</u> Sufficient choline intake supports myelin sheath integrity and production of acetylcholine, improving sensory tolerance and executive function in ADHD. Taking more than the RDA does not appear beneficial.
- <u>Cognitive function:</u> Moderate intake of dietary choline is associated with a lower risk of low cognitive function. Taking choline in excess of the RDA does not appear beneficial. In pregnancy, taking 550–1,000 mg daily of choline from supplements in addition to diet may improve cognitive outcomes in children.
- <u>Memory:</u> Taking 2,000 mg of choline for 2 weeks may improve memory in individuals on long-term total parenteral nutrition.

<u>Toxicity:</u> The upper limit is set at 3,500 mg daily. Symptoms of choline toxicity include fishy body odor, vomiting, excessive sweating and salivation, low blood pressure, and liver toxicity. Choline has no known interactions with medications.

Vitamins *for Mental Health*

Vitamin C (Ascorbic Acid)

<u>RDA:</u> 75–90 mg daily

<u>Found in:</u> citrus fruits, strawberries, bell peppers, kiwi, parsley, spaghetti squash, cantaloupe, broccoli, Brussels sprouts, tomatoes, onions, coconut milk, blueberries, and potatoes. Heating, long food storage times, or cooking in water reduce vitamin C content.

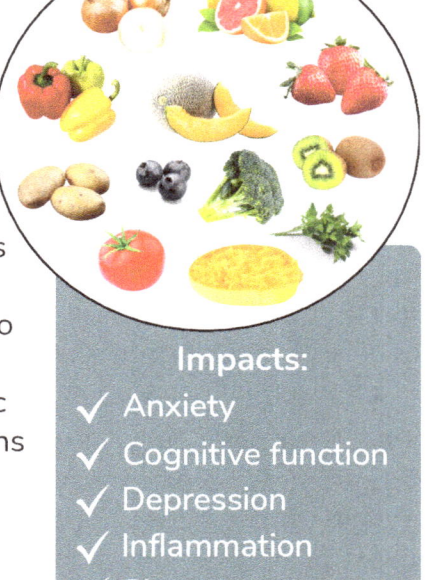

<u>How it works:</u> Vitamin C helps neurons mature and helps form the myelin sheath. It acts as an antioxidant and regenerates other antioxidants, such as vitamin E. It's also needed to make some neurotransmitters and aids in glutamatergic, dopaminergic, cholinergic, and GABAergic transmission and related behaviors. The brain and neurons maintain a higher level of vitamin C than the fluid that surrounds them, which aids in optimal cell processing.

Impacts:
- ✓ Anxiety
- ✓ Cognitive function
- ✓ Depression
- ✓ Inflammation
- ✓ Sleep

<u>At risk for deficiency:</u> Groups at risk include those with limited food variety for many weeks, severe intestinal malabsorption, some types of cancer, and end-stage renal disease. People who smoke need 35 mg additional vitamin C daily. Overt deficiency results in scurvy, with symptoms of fatigue, malaise, and gum inflammation. Scurvy increases infection risk, impairs wound healing, and weakens connective tissues.

<u>Dietary supplements:</u> Supplements are available in several forms, but ascorbic acid is the preferred type due to cost and relatively similar absorption and bioavailability. Take vitamin C with food for best absorption.

- <u>Anxiety and depression</u>: A small study showed that taking high doses of 250–500 mg of vitamin C with meals 2–3 times per day may help reduce symptoms of anxiety and depression.
- <u>Cognitive function, inflammation and sleep:</u> Sufficient vitamin C is associated with a lower risk of developing Alzheimer's disease. It acts as an antioxidant to reduce inflammation. Its role in neurotransmitter production provides a calming effect for sleep. Taking more than RDA does not appear beneficial.

<u>Toxicity:</u> The upper limit is set at 2,000 mg daily. High doses of oral vitamin C can cause gastrointestinal distress. Avoid chronic high doses in renal disease and hereditary hemochromatosis.

Vitamins *for Mental Health*

Vitamin D (Calciferol)

<u>RDA:</u> 15–20 mcg (600–800 IU) daily

<u>Found in:</u> fatty fish, egg yolks, fortified dairy or dairy alternatives, beef liver, and mushrooms. Vitamin D is also made by the skin when it's exposed to UV light from sunshine. Very long cooking times can degrade vitamin D in foods.

<u>How it works:</u> Vitamin D can be activated by an enzyme in the brain, especially in neurons in the amygdala and glial cells in the hypothalamus. This local activation indicates vitamin D's importance for brain health. Vitamin D plays many other roles in the body, including reducing inflammation, modulating cell growth, immune function, and glucose metabolism.

Impacts:

✓ ADHD

✓ Anxiety

✓ Cognitive function

✓ Depression

<u>At risk for deficiency:</u> Groups at risk include those following a vegan, vegetarian, dairy-free, gluten-free, or fish-free diet, breastfed infants, older adults, those with limited sun exposure, living north of 37° latitude (which runs just south of San Francisco, California across to just south of Richmond, Virginia), people with dark skin, those with fat malabsorption, obesity, or history of gastric bypass surgery. Severe deficiency can cause hypocalcemia and secondary hyperparathyroidism, causing muscle weakness, cramps, fatigue, and depression. Long-term deficiency can cause osteomalacia in adults and rickets in children. Vitamin D insufficiency is more mild but very common. Low vitamin D levels are associated with depression, cardiovascular disease, type 2 diabetes, metabolic syndrome, some types of cancer, and some types of autoimmune diseases, such as rheumatoid arthritis and inflammatory bowel disease.

<u>Dietary supplements:</u> Vitamin D3 (cholecalciferol), the active form of the vitamin, is more effective in raising serum levels than vitamin D2 (ergocalciferol). To correct a deficiency, your healthcare provider may prescribe a high weekly dose of vitamin D for up to several months. Once blood levels return to normal it's common to return to a lower daily maintenance dose of vitamin D.

Vitamin D (Calciferol) (continued)

<u>Dietary supplements (continued):</u> Vegan supplements are available from lichen. Take this fat-soluble vitamin with food containing fat for best absorption.

- <u>ADHD:</u> Clinical practice guidelines* weakly recommend taking 1,500–4,000 IU** of vitamin D daily for adjunctive use in children with ADHD, especially those with insufficient intake or skin exposure to sunlight.
- <u>Anxiety:</u> Taking 50,000 IU** of vitamin D once weekly for 3 months in addition to medication may moderately reduce symptoms for adults with generalized anxiety disorder compared to using medication alone.
- <u>Cognitive function:</u> Healthy adults with low vitamin D levels tend to have worse cognitive performance, more cognitive decline, and a higher risk of developing Alzheimer's disease compared to healthy adults with high vitamin D levels. In the absence of a deficiency, taking more vitamin D than the RDA does not appear beneficial to cognitive function.
- <u>Depression:</u> Clinical practice guidelines* weakly recommend taking 1,500–4,000 IU** of vitamin D daily for adjunctive or monotherapy in patients with depression, especially those with insufficient intake or inadequate skin exposure to sunlight. Research results have been mixed with a high amount of variability between studies. The most potential benefit appears to be seen in adults with depression who take a one-time high dose of 150,000–500,000 IU** of vitamin D3 (cholecalciferol). A single high dose of 100,000 IU** of vitamin D2 (ergocalciferol) may improve symptoms of seasonal affective disorder (SAD). Taking vitamin D supplements does not appear to reduce the risk of developing depression.

<u>Toxicity:</u> The upper limit is set at 100 mcg (4,000 IU) daily, although a person with a deficiency may take an initial higher dose daily or weekly under medical supervision until blood levels recover, then they can return to a maintenance dose. Toxicity from food and supplements causing high blood levels of vitamin D can cause high blood calcium levels, renal failure, calcification of soft tissues, cardiac arrhythmias and in extreme cases, death. Extensive time in tanning beds can cause elevated serum levels.

*Clinical practice guidelines come from the World Federation of Societies of Biological Psychiatry (WFSBP) and the Canadian Network for Mood and Anxiety Treatments (CANMAT).

**Use caution if taking doses higher than the upper limit as this may result in adverse events or side effects. Consult with your medical team when starting or changing a dose of a supplement.

Vitamins *for Mental Health*

Vitamin E (Alpha-Tocopherol)

<u>RDA:</u> 15 mg daily

<u>Found in:</u> nuts, sunflower seeds, vegetable oils, leafy greens, wheat germ, pumpkin, red bell pepper, broccoli, and fortified grains. Vitamin E is often added to food as a preservative due to its antioxidant effects.

<u>How it works:</u> Vitamin E is located mainly in cell membranes, where it enhances stability to protect cells from free radicals. It reduces oxidative damage during fat metabolism. Vitamin E prevents the production of free radicals that damage cells, which may prevent damage to neurons that leads to cognitive decline and neurodegenerative diseases.

<u>At risk for deficiency:</u> Overt deficiency is rare especially in adults. Groups at risk include those with fat malabsorption disorders, untreated Crohn's disease, cystic fibrosis, bariatric surgery, food insecurity, a very low-fat diet, or rare genetic disorders. Deficiency can cause hemolytic anemia, a condition where red blood cells rupture.

Impacts:
- ✓ Anxiety
- ✓ Inflammation
- ✓ Cognitive function
- ✓ Sleep

<u>Dietary supplements:</u> Naturally-occurring vitamin E is labeled as D-alpha-tocopherol and is twice as potent as its synthetic counterpart, labeled DL-alpha-tocopherol. Other forms of vitamin E are not as biologically active. Supplements can be taken at any time of day and should be taken with food containing fat for best absorption. Vitamin E may need to be taken separately from antidepressant and antipsychotic medication as it can interfere with their absorption.

- <u>Anxiety, cognitive function, and sleep</u>: Sufficient Vitamin E is necessary to support cell structure and for antioxidant activity to maintain brain health. It has been shown to slow cognitive decline but not the onset of Alzheimer's disease. Taking more vitamin E than the RDA does not appear to be beneficial.
- <u>Inflammation:</u> Vitamin E is naturally anti-inflammatory and has the ability to reduce oxidative damage. Taking more than the RDA does not appear beneficial.

<u>Toxicity:</u> The upper limit is set at 1,000 mg daily. High doses of supplemental vitamin E may increase the risk of hemorrhagic stroke and prostate cancer. No adverse effects have been found from consuming vitamin E from food.

Vitamins *for Mental Health*

Vitamin K (Phylloquinone or Menaquinone)

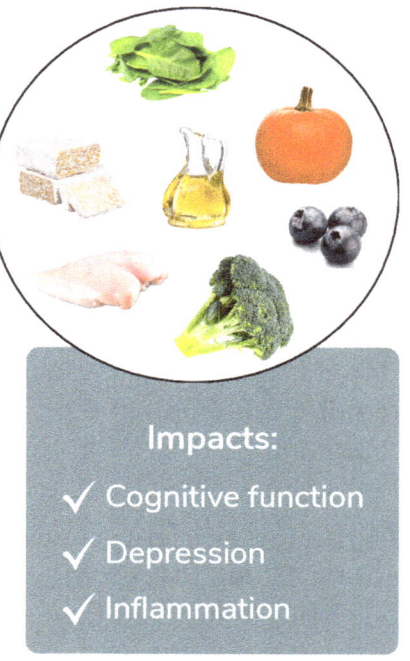

AI*: 90–120 mcg daily

<u>Found in:</u> leafy greens, broccoli, fermented soy (natto, tempeh), pumpkin, blueberries, vegetable oils, and chicken. Bacteria in the gut also produce vitamin K in healthy adults.

<u>How it works:</u> Vitamin K helps make key fats that are needed for brain cell growth and the formation of the myelin sheath. It activates special proteins that reduce brain inflammation, protects memory-related neurons, and may help prevent brain cell damage.

<u>At risk for deficiency:</u> Groups at risk include those with a history of bariatric surgery, malabsorptive disorders, or babies not given vitamin K at birth. The main symptom of deficiency is bleeding, which can be life-threatening in newborns and infants. Deficiency can also weaken bones.

Impacts:

✓ Cognitive function

✓ Depression

✓ Inflammation

<u>Dietary supplements:</u> Vitamin K1 supplements are available as phylloquinone or phytonadione. Vitamin K2 is available as MK-4 or MK-7; all types seem to be similar in bioavailability. Take supplements with food containing fat for best absorption. Excessive vitamin A supplementation may interfere with vitamin K absorption.

- **<u>Cognitive function:</u>** Adults with metabolic syndrome and cognitive impairment who eat more dietary vitamin K seem to have a slower rate of cognitive decline than those who eat very little. Higher vitamin K levels in the brain are associated with a lower neurofibrillary tangle burden, a hallmark of Alzheimer's disease.
- **<u>Depression:</u>** Population research shows that eating more vitamin K (as much as 232 mcg daily from the diet) is associated with a lower likelihood of having depressive symptoms. Using vitamin K supplements to prevent or treat clinical depression has not been studied.
- **<u>Inflammation:</u>** Adequate intake of vitamin K is necessary for anti-inflammatory functions but taking more than the RDA does not appear to be beneficial.

<u>Toxicity:</u> No upper limit has been established because there have been no adverse effects observed from consuming high doses from food or supplements. Vitamin K is rapidly metabolized and excreted; small amounts circulate in the blood.

*AI (Adequate Intake) listed here because an RDA has not been established.

Minerals *for Mental Health*

Calcium

<u>RDA:</u> 1,000–1,200 mg daily

<u>Found in:</u> dairy products, chia seeds, broccoli, green leafy vegetables, beans, lentils, and fortified non-dairy milk.

<u>How it works:</u> Calcium helps control vasoconstriction and vasodilation (opening and closing of blood vessels) and nerve impulse transmission. Calcium activity is abnormal in mood disorders and mood-stabilizing treatments may regulate calcium ion hyperactivity.

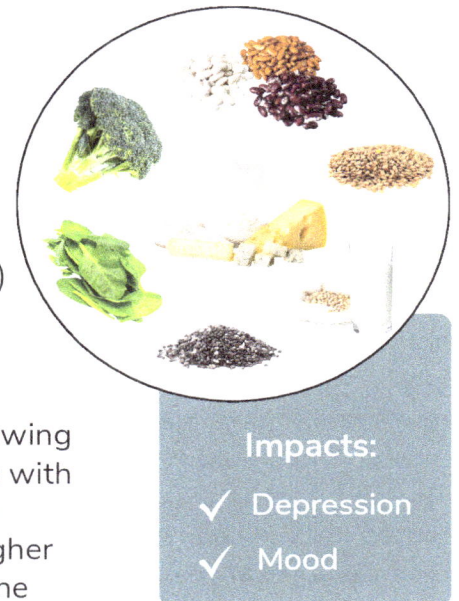

Impacts:

✓ Depression

✓ Mood

<u>At risk for deficiency:</u> Groups at risk include those following dairy-free, vegan, vegetarian, or gluten-free diet, those with undiagnosed or untreated celiac disease, or those with vitamin D deficiency. Postmenopausal women have higher calcium needs. Calcium deficiency leads to reduced bone strength and osteoporosis. Low blood calcium levels are usually related to a secondary deficiency or impaired hormone production and can increase the risk of symptoms of depression and bipolar disorder.

<u>Dietary supplements:</u> Look for the "elemental calcium" amount on a supplement label, which indicates the amount of calcium in the supplement rather than the weight of the compound. Calcium carbonate is usually the best value and is well-tolerated; it's best taken with food. Calcium citrate is more readily absorbed, but is often more expensive; take calcium citrate on an empty stomach. All calcium supplements should be taken several hours apart from iron or zinc supplements, tetracycline antibiotics, or levothyroxine. The body reduces the absorption of calcium after intake of 500 mg. For maximum absorption, spread calcium intake throughout the day, taking no more than 500 mg calcium from combined food and supplements at one time.

- **Depression and mood:** Adequate calcium intake is necessary for nerve impulse transmission and blood vessel functions. In pregnancy and postpartum, early research shows that taking 2,000 mg of calcium daily beginning at 11–21 weeks gestation may reduce depression at 12 weeks postpartum.

<u>Toxicity:</u> The upper limit is set at 2,500 mg from both food and supplements. High calcium intake increases the risk of kidney stones, prostate cancer, constipation, heart problems, and can decrease absorption of minerals like iron and zinc.

Minerals *for Mental Health*

Iron

<u>RDA:</u> 8 mg daily for men and non-menstruating people; 18 mg daily for menstruating people

<u>Found in:</u> Heme iron is the most bioavailable form; it's found in red meat, fish, oysters, clams, and poultry. Nonheme iron is less bioavailable and is found in beans, lentils, leafy greens, nuts, seeds, dried fruit, tofu, whole or enriched grains, coconut milk, and hemp seeds. Eating a source of vitamin C with nonheme iron increases absorption.

<u>How it works:</u> Iron supports brain development, including brain myelination, and is essential for several neurotransmitters, such as serotonin, norepinephrine, epinephrine, and dopamine.

<u>At risk for deficiency:</u> Groups at risk include those following a gluten-free or low-meat-intake diet, those with malabsorptive disorders, parasites, surgery, blood loss or donation, or cancer.

<u>Dietary supplements:</u> Ferrous iron is more bioavailable than ferric iron. The dose on the Supplement Facts panel reflects elemental iron. Take iron with food to reduce digestive side effects, but separately from calcium, coffee, tea, high-fiber foods, or foods with phytates (grains, legumes, or nuts) that can inhibit absorption. Store supplements away from children and pets to avoid overdose.

Impacts:
- ✓ ADHD
- ✓ Depression
- ✓ Cognitive function
- ✓ Sleep

- <u>ADHD and cognitive function:</u> Correcting a deficiency can improve focus, verbal learning, and memory. In the absence of a deficiency it does not seem beneficial.
- <u>Depression:</u> Adequate iron levels support energy, sleep, and neurotransmitter production. Taking iron in the absence of a deficiency does not seem beneficial.
- <u>Sleep:</u> Taking 325 mg* of ferrous sulfate twice daily plus 100 mg of vitamin C twice daily for 12 weeks may reduce symptoms of restless leg syndrome in those with low-normal serum ferritin, but should be used with caution due to the risk of toxicity. The American Academy of Neurology provides additional specific dose recommendations for treating restless leg syndrome.

<u>Toxicity:</u> The upper limit is set at 45 mg daily. Taking 25 mg of iron or more can reduce zinc absorption and cause digestive side effects. Extremely high doses (above 130 mg) can cause severe digestive side effects and bleeding, leading to death. Those with hereditary hemochromatosis need treatment to prevent iron toxicity.

*Use caution if taking doses higher than the upper limit as this may result in adverse events or side effects. Consult with your medical team when starting or changing a dose of a supplement.

Minerals *for Mental Health*

Magnesium

<u>RDA:</u> 310–420 mg daily

<u>Found in:</u> leafy greens, nuts, beans, lentils, avocados, fish, shrimp, seeds, soy, coffee, tea, cocoa, oats, barley, peanut butter, dairy, blackstrap molasses, corn, peas, carrots, brown rice, parsley, and coconut milk. Magnesium can be lost in the process of boiling food.

<u>How it works:</u> Magnesium elicits a calming effect in two ways, by blocking NMDA receptors, which reduces neuron excitability, and working as a GABA agonist and binding to GABA receptors. Magnesium also regulates the synthesis and release of several neurotransmitters and plays an important role in nerve conduction through active transport of ions like potassium and calcium. It serves as a cofactor for many different biochemical reactions in the body, including energy production and DNA synthesis, among others. In the pancreas, magnesium plays a role in insulin production.

Impacts:
- ✓ ADHD
- ✓ Anxiety
- ✓ Depression
- ✓ Sleep

<u>At risk for deficiency:</u> Groups at risk include those following a dairy-free or Standard American Diet, those with untreated celiac or inflammatory bowel disease, resection of the small intestine, type 2 diabetes, insulin resistance, alcohol use disorder, or older adults. Some ADHD medications can deplete magnesium. Over half of adults in the US consume less than the recommended amount of magnesium. Insufficient magnesium intake is more common than overt deficiency. Low intake of magnesium is associated with increased risk of obesity, diabetes, cardiovascular disease, metabolic syndrome, and osteoporosis. Supplemental magnesium may be beneficial because it is correcting a deficiency, rather than high doses of magnesium itself providing benefit.

<u>Dietary supplements:</u> To enhance absorption, take magnesium with vitamin D, lactose (found in dairy milk), or fructose (found in table sugar and fruit). Avoid taking supplements at the same time as consuming foods with phytate (seeds, nuts, legumes, whole grains, or green leafy vegetables), fiber, calcium, very high doses of zinc, or excessive unabsorbed fatty acids that can inhibit absorption.

Magnesium (continued)

Dietary supplements (continued): For digestive uses, take supplements with food and consider taking them earlier in the day. For sleep or relaxation, take supplements before bed for a potential calming effect and best absorption overnight. There are multiple types of magnesium that have different absorption, side effects, and benefits. The information on page 211 reviews common forms of magnesium to help you choose the best type for you based on your needs.

- **ADHD:** Lower levels of magnesium in blood and hair may be associated with a higher rate of ADHD. Taking 6 mg of magnesium per kg body weight (equal to 490 mg** for a 180 lb person) for 6 months may improve hyperactivity and emotional aspects of ADHD, but results from two small clinical trials in children are mixed. It may be beneficial to combine with vitamin D supplementation.
- **Anxiety and depression:** Sufficient magnesium is needed for neurotransmitter production and GABA-regulating benefits to manage anxiety. Early-stage research shows that taking 2 g of magnesium chloride daily for 6 weeks may reduce symptoms of anxiety and depression, but the study did not have a control group and other findings show mixed results. Clinical practice guidelines* currently state that taking magnesium in doses of 100–400 mg** daily is not recommended for adjunctive or monotherapy use in patients with depression.
- **Sleep:** Taking 500–700 mg** of magnesium before bed may reduce the time to fall asleep, but does not necessarily improve sleep quality. Studies used magnesium oxide and magnesium citrate, but other forms may be beneficial with fewer digestive side effects. It may be beneficial to combine magnesium with other ingredients such as L-theanine, tart cherry juice, and/or and melatonin.

Toxicity: The upper limit is set at 350 mg for magnesium from supplements and medication, due to side effects including diarrhea, nausea, and abdominal cramping. Extremely high doses have caused fatalities by causing loss of reflexes and respiratory depression. Toxicity risk increases with impaired renal function. There is not an upper limit set for food sources of magnesium because it would be difficult to eat enough food to cause toxicity and the kidneys excrete excess amounts.

*Clinical practice guidelines come from the World Federation of Societies of Biological Psychiatry (WFSBP) and the Canadian Network for Mood and Anxiety Treatments (CANMAT).

**Use caution if taking doses higher than the upper limit as this may result in adverse events or side effects. Consult with your medical team when starting or changing a dose of a supplement.

Minerals *for Mental Health*

Magnesium citrate: is a commonly used form. It dissolves in water, is easily absorbed, inexpensive, and has a high bioavailability. It's used to replenish low magnesium levels and to treat constipation at higher doses.

Magnesium chloride: dissolves in water and is well-absorbed. It's used orally to replenish low magnesium levels and may decrease symptoms of anxiety and depression. It's used topically in skin creams to relieve muscle soreness.

Magnesium glycinate: dissolves in water and is easily absorbed. Magnesium glycinate may have more calming and antidepressant effects than other forms of magnesium. It may help improve sleep and reduce anxiety, depression, and stress. Glycine has antioxidant properties and also may help with sleep and mental health.

Magnesium lactate: dissolves in water, is easily absorbed, and has fewer digestive side effects. It may help with symptoms of stress and anxiety. Magnesium lactate is also used as a food additive as a preservative and flavoring agent.

Magnesium L-threonate: is easily absorbed and has been shown to increase magnesium concentrations in brain cells in animal models. It may help with learning, memory, managing depression, Alzheimer's disease, and memory loss.

Magnesium malate: is well-absorbed as a dietary supplement and is used to replenish magnesium levels. It has fewer digestive and laxative effects. It may help with fibromyalgia and chronic fatigue syndrome.

Magnesium oxide: is poorly absorbed. It has laxative effects and is most often used to treat heartburn, indigestion, and constipation. It may help with symptoms of depression and reduce the time to fall asleep.

Magnesium taurate: is generally well-tolerated with fewer side effects than other magnesium forms. It may promote healthy blood pressure and blood glucose levels, lower anxiety, and help with recovery after traumatic brain injuries.

Minerals *for Mental Health*

Selenium

<u>RDA:</u> 55 mcg daily

<u>Found in:</u> Brazil nuts, fish, shrimp, poultry, pork, beef, organ meats, sunflower seeds, grains, dairy, eggs, oats, brown rice, mushrooms, and lentils.

<u>How it works:</u> Selenium is a component of selenoproteins, which help reduce oxidative stress and inflammatory processes, thus helping protect against neurodegenerative diseases. It may play a role in healthy brain function; low blood levels are associated with Alzheimer's disease and lower cognitive scores.

Impacts:

✓ Anxiety

✓ Cognitive function

✓ Depression

✓ Inflammation

<u>At risk for deficiency:</u> Groups at risk include those following vegetarian or vegan diets, living in selenium-deficient regions, on long-term hemodialysis, or with HIV.
Overt deficiency is rare but has been seen in parts of China where selenium levels in the soil are very low.
Selenium deficiency could worsen iodine deficiency.

<u>Dietary supplements:</u> Available supplement forms include selenomethionine, selenium-enriched yeast, selenite, and selenate, which are all well-absorbed. Take selenium with vitamin E for increased antioxidant activity.

- <u>Anxiety, depression, inflammation:</u> Sufficient selenium is needed for reducing oxidative stress to maintain brain health. Taking more than the RDA does not appear beneficial.
- <u>Cognitive function:</u> Lower levels of selenium are associated with greater risk of poor cognitive scores. Taking 200 mcg of selenium for Alzheimer's disease and dementia has shown mixed results. Instead, focus on consuming the RDA.

<u>Toxicity:</u> The upper limit is set at 400 mcg. Selenium toxicity (selenosis) can occur from supplements and dietary sources, such as consuming Brazil nuts regularly. Brazil nuts contain about 90 mcg of selenium, so limit intake to less than 5 per day, eaten only occasionally. Up to 90% of selenium is absorbed, regardless of the body's selenium status. Symptoms of excess intake include garlic odor on the breath and metallic taste in the mouth. Chronic selenosis symptoms include hair loss, brittle nails, skin rash, nausea, diarrhea, fatigue, irritability, and nervous system abnormalities.

Minerals *for Mental Health*

Zinc

<u>RDA:</u> 8–11 mg daily

<u>Found in:</u> oysters, crab, shrimp, beef, pumpkin seeds, pork, turkey, cheese, lentils, tofu, wheat germ, hemp seeds, and fortified grains. Phytates in some plants (seeds, nuts, legumes, whole grains) bind zinc and reduce absorption. Fermenting foods or soaking beans, grains, and seeds increases zinc's bioavailability.

<u>How it works:</u> Zinc binds to one of the NMDA subreceptors, which dampens the NMDA receptor. This reduces overactive glutamate, increasing GABA in the brain. Zinc is also involved in the serotonergic system, increases levels of BDNF in the areas of the brain that control emotions, and is involved in DNA synthesis.

<u>At risk for deficiency:</u> Groups at risk include those following a vegan, vegetarian, or gluten-free diet, those with bariatric surgery, newly diagnosed or untreated celiac disease, ulcerative colitis, or Crohn's disease, pregnant or lactating people, those with sickle cell disease, alcohol use disorder, or HIV.

Impacts:
- ✓ Anxiety
- ✓ Cognitive function
- ✓ Depression

<u>Dietary supplements:</u> Zinc citrate and zinc gluconate are slightly better absorbed than zinc oxide. Supplements are best absorbed on an empty stomach, but taking them with a small meal (without calcium, iron, or phytates) can help reduce nausea.

- <u>Anxiety:</u> Sufficient zinc is needed for the sertonergic system and to regulate GABA, which helps manage anxiety with its calming effect. Taking more zinc than the RDA does not appear beneficial.
- <u>Cognitive function:</u> Early-stage research shows that taking 30 mg of zinc daily for 12 weeks may improve cognitive function and executive processing.
- <u>Depression:</u> Oral zinc seems to be beneficial when used in combination with antidepressant treatments. Dosing varies between 7–25 mg daily for 12 weeks.

<u>Toxicity:</u> The upper limit is set at 40 mg daily. Zinc from food is unlikely to cause toxicity. Short-term high zinc intake can cause nausea, dizziness, headaches, gastric distress, vomiting, and loss of appetite. Chronic high intake of more than 50 mg daily can reduce copper absorption, reduce immune function, and lower HDL cholesterol. Some denture adhesive creams contain zinc and long-term use can lead to toxicity.

Phytonutrients *for Mental Health*

Phytonutrients, also called phytochemicals, are compounds that plants produce as a defense system. There are over 10,000 different types of phytonutrients that have a wide range of benefits in humans. They are found in fruits, vegetables, tea, coffee, herbs, and spices and are often referred to by their individual names, such as polyphenols or flavonoids. Phytonutrients serve many functions; they are precursors to some vitamins, provide powerful anti-inflammatory and antioxidative properties, and prevent damage to DNA, among many other effects.

 Although phytonutrients are not well-studied in areas of mental health, reducing inflammation and oxidation generally improves memory and cognition. There is not a way to specifically measure the levels of phytonutrients in the body, but people at risk for insufficient intake include those eating a Standard American Diet or any eating pattern that is low in whole plant foods, especially colorful fruits and vegetables.

Eating patterns that are high in phytonutrients are usually rich in fruits and vegetables, which have many of the micronutrients necessary for optimal physical and mental health. It's not clear if standalone phytonutrient supplements are as effective as those found in food. There is no danger of eating too many phytonutrients from food, but very high doses of dietary supplements can cause various problems and potential medication interactions. We are highlighting a few of the most well-studied phytonutrients, but this is not an exhaustive list.

Common Phytonutrients

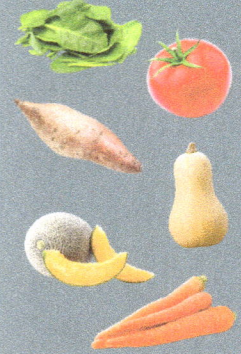

Beta-Carotene: is found in orange, yellow, and green fruits and vegetables, such as carrots, spinach, lettuce, tomatoes, sweet potatoes, broccoli, cantaloupe, and winter squash. The body converts beta-carotene to vitamin A. Eating patterns high in beta-carotene are associated with a lower risk of depression. It works as an antioxidant and may reduce levels of the inflammatory cytokines interleukin-6 (IL-6) and tumor necrosis factor-alpha (TNF-alpha), which are increased in depression.

Phytonutrients *for Mental Health*

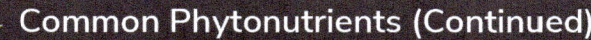

Common Phytonutrients (Continued)

<u>Lycopene:</u> is a powerful antioxidant found in red and orange fruits and vegetables, including tomatoes, red peppers, carrots, beets, watermelon, and apricots. Cooking tomatoes and consuming these foods with a source of fat increases the bioavailability. Diets rich in lycopene are associated with a lower risk of depression and improved sleep, but lycopene supplements have shown mixed results.

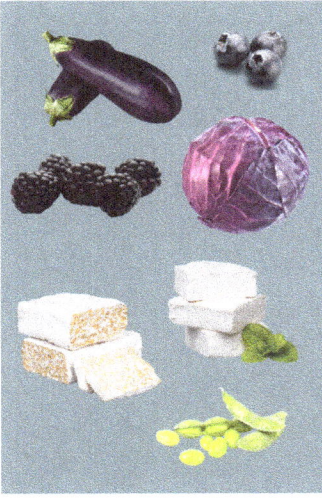

<u>Flavonoids:</u> have six subcategories. The two most well-known are anthocyanins in blue and purple foods such as blueberries, blackberries, eggplant, or purple cabbage; and isoflavones, found in soy. Anthocyanins have antioxidant effects, likely leading to improved brain function, reduced inflammation, and promotion of heart health. A higher intake of dietary anthocyanins has been associated with a lower risk of depression, prevention or delay of the progression of Parkinson's disease, and improved sleep. Isoflavones in soy may improve sleep and diets high in soy are associated with a reduced risk of depression.

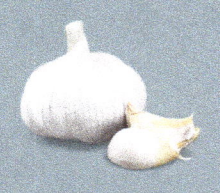

<u>Allicin:</u> is found in garlic and activated when a bulb is crushed. Among its many other health benefits, it works as an antioxidant, maintains levels of neurotransmitters, and reduces inflammatory cytokines, all of which may protect cognitive function. Allicin protects against neuroinflammation and is associated with a lower risk of Alzheimer's disease. Effective therapeutic doses of allicin supplements have not been established.

Phytonutrients *for Mental Health*

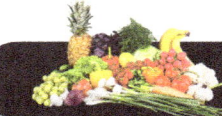

Common Phytonutrients (Continued)

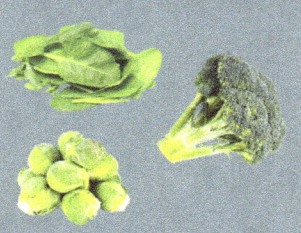

<u>Chlorophyll:</u> is found in green leafy vegetables, broccoli, and Brussels sprouts. It's broken down in processing and cooking, so minimally-processed or raw vegetables are a better source. It works as an antioxidant to reduce oxidative damage and may help preserve neurons that could prevent or slow the progression of neurodegenerative diseases.

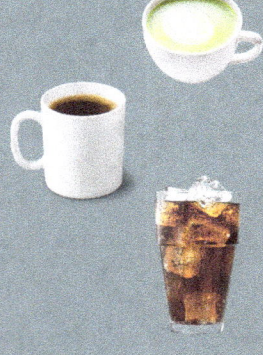

<u>Caffeine:</u> is a natural stimulant found in coffee, tea, cacao, and yerba mate leaves. It can also be added to energy drinks, supplements, and beverages. Moderate consumption of 3–4 cups of coffee (300–400 mg) or less boosts alertness, energy, and may reduce the risk of Alzheimer's and Parkinson's diseases. Lower doses may reduce the risk of depression by stimulating dopamine production. The FDA considers 400 mg daily to be safe; toxic effects including seizures can occur with rapid ingestion of 1200 mg. Consuming too much caffeine can cause increased heart rate, heart palpitations, high blood pressure, sleep disruptions, anxiety, and gastrointestinal distress. Decaffeinated products contain a small amount of caffeine; to avoid it completely, look for "caffeine-free" on the label.

Approximate Caffeine Amounts in Common Beverages

- 8 oz brewed coffee: 96 mg
- 1 oz espresso: 63 mg
- 8 oz black tea: 48 mg
- 8 oz decaf tea or coffee: 2–10 mg
- 8 oz green tea: 29 mg
- 8 oz yerba mate: 80 mg

- 1 oz chocolate bar: 12 mg
- 8 oz soda: 35 mg
  - 12 oz soda: 52 mg
- 8 oz energy drink: 79 mg
- 2 oz energy shot: 200 mg
- Supplements: 100–200 mg per dose

Additional Dietary Supplements *for Mental Health*

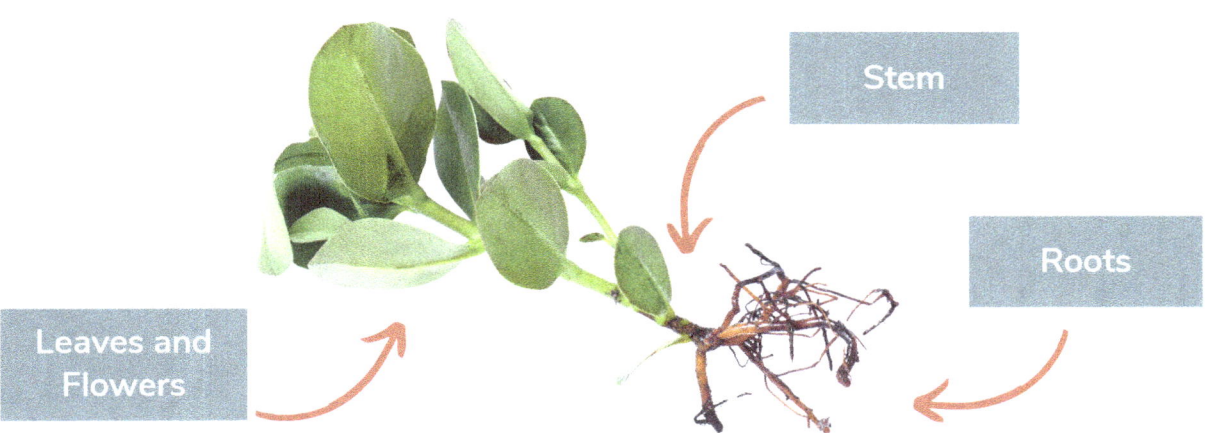

Plants and their extracts have been used for thousands of years in many different cultures for their medicinal properties. Many modern pharmaceutical medications were originally derived from plants. Different plant parts may be used for their therapeutic effect, including leaves, stems, roots, flowers, or seeds. These can be used to make teas, tinctures, extracts, tablets, or capsules.

The quality of research to support health claims of herbal and other dietary supplements varies widely. Some research is mostly in animal or cell models, making it difficult to generalize their results to humans. Many studies have a small sample size and show promising results, but more robust trials are needed to show safety and efficacy. A common challenge for dosing recommendations is that many studies use different doses, herbal preparations, and timing, or are paired with other herbs. We have provided suggested doses for herbs, including standardization of the active compound for supplements when the information is available.

Herbal supplements are often considered as "natural" treatments, but this does not mean they are harmless. Some herbs even have life-threatening interactions with medications as seen with St. John's Wort (see page 234 for more information). None of these dietary supplements have been tested as thoroughly as FDA-approved pharmaceutical medications. See pages 170-173 for information about how to choose a quality dietary supplement.

This is not an exhaustive list of all herbal supplements with potential benefits for mental health. The ones included have the most research to date, but their inclusion is not an endorsement or recommendation to take them. Instead, use this information to work with your mental health team to determine your treatment plan.

Additional Dietary Supplements *for Mental Health*

Ashwagandha (*withania somnifera*)

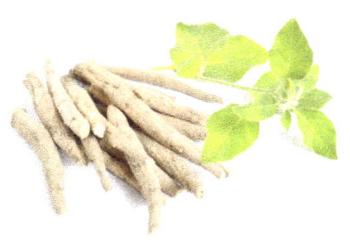

Also known as: winter cherry, Indian ginseng (does not belong to ginseng family), dunal, solanacea

How it works: Ashwagandha has been traditionally used in Ayurvedic and Unani medicine systems as an adaptogen. It may decrease the stress response from the HPA axis by reducing cortisol and corticosteroid release.

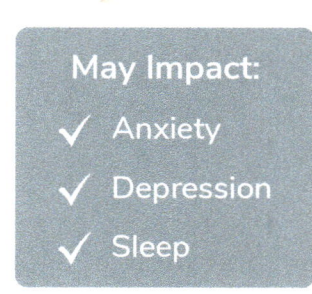

May Impact:
- ✓ Anxiety
- ✓ Depression
- ✓ Sleep

Dietary supplements: Dosing suggestions are challenging with ashwagandha root supplements because preparations are often not standardized in the research literature and doses can range from 120–12,000 mg daily.

- **Anxiety:** Taking 600–12,000 mg of oral ashwagandha daily for up to 10 weeks may moderately improve anxiety scores, especially for someone experiencing chronic stress and anxiety disorder. For those with generalized anxiety disorder, clinical practice guidelines* provisionally recommend taking 300–600 mg of ashwagandha root extract daily, standardized to 5% withanolides (the active compound). It may be used alone or in combination with medication.
- **Depression:** Taking 500 mg of oral ashwagandha root extract daily may reduce the severity of depression symptoms, but research is limited.
- **Sleep:** Taking 120–1,250 mg of oral ashwagandha root extract daily in divided doses may modestly improve sleep in those with or without insomnia.

Side effects: may include mild drowsiness and sedation. Other possible side effects include upset stomach, loose stools, and nausea.

Caution: Ashwagandha appears to be safe and well-tolerated for up to 3 months of use for most people. Safety for long-term use has not been well-studied. Several case reports show that it can cause acute liver injury, affect thyroid function, possibly cause spontaneous abortion, and increase testosterone levels. It may interact with benzodiazepines, CNS depressants, immunosuppressants, thyroid, blood glucose, blood pressure, or other medications, It is not recommended for use in pregnancy, breastfeeding, thyroid disease, liver disease, or for people with prostate cancer.

*Clinical practice guidelines come from the World Federation of Societies of Biological Psychiatry (WFSBP) and the Canadian Network for Mood and Anxiety Treatments (CANMAT).

Additional Dietary Supplements *for Mental Health*

Chamomile (*matricaria recutita*)

Also known as: chamomilla recutita, matricaria chamomilla, German chamomile; **not to be confused with** Roman chamomile

How it works: Chamomile has been traditionally used as a medicinal herb in ancient China, Egypt, Greece, and Rome. The FDA gives it a GRAS rating in the US. The flavonoids in chamomile may help reduce anxiety by binding to GABA receptors and affecting dopamine and serotonin transmission. Research in animals suggests that it may increase cAMP levels, which can improve message transmission to cells.

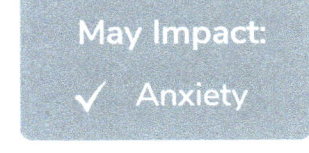

May Impact:

✓ Anxiety

Dietary supplements: Chamomile is available in oral forms as tea or in capsules. Extracts should be standardized to contain 1.2% apigenin (an active compound). It is also used in aromatherapy, topically, and as a mouthwash. Although there is interest in using chamomile for insomnia and ADHD, there is insufficient reliable evidence regarding its benefit in these conditions.

- **Anxiety:** Aromatherapy is typically used at 7 drops of chamomile essential oil 10% for 12 hours nightly, but research is limited and has mixed results as to how effective this is. Oral supplements are usually dosed at 250–2,000 mg daily or 1–2 cups of tea daily. Symptoms may return after stopping the supplement and clinical practice guidelines* do not currently recommend oral supplements of German chamomile as a treatment for generalized anxiety disorder.

Side effects: from teas, food, and topical treatments are uncommon, but may include nausea, dizziness, and allergic reactions. Chamomile can cause eye irritation if it's used topically near the eye.

Caution: Chamomile from food and teas is likely to be safe. Oral supplements of chamomile appear to be safe for doses up to 1,500 mg for 26 weeks. People with allergies to ragweed, chrysanthemums, marigolds, or daisies may also be allergic to chamomile. It may interact with some medications, including central nervous system depressive agents, anti-inflammatory medication, aspirin, or reduce the effectiveness of birth control pills. It is not recommended for use in pregnancy.

*Clinical practice guidelines come from the World Federation of Societies of Biological Psychiatry (WFSBP) and the Canadian Network for Mood and Anxiety Treatments (CANMAT).

Additional Dietary Supplements *for Mental Health*

Ginseng (panax ginseng)

<u>Also known as:</u> Korean ginseng, Manchurian ginseng, Asian ginseng; **Not to be confused with** Siberian ginseng, Brazilian ginseng, American ginseng, Desert ginseng, Chinese ginseng, or Indian ginseng (ashwagandha)

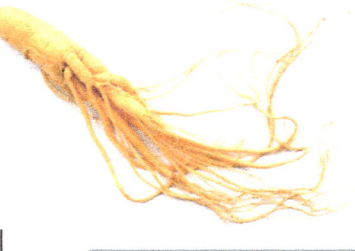

<u>How it works:</u> Panax ginseng is used in traditional Chinese medicine as an adaptogen. It appears to increase neuron cell survival and improve neurite growth, which may help with cognitive function. Panax ginseng may also protect neurons in the hippocampus and may delay neuronal death if blood flow is temporarily restricted, such as with a stroke.

<u>Dietary supplements:</u> Oral Panax ginseng supplements are sometimes standardized to ginsenoside concentration, but amounts vary widely between 1–8%. Panax ginseng is also available as a tea.

> **May Impact:**
> ✓ ADHD
> ✓ Alzheimer's disease
> ✓ Cognitive function

- <u>ADHD:</u> A small study showed that when combined with 500 mg of omega-3 fatty acid supplements daily, taking 3 mg of Panax ginseng extract daily may improve symptoms of ADHD in children. Panax ginseng's effect on its own is unclear.
- <u>Alzheimer's disease:</u> Early-stage research shows that taking Panax ginseng root at 4,500–9,000 mg daily for 12 weeks can improve cognitive performance.
- <u>Cognitive function:</u> Taking 200–400 mg of oral Panax ginseng daily in either single or divided doses for 8–12 weeks seems to improve abstract thinking, attention, arithmetic skills, and reaction time in middle-aged adults, but not young adults. Memory benefits appear to be dependent on its combination with ginkgo.

<u>Side Effects:</u> may include diarrhea, nausea, vomiting, cramps, headaches, alterations in blood pressure, skin irritations, and vaginal bleeding.

<u>Caution:</u> Supplements of Panax ginseng generally appear to be safe for up to 6 months with a low incidence of harm. High doses or long-term use of 3 g or more per day may cause high blood pressure, nervousness, sleeplessness, diarrhea, or skin eruption. Doses of over 15 g per day have been associated with depersonalization, confusion, and depression. Avoid taking with caffeine due to its stimulant effect. Panax ginseng can interact with a variety of medications, including diuretics, insulin, blood thinners, and hormone replacement therapy, among others. Oral Panax ginseng may be unsafe during pregnancy.

Additional Dietary Supplements *for Mental Health*

Gingko (*ginko biloba*)

<u>Also known as:</u> fossil tree, maidenhair tree, EGb-761 extract
<u>How it works:</u> Gingko has a long history of use in Chinese
medicine. It's rich in polyphenols, including flavonoids and
terpenoids. Flavonoids protect the nerves, heart muscle, blood
vessels, and retina from damage. Gingko flavonoids may also
have similar effects to GABA, providing anti-anxiety properties.
Terpenoids in gingko biloba improve blood flow by dilating blood
vessels and reducing the stickiness of platelets. Gingko was
originally thought to help reduce dementia because it improves
blood flow to the brain. New research suggests it may also
protect nerve cells that are damaged in Alzheimer's disease.

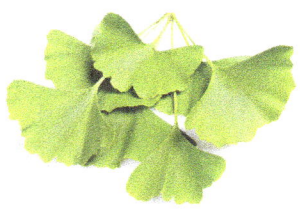

May Impact:
✓ Anxiety
✓ Cognitive function

<u>Dietary supplements:</u> Gingko is available in capsules, tablets, liquid extracts, and as
dried leaves for teas. The supplement form is also called EGb-761 extract and should
be a 50:1 concentrated extract. Supplements should be standardized to 24–32%
flavone glycosides (flavonoids or heterosides) and 6–12% terpene lactones
(terpenoids). Take supplements with meals. Gingko has been considered for ADHD
and depression, but studies have shown mixed results or are of poor quality.

- <u>Anxiety:</u> Taking 240–480 mg of EGb-761 daily for at least 4 weeks may modestly
  reduce symptoms of anxiety in people with generalized anxiety disorder or
  adjustment disorder with anxiety.
- <u>Cognitive function:</u> Oral supplements of EGb-761 taken daily at 240 mg for
  24 weeks may improve the symptoms of Alzheimer's disease, vascular, or mixed
  dementia. Taking 240–600 mg of gingko extract daily may help with some aspects
  of cognitive function in healthy adults, but research has been mixed and of poor
  quality. Gingko does not appear to prevent or slow the progression of dementia,
  nor improve memory or attention in older adults with normal mental function.

<u>Side effects:</u> may include stomach upset, headaches, skin reactions, and dizziness.
<u>Caution:</u> Gingko biloba is likely safe for long-term use. Extracts are often adulterated
with contaminants and not all tests can detect poor quality supplements. Fresh or
roasted seeds or the whole, crude gingko plant should not be consumed, as these are
toxic and potentially deadly. Gingko has several possible drug interactions including
antidepressants, anticonvulsants, anticoagulants, blood glucose lowering medications,
blood pressure medications, diuretics, NSAIDs, cylosporine, and benzodiazepines.
Gingko should not be taken during pregnancy.

Additional Dietary Supplements *for Mental Health*

Kava (*piper methysticum*)

<u>Also known as:</u> ava pepper, kawa, intoxicating long pepper, and yangona; **not to be confused with** Indian Long Pepper.

<u>How it works:</u> Kava is traditionally used by Pacific Islanders in ceremonies and cultural practices. Kava has been used as a short-term treatment for anxiety, insomnia, and stress. Kavalactones are a bioactive compound found in the kava root that cross the blood-brain barrier. They may work by affecting signaling via glutamine, GABA, dopamine, and serotonin. Kava works as a depressant by reducing the messages between the brain and body. It has been used in Australia as a harm-reduction alternative to alcohol. Kava is also used recreationally to relax the body and induce mild euphoria.

May Impact:
✓ Anxiety
✓ Sleep

<u>Dietary supplements:</u> Supplements are made from the root or stump of the kava shrub and are available in different forms, including drinks, powders, capsules, extracts, or drops. Supplements should be standardized to 70% kavalactones.

- <u>Anxiety:</u> Oral supplements dosed at 150–400 mg daily for at least 5 weeks may reduce symptoms of non-psychotic anxiety; clinical practice guidelines* recommend the use for acute or short-term treatment. Kava may not be beneficial for generalized anxiety; clinical practice guidelines* recommend against its use.
- <u>Sleep:</u> One small study found that taking 200 mg daily of oral kava for 4 weeks may reduce sleep disturbances for those with non-psychotic anxiety disorders.

<u>Side effects:</u> At lower doses, side effects may include headaches, mild sleepiness, numbness in the mouth or throat, reduced appetite, memory problems, or tremors. High doses can cause drowsiness, nausea, loss of muscle control, mild fever, pupil dilation, red eyes, dry, scaly skin, tremor, and liver damage.

<u>Caution:</u> Long-term use of kava may have similar side effects as those seen with long-term use of benzodiazepines. High doses of 1,000 mg daily or more for longer than a month are more likely to result in liver damage. The FDA issued a warning about kava in 2002 when it was linked with reports of severe liver damage, even in short-term use. Kava can interact with CNS depressants such as alcohol or benzodiazepines and some antipsychotic medication. Do not consume kava with alcohol, while operating heavy machinery, or if pregnant or breastfeeding.

*Clinical practice guidelines come from the World Federation of Societies of Biological Psychiatry (WFSBP) and the Canadian Network for Mood and Anxiety Treatments (CANMAT).

Additional Dietary Supplements *for Mental Health*

Lavender (*lavandula angustifolia*)

<u>Also known as:</u> English lavender, French lavender

<u>How it works:</u> Lavender has been used since ancient times in aromatherapy and as a topical treatment for relaxation and various mood disorders. The FDA gives it a GRAS rating for use in food. It may reduce anxiety by blocking calcium from entering certain nerve cells, thus dampening the stress response of the central nervous system. Lavender can also block serotonin transporters, allowing more serotonin to remain in the blood for the brain to use. Aromatherapy appears to work via the limbic system in the brain. Additionally, it appears to have an antioxidant effect and may be neuroprotective.

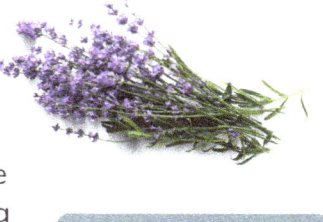

May Impact:
- ✓ Anxiety
- ✓ Depression
- ✓ Sleep

<u>Dietary supplements:</u> Supplemental forms of lavender include topical administration via massage, bath, or other methods; aromatherapy; or oral ingestion of an essential oil preparation called Silexan or dried lavender flower powder. Look for "essential oil" and not just "lavender oil" on the label for a pure, concentrated oil. Lavender oil should contain 25%–46% linalyl acetate and 20%–45% linalool for a therapeutic effect.

- <u>Anxiety and depression:</u> Clinical practice guidelines* state that taking 80–160 mg of oral lavender essential oil or 500–1,500 mg of dried lavender flower twice daily as either monotherapy or adjunct therapy is provisionally recommended for generalized anxiety disorder and weakly recommended for major depressive disorder. Most research has studied this dose for 6–10 weeks. Aromatherapy using lavender oil concentrated at 2–100% may help with anxiety in acute or situation-based anxiety, such as at the dentist office, but more research is needed.

- <u>Sleep:</u> Lavender aromatherapy may improve some subjective measures of sleep, but studies have conflicting results and improvements appear to be minimal.

<u>Side effects:</u> may include mild, transient nausea, diarrhea, and bloating with oral supplements. Topical use may cause skin reactions in those allergic to lavender.

<u>Caution:</u> Oral lavender essential oil generally appears to be safe, although little is known about its long-term use. A few instances of an increase in breast gland tissue in young boys while using topical lavender have been reported. Use oral supplements with caution if taking central nervous system depressant medications.

*Clinical practice guidelines come from the World Federation of Societies of Biological Psychiatry (WFSBP) and the Canadian Network for Mood and Anxiety Treatments (CANMAT).

Additional Dietary Supplements *for Mental Health*

Lemon Balm (*melissa officinalis*)

<u>Also known as:</u> balm mint; blue balm, **not to be confused** with lemon, lemon grass, or lemon basil

<u>How it works:</u> Lemon balm has been used to treat digestive issues, anxiety, mood, improve sleep, and heal wounds. The FDA lists it as GRAS. Phytonutrients in lemon balm, specifically rosmarinic acid, may provide a calming effect by inhibiting GABA-transaminase to increase GABA levels in the brain. Aromatherapy may reduce acetylcholine breakdown and also may act on GABA receptors. Lemon balm has anti-inflammatory, antioxidant, and anti-microbial properties, and may have a prebiotic effect.

May Impact:
- ✓ Anxiety
- ✓ Depression
- ✓ Memory
- ✓ Sleep

<u>Dietary supplements:</u> Lemon balm extracts have been studied the most and should be standardized to more than 7% rosmarinic acid and more than 15% hydroxycinnamic acid. It has been considered for cognitive decline, Alzheimer's disease, and ADHD, but there is not enough data to know if it is beneficial. Lemon balm extracts differ from lemon balm oil, which is moderately toxic.

- <u>Anxiety:</u> Studies using 600–3,000 mg of lemon balm extract daily for 3–56 days show mixed results for reducing anxiety, partly due to inconsistent study methods. A single dose of 300–600 mg of lemon balm extract may increase calmness, alertness, and reduce anxiety in acute stress. Lemon balm may be more effective when combined with valerian, passion flower, and/or butterbur.
- <u>Depression:</u> Taking 1,200–3,000 mg of oral lemon balm extract daily for 3–56 days may moderately improve depression symptoms. Aromatherapy for 30 minutes a day may also be beneficial.
- <u>Memory:</u> A single dose of 1,600 mg of oral lemon balm extract may have an acute effect on improving working memory, but the studies to date have been small.
- <u>Sleep:</u> Taking 80 mg of lemon balm extract in combination with 160 mg of valerian may may improve the quality and quantity of sleep, but it's not clear if these results can be attributed to lemon balm, valerian, or the combination.

<u>Side effects:</u> No serious side effects have been reported. It may reduce alertness.

<u>Caution:</u> Extracts appear to be safe even at high doses of 5,000 mg daily for 20 days. Lemon balm may reduce the effectiveness of SSRI medications or interact with sedative, thyroid, or HIV medications. Do not take it if pregnant or breastfeeding; use it with caution in glaucoma or thyroid conditions.

Additional Dietary Supplements *for Mental Health*

Melatonin

<u>Food Sources:</u> fish (especially salmon and sardines), eggs, milk, pistachios, almonds, goji berries, tart cherries, and mushrooms

<u>How it works:</u> Darkness triggers the pineal gland to produce melatonin, a neurohormone that regulates circadian rhythm and sleep patterns. It's produced from serotonin and sends information about light and darkness to the body, causing sleepiness and helping the body stay asleep during the night. Light inhibits its production and natural levels of melatonin drop to undetectable levels in the morning.

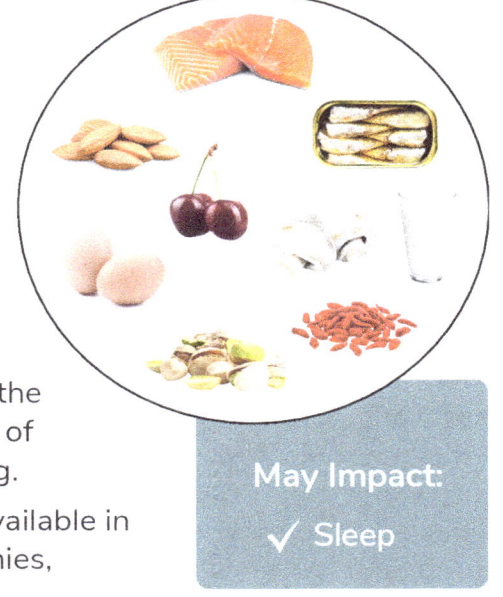

May Impact:

✓ Sleep

<u>Dietary supplements:</u> Melatonin supplements are available in a variety of forms, including tablets, capsules, gummies, liquid drops, lozenges, patches, and sprays.

- <u>Sleep:</u> Studies have used various doses of melatonin, from 0.3–5 mg daily. It's most common to start with a low dose and gradually increase as needed. Taking 1–3 mg of melatonin within 30 minutes of bedtime may help reduce the time it takes to fall asleep. Supplemental melatonin starts to work in 20–40 minutes, has a peak effect at about 1 hour, and levels decrease 4–8 hours after the dose. The supplemental form of melatonin may help shorten the time to fall asleep, but data regarding the quality of sleep is mixed and people often return to their baseline sleep patterns after stopping supplementation.
Taking supplemental melatonin may be especially helpful for delayed sleep-wake phase disorder, blind people, and shift workers, or to reduce symptoms of jet lag. Clinical practice guidelines* weakly recommend against using melatonin to treat insomnia due to a lack of efficacy in improving sleep onset, maintenance, or quality using a dose of 2 mg daily; some research shows that taking a higher dose of 3–5 mg of melatonin may reduce the time it takes to fall asleep and increases the total sleep time. Older adults may see more consistent benefits, as the body decreases production of melatonin with increasing age and some elderly patients may be deficient in melatonin.

*Clinical practice guidelines come from an American Academy of Sleep Medicine task force.

Additional Dietary Supplements *for Mental Health*

Melatonin (continued)

<u>Side effects:</u> are typically mild but may include daytime drowsiness, nausea, headache, dizziness, vivid dreams or nightmares, stomach cramps, and mood changes, including bouts of depression and irritability. Avoid driving or using machinery within 5 hours of a dose.

<u>Caution:</u> Taking supplemental melatonin can signal the body to produce less of the endogenous hormone, so it should be used with caution in young people and children. Melatonin supplements appear to generally be safe for use in adults at a dose of 8 mg daily for up to 6 months or at 10 mg daily for up to 2 months. Always choose a synthetic supplement with a reputable third-party certification to avoid contamination with serotonin and ensure an accurate and consistent dose; melatonin content can vary significantly between batches of supplements, with some containing as much as five times the dose listed on the label. Use melatonin with caution if taking caffeine, contraceptive medication, or fluvoxamine as these can theoretically increase levels of melatonin. Melatonin may interfere with immunosuppressant drugs. Older adults produce less endogenous melatonin hormone, but both the natural and synthetic version remain active for longer. It should be used with caution in people with depression as it may worsen existing symptoms. Avoid the use of melatonin in people with liver or kidney damage due to their decreased ability to metabolize the hormone.

Melatonin Use in Children

Melatonin supplementation may help with sleep disorders, ADHD, or autism spectrum disorder, but most experts recommend avoiding its use as a general sleep aid or to induce sleep in otherwise healthy children. Taking supplements of melatonin can signal the body to produce less of the endogenous hormone. For this reason, long-term use of melatonin should be avoided in children and young people. It may be best to avoid taking melatonin for longer than 3 months and to limit the dose to a maximum of 3 mg daily in children or 5 mg daily in adolescents. In children, side effects may include headache, drowsiness, dizziness, agitation, or nighttime bedwetting. Discuss sleep concerns with your child's medical team before starting dietary supplements.

Additional Dietary Supplements *for Mental Health*

Functional Mushrooms

<u>How they work:</u> Functional mushrooms are types of fungi that are purported to have natural health benefits. They should not be confused with psychedelic mushrooms, which contain psilocybin or other hallucinogens. Some functional mushrooms are eaten as a food. As a dietary supplement, functional mushrooms have been used medicinally in many cultures for centuries. Mushrooms contain many phytonutrients and so can reduce inflammation and work as an antioxidant. Many are used as adaptogens. While there is some promising research about the benefits of functional mushrooms, most studies have been done in cell or animal models and there is very limited human data.

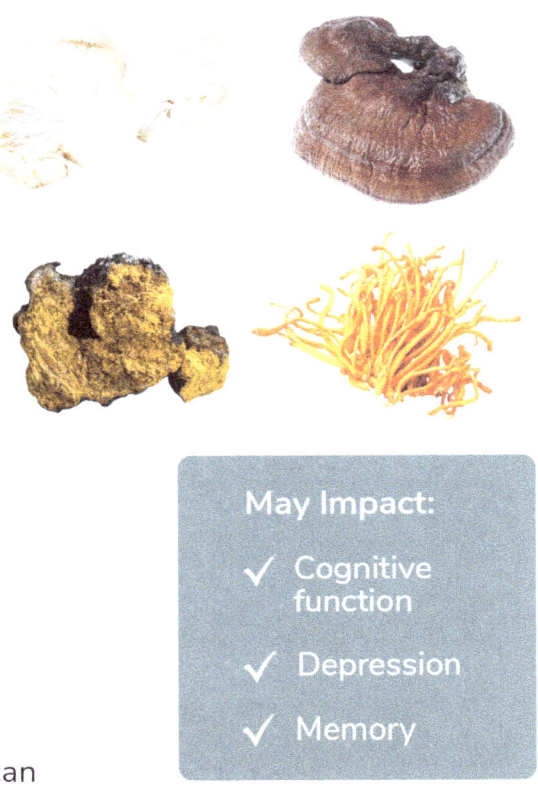

May Impact:

✓ Cognitive function

✓ Depression

✓ Memory

<u>Dietary supplements:</u> are available in powders, capsules, tinctures, and functional foods. Some can be eaten as whole foods. Dosing varies based on the type of mushroom used. See the following pages for examples of common functional mushrooms used in dietary supplements.

<u>Side effects:</u> may include upset stomach, nausea, diarrhea, constipation, dizziness, dry mouth, itching, and skin rash. Some mushrooms are toxic and can result in severe side effects.

<u>Caution:</u> There are many different types of mushrooms that have a wide range of effects. Most functional mushrooms appear to be safe, but can interact with a wide variety of medications. Many functional mushroom products contain more than one ingredient so be careful to check for multiple medication reactions.

Additional Dietary Supplements *for Mental Health*

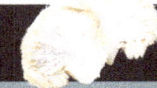

Lion's Mane (Hericium erinaceas)

How it works: Lion's mane is purported to improve cognition by increasing nerve growth factor to stimulate nerve growth. It may reverse stress-related changes to neurotransmitters such as dopamine and serotonin.

Dietary supplements: You can eat fresh lion's mane as you would other types of mushrooms. As a dietary supplement, early-stage research shows that taking 1.05 g of lion's mane mycelia, standardized to contain 5 mg/g of erinacrine A (an active compound) daily for 49 weeks may improve some symptoms in patients with mild Alzheimer's disease. It does not appear to improve cognitive function in healthy adults, even when taking up to 10 g daily. There is interest in using it for anxiety and depression, but there is insufficient evidence for its use.

Caution: Taking 1 g daily for up to 16 weeks appears to be safe for most people. Side effects may include gastrointestinal discomfort, nausea, and diarrhea. Use lion's mane with caution with autoimmune disorders. Avoid taking it if you are pregnant or breastfeeding.

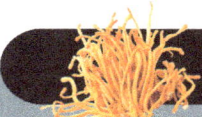

Cordyceps (cordyceps *miliaris*, cordyceps *sinensis*)

How it works: Cordyceps are a parasitic fungi that grow on specific insects. They are used in traditional Chinese medicine for anti-aging and pro-vitality effects. Cordyceps are rich in antioxidants and thought to have neuroprotective effects, which may lead to benefits in learning and memory. Most often cordyceps are used for their adaptogenic properties.

Dietary supplements: Supplements are available in capsules, powders, extracts, and gummies. There is not enough reliable research to determine if supplemental cordyceps are beneficial for mental health conditions.

Caution: Supplements appear to be safe in doses of 3–6 g daily for up to a year. Side effects may include abdominal discomfort, constipation, and diarrhea. Cordyceps may interact with anticoagulant or immunosuppressant medication.

Additional Dietary Supplements *for Mental Health*

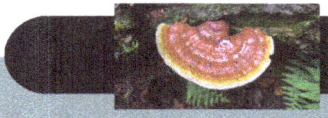

Reishi (*Ganoderma lucidum*)

How it works: Reishi may help neural function, protect against nerve damage, and protect against some stressors, such as low oxygen or cold exposure. It may have immune-boosting and antioxidant effects.

Dietary supplements: Reishi supplements are available as an extract or whole powdered mushroom in a pill. The usual dose is 1.4–5.4 g of whole powdered reishi mushroom daily or extracts of 6 mg daily or less. There is interest in using reishi for Alzheimer's disease, sleep, and stress, but there is insufficient evidence for its use in these conditions.

Caution: Reishi extracts of 6 mg daily appear to be safe for up to a year. Powdered reishi appears to be safe in typical doses for up to 16 weeks. Side effects may include dizziness, dry mouth, itching, nausea, rash, and stomach upset. Reishi may increase the risk of bleeding and can interact with anticoagulants, blood glucose, and blood pressure medication.

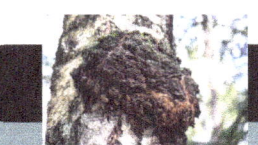

Chaga (*inonotus obliquus*)

How it works: Chaga is a parasitic fungus that grows on the trunks of trees. It contains a multitude of compounds that exert anti-inflammatory, antioxidant, and other effects, but the exact underlying mechanisms are still poorly understood.

Dietary supplements: Supplemental chaga is available as a tincture or used in teas or concentrates. Almost no research has been done in humans, so there is not enough reliable information to provide recommendations for a safe dose.

Caution: Use chaga with caution if you have a history of kidney stones due to its high levels of oxalate. There are several case studies of kidney toxicity with very high doses of chaga or long duration of supplementation. Chaga may interact with anticoagulants, blood glucose, and immunosuppressant medications. Avoid using chaga if you are pregnant or breastfeeding.

Additional Dietary Supplements *for Mental Health*

Passion Flower (*Passiflora incarnata*)

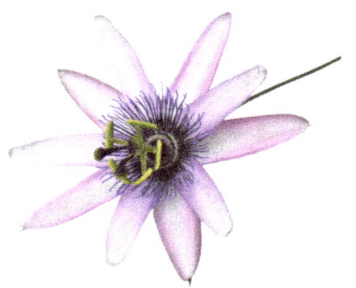

<u>Also known as:</u> maypop, apricot vine, passiflora

<u>How it works:</u> Passion flower has been traditionally used as a sedative, and recently to treat anxiety, insomnia, and seizures. The FDA gives it a GRAS rating for use as a food additive, but has removed it as an over-the-counter sleep medication due to lack of evidence to support its efficacy. Passion flower may inhibit the uptake of GABA into neuronal synapses, thus increasing its levels in the brain.

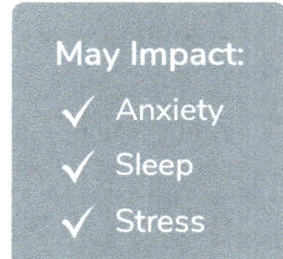

May Impact:
- ✓ Anxiety
- ✓ Sleep
- ✓ Stress

<u>Dietary supplements:</u> Passion flower supplements are available in infusions, teas, extracts, and tinctures. Although there is interest in using it for ADHD, there is not enough research to determine if it is beneficial.

- <u>Anxiety:</u> Early-stage research shows that taking 90–400 mg of a dried alcoholic extract of passion flower once or twice daily for 2–8 weeks may reduce symptoms of non-specific anxiety. Taking 15–45 drops of oral passion flower extract once daily for 28 days may reduce anxiety symptoms to a similar degree as some medication. These findings are limited by small study size and lack of consistency in control groups. It may be beneficial to use passion flower in combination with valerian root.
- <u>Stress:</u> One study showed that taking 600 mg of passion flower daily at bedtime for 30 days may reduce stress, but researchers did not measure how other stressors changed during the study. Combining passion flower with lemon balm, valerian, and butterbur may be beneficial.
- <u>Sleep:</u> Taking 60–600 mg of passion flower extract daily at bedtime for 14–30 days may increase total sleep time and reduce the time to fall asleep. Combining it with with lemon balm, valerian, and/or butterbur may be beneficial.

<u>Side effects:</u> may include drowsiness, confusion, hypersensitivity, sedation, and uncoordinated movement.

<u>Caution:</u> Passion flower appears to be safe at doses of up to 800 mg daily for 8 weeks when taken as alcohol-extracted dried leaves. High doses of 3.5 g for even short periods of time may be unsafe. It may interact with sedatives, monoamine oxidase inhibitors, and blood thinners. Avoid taking it if you are pregnant or breastfeeding.

Additional Dietary Supplements *for Mental Health*

Rhodiola *(rhodiola rosea)*

<u>Also known as:</u> rhodiola, arctic root, golden root, rose root, king's crown

<u>How it works:</u> Rhodiola has been traditionally used in Russia and Scandinavia to treat anxiety, fatigue, and depression. Today it's used as an adaptogen. There are over 140 identified phytochemicals in rhodiola. These appear to work by stimulating receptors for serotonin, dopamine, and acetylcholine. It also may increase the levels and activity of several neurotransmitters, including serotonin and some endorphins. Rhodiola appears to allow dopamine and serotonin to move more freely in the brain by increasing permeability of the blood-brain barrier.

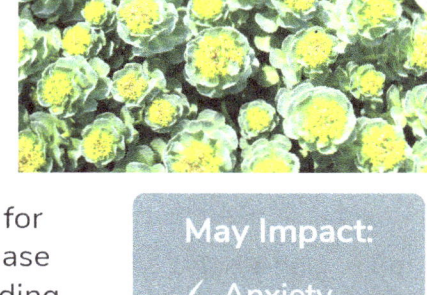

May Impact:

✓ Anxiety

✓ Depression

✓ Fatigue

✓ Stress

<u>Dietary supplements:</u> Rhodiola root extracts should contain 3% rosavin and 1% salidroside. Take supplements on an empty stomach and avoid taking it at bedtime as it may have a stimulating effect.

- <u>Anxiety:</u> Early-stage research in college students shows that taking 200 mg of oral dried rhodiola extract twice daily for 2 weeks may reduce levels of anxiety, anger, confusion, negative mood, and stress. More research is needed to determine rhodiola's effectiveness for treating generalized anxiety disorder.
- <u>Depression:</u> Taking 340–680 mg of oral rhodiola extract daily for 6–12 weeks may reduce symptoms of depression when taken alone or in combination with sertraline. However, clinical practice guidelines* state that rhodiola is not recommended for major depressive disorder based on mixed evidence.
- <u>Fatigue and stress:</u> Early-stage research shows that taking 50–660 mg of rhodiola root extract 1–2 times daily for up to 12 weeks may reduce perceived levels of stress, burnout, fatigue, and increase attention and subjective well-being. A more common dose for stress is 200 mg twice daily for 4–12 weeks.

<u>Side effects:</u> may include dizziness, and increased or decreased saliva production.

<u>Caution:</u> Taking 300 mg of rhodiola extract twice daily for up to 12 weeks appears to be safe. Use it with caution in pregnancy or lactation, if taking antidepressants, blood thinners, immunosuppressants, blood glucose, or blood pressure lowering medication.

*Clinical practice guidelines come from the World Federation of Societies of Biological Psychiatry (WFSBP) and the Canadian Network for Mood and Anxiety Treatments (CANMAT).

Additional Dietary Supplements *for Mental Health*

SAMe (S-adenosyl-L-methionine)

Also known as: SAM, SAM-e, sammy, samyr

How it works: SAMe is a compound naturally produced by the body. It serves as a methyl group donor in a process called methylation, by which SAMe helps make and manage important compounds including hormones, neurotransmitters, DNA, and more. A deficiency of vitamin B12 (folate) can result in decreased levels of SAMe concentration in the body.

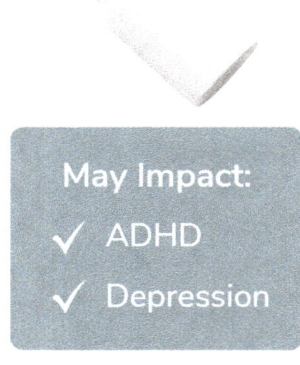

May Impact:
✓ ADHD
✓ Depression

Dietary supplements: SAMe is available as an oral, intravenous, or intramuscular supplement. Take oral SAMe in 1–3 divided doses on an empty stomach, either 30–60 minutes before a meal or 2 hours after eating. Oral supplements have a much lower bioavailability than intramuscular forms. There is interest in using SAMe for Alzheimer's disease, but there is not enough research about its effects in this condition to determine if it is beneficial.

- **ADHD:** Gradually increasing the dose up to taking 800 mg of SAMe 3 times daily for 4 weeks may reduce ADHD symptoms in adults, but this was only shown in one small clinical trial and more study is needed.
- **Depression:** Clinical practice guidelines* weakly recommend taking 1,600–3,200 mg of oral SAMe daily as an adjunct treatment for major depressive disorder, but they do not recommend lower doses for monotherapy. Other practice guidelines* suggest that SAMe can be considered for those with depression who prefer complimentary or alternative therapies. Research results have been mixed due to small sample sizes, short treatment periods, and potentially flawed study designs.

Side effects: Supplemental oral SAMe is usually well tolerated at typical doses, but side effects may include decreased appetite, diarrhea, dizziness, dry mouth, flatulence, headache, insomnia, nausea, nervousness, sweating, and vomiting.

Caution: SAMe can be safely taken for up to 2 years at typical doses. It may interact with levodopa and reduce its effectiveness. Use SAMe with caution if you are taking SSRI medications, as it can increase the risk of serotonin syndrome.

*Clinical practice guidelines come from the World Federation of Societies of Biological Psychiatry (WFSBP) and the Canadian Network for Mood and Anxiety Treatments (CANMAT). Other practice guidelines come from the American Psychiatric Association.

Additional Dietary Supplements *for Mental Health*

Saffron (crocus sativus)

<u>Also known as:</u> autumn crocus, azafron, kashmira

<u>How it works:</u> Saffron is the most expensive spice in the world and has been used medicinally for centuries. The FDA gives it a GRAS rating. Saffron and its active compound crocin are powerful antioxidants that may reduce oxidative stress in the brain. Saffron may prevent the reuptake of dopamine, serotonin, and norepinephrine, thus increasing their effect by allowing them to remain available to the brain for longer. It may also help calm the HPA axis and reduce cortisol levels.

May Impact:
- ✓ ADHD
- ✓ Alzheimer's disease
- ✓ Anxiety
- ✓ Depression
- ✓ Sleep

<u>Dietary supplements:</u> The active compound crocin is sometimes listed on supplement labels. Most studies use extracts containing about 0.15 mg safranal and/or 1.75 mg crocin per 15 mg extract.

- <u>ADHD:</u> Early-stage research suggests that 20–30 mg daily of oral saffron may be beneficial either by itself or with methylphenidate (Ritalin©).
- <u>Alzheimer's disease:</u> Taking 30 mg of saffron extract daily in single or divided doses may improve cognitive ability and slow Alzheimer's disease progression.
- <u>Anxiety:</u> Early-stage research suggests that taking 50 mg of saffron extract twice daily for 12 weeks may improve symptoms of anxiety.
- <u>Depression:</u> Taking 30 mg of saffron extract or 100 mg of dried saffron stigma for 6–12 weeks may improve symptoms of depression. Taking 15 mg of crocin twice daily for 4 weeks may be beneficial as an adjunct therapy with SSRI medication.
- <u>Sleep:</u> Taking saffron or crocin may improve sleep quality, but doses in studies have varied between 5–100 mg daily and the validity of these findings may be limited due to funding by the supplement manufacturers.

<u>Side effects:</u> may include nausea, vomiting, change in appetite, dry mouth, headache, anxiety, and drowsiness.

<u>Caution:</u> Safe doses include: saffron extract up to 100 mg daily for 3 months; saffron powder up to 300 mg daily for 10 days; crocin up to 30 mg daily for 12 weeks. Saffron doses of 1.2–2 g may cause vomiting, diarrhea, bleeding, and kidney damage; over 5 g can cause more severe symptoms; and 12–20 g may cause death. Saffron is prone to contamination due to its high cost; choose a supplement with a third-party certification to ensure purity and potency. It may interact with caffeine, blood glucose, blood pressure, or sedative medications. Avoid supplemental forms in pregnancy.

Additional Dietary Supplements *for Mental Health*

St. John's Wort *(hypericum perforatum)*

<u>Also known as:</u> klamath weed, enola weed, or goatweed

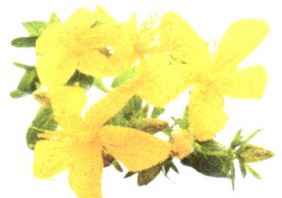

<u>How it works:</u> St. John's wort is used in traditional Chinese medicine and in some European countries to treat depression. It works as a reuptake inhibitor of serotonin, dopamine, and norepinephrine (similar to SSRI medication) and may decrease the uptake of GABA and L-glutamate in the neural synapses to provide mood-balancing effects. St. John's wort may also increase the brain's ability to change connections between neurons (neuroplasticity) and help create new neurons.

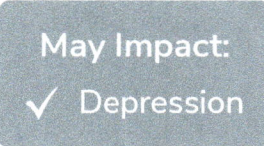

May Impact:
✓ Depression

<u>Dietary supplements:</u> St. John's wort is available as a tea using dried flowers or oral supplements of ground flowers or dried leaves. It can be infused into oil for topical use. St. John's wort has been suggested for use in anxiety, memory, and ADHD, but there is not enough evidence to determine if it is beneficial in these conditions.

- **Depression:** Clinical practice guidelines* state that taking 600–1,800 mg daily of St. John's wort using standardized doses (3:1 to 7:1 extracts, standardized to approximately 0.2–0.3% hypericin and/or 5–6% hyperforin) may be as effective and better tolerated than medications for depression and is recommended as a monotherapy for mild to moderate forms of major depressive disorder.

<u>Side effects:</u> may include diarrhea, abdominal pain, nausea, vomiting, trouble sleeping, anxiety, dry mouth, dizziness, fatigue, headache, and sexual dysfunction. Topical supplements may cause photosensitivity or photodermatitis with sun exposure. Rare but serious adverse effects include suicidal ideation and psychosis.

<u>Caution:</u> DO NOT USE WITHOUT FIRST CONSULTING YOUR MENTAL HEALTH TEAM. When taken with certain antidepressants, St. John's Wort can cause serotonin syndrome, a life-threatening increase in serotonin levels. The extract appears safe in doses up to 900 mg daily for 12 weeks when used appropriately. Supplement potency can vary significantly; choose a supplement with a reputable third-party certification. St. John's wort can reduce the effectiveness of hormonal contraceptives, statins, blood thinners, HIV medication, immunosuppressants, some types of cancer medication, anti-seizure medication, and others. Use caution in pregnancy and lactation.

*Clinical practice guidelines come from the American College of Physicians. Dosing guidelines come from the World Federation of Societies of Biological Psychiatry (WFSBP) and the Canadian Network for Mood and Anxiety Treatments (CANMAT).

Additional Dietary Supplements *for Mental Health*

Turmeric (*Curcuma aromatica, curcuma longa*)

Also known as: curcuma; **not to be confused with** Javanese turmeric

How it works: The FDA gives turmeric a GRAS rating for food use. Curcumin is the active compound in turmeric. It can stimulate the growth of new neurons and has antioxidant and anti-inflammatory properties, potentially protecting brain cells from damage. It may help reduce the buildup of amyloid plaques and tau tangles in the brain, which are hallmarks of Alzheimer's disease. Turmeric also may increase levels of DHA in the brain.

Dietary supplements: Turmeric extracts should be standardized to 80–95% curcuminoids. Curcumin is also available as a supplement and its dose is often found on supplement labels.

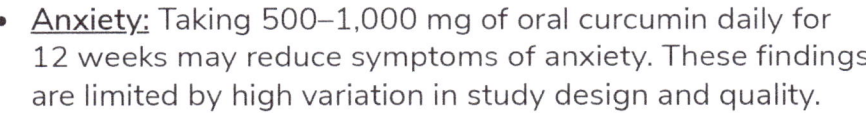

May Impact:
- ✓ Anxiety
- ✓ Cognitive function
- ✓ Depression
- ✓ Inflammation

- **Anxiety:** Taking 500–1,000 mg of oral curcumin daily for 12 weeks may reduce symptoms of anxiety. These findings are limited by high variation in study design and quality.
- **Cognitive function:** Taking 90 mg of oral curcumin twice daily for 18 months may improve long-term memory and attention in elderly patients with cognitive decline. Although there is interest in using turmeric to treat Alzheimer's disease, current research has not shown a benefit of supplementation.
- **Depression:** Taking 1 g of oral curcumin daily for 6 weeks or more may improve the symptoms of depression when taken alone or in combination with antidepressant medications. Clinical practice guidelines* provisionally recommend taking 500–1,000 mg of curcumin extract daily either alone or in combination with other therapies for use in mild to moderate depression.
- **Inflammation:** Turmeric extract is most commonly used at a dose of 1.5 g daily for up to 3 months. Taking 180–500 mg of curcumin daily for 6–12 weeks may improve some measures of inflammation, such as reducing osteoarthritis pain.

Side effects: may include digestive discomfort, nausea, and vomiting.

Caution: Turmeric extract and curcumin are likely to be safe at these doses: 8 g daily for 2 months, 3 g daily for 3 months, or 1.5 g daily for 12 months. Large doses may harm the liver. It has multiple potential interactions, such as with chemotherapy drugs, blood thinners, and blood glucose lowering medication, among others. In pregnancy and lactation, food sources appear safe but supplements should be avoided.

*Clinical practice guidelines come from the World Federation of Societies of Biological Psychiatry (WFSBP) and the Canadian Network for Mood and Anxiety Treatments (CANMAT).

Additional Dietary Supplements *for Mental Health*

Valerian (*valeriana officinalis*)

<u>Also known as:</u> all-heal, garden heliotrope, St. George's Herb, valeriana edulis, valeriana wallichii, or valeriana fauriei; **not to be confused with** red-spur valerian

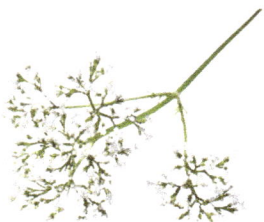

<u>How it works:</u> Valerian is used in Europe for sleep and nervous tension. It contains multiple compounds and the way it works is not fully understood. Valerenic acid is one of the main bioactive compounds that may stimulate the GABA receptor response. Other compounds may inhibit the breakdown of GABA, allowing it to remain available to the brain and providing calming effects.

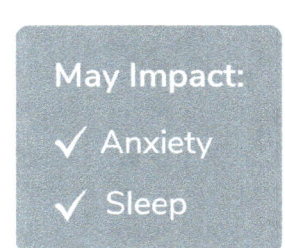

May Impact:

✓ Anxiety

✓ Sleep

<u>Dietary supplements:</u> Dried valerian roots are prepared as teas or tinctures. Dried plant materials, including stems and extracts, are found in capsules or tablets. Some extracts are standardized to 0.25%–1% valerenic acid. Valerian is often used with other herbs such as passion flower.

- <u>Sleep:</u> The European Medicines Agency recommends taking 400–600 mg of valerian extract or 0.3–3 g powdered valerian root up to 3 times daily to aid sleep or for the relief of mild nervous tension. Other research suggests that taking 300–600 mg daily of valerian whole root extract appears to modestly improve sleep quality, but it may take up to 4 weeks to provide benefit. For tea, steep 2–3 g of dried herbal valerian root for 10–15 minutes. Valerian does not appear to improve the time it takes to fall asleep, sleep duration, or severity of insomnia.
- <u>Anxiety:</u> Studies have shown mixed results of the effectiveness of valerian on anxiety symptoms. Whole root preparations appear to work better than valerian extracts. One study in patients on hemodialysis used a dose of 530 mg daily for 1 month and showed an improvement in anxiety scores.

<u>Side effects:</u> may include drowsiness, diarrhea, upper abdominal pain, nausea, heartburn, headache, dizziness, vivid dreams, or itchy skin.

<u>Caution:</u> Abruptly stopping valerian after chronic use has been associated with cases of heart failure and hallucinations; taper doses down slowly to avoid symptoms of withdrawal, including elevated heart rate, anxiety, irritability, and insomnia. Doses of 300–600 mg daily for up to 6 weeks appear safe; long-term safety data is not available. Valerian may interact with alcohol, benzodiazepines, and other sedatives. Avoid taking valerian if you are pregnant or breastfeeding.

Troubleshooting Guide for Common Challenges in Mental Health

Common Blocks When Getting Started

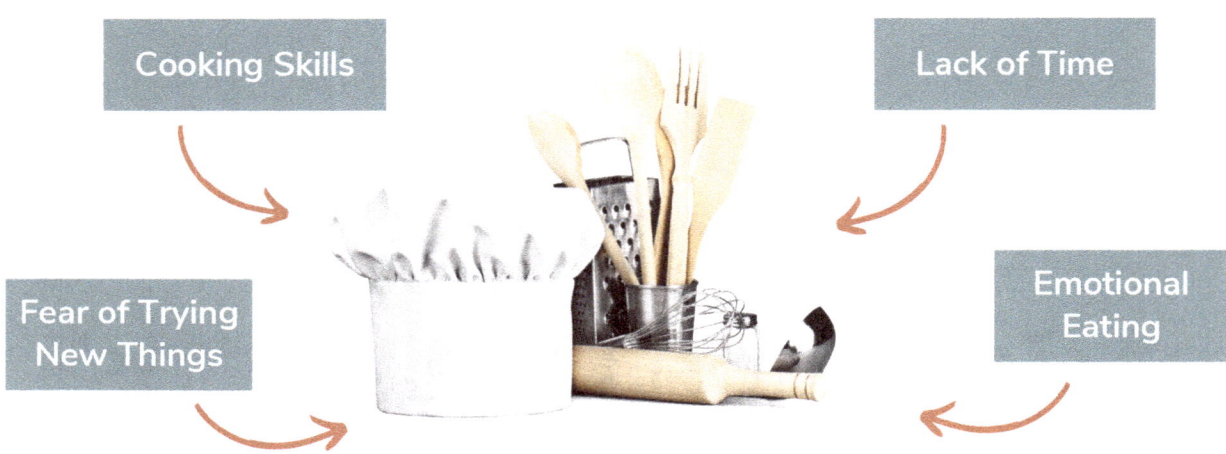

Cooking Skills

Lack of Time

Fear of Trying New Things

Emotional Eating

Some of the biggest challenges with nutrition are not about knowledge, but rather about how to overcome barriers to successfully implement new habits for your lifestyle. If it were easy to cook at home and nourish your body, everyone would do it.

Unfortunately, we know that many things are challenging when changing your nutrition and health habits, including specific challenges with mental health needs. If you've never been taught to cook, following a recipe can feel intimidating. If you're cooking for one person, you need to adjust your recipes so you don't cook too much. If you struggle with staying on task, strategies for staying focused may be helpful. If you often use food as a coping mechanism for stress, you'll need to learn to meet your root needs using the right tools, including options beyond food.

You might find that you identify with some common blocks even if you've never had a formal diagnosis, and you might benefit from these helpful strategies. If you find these mental blocks often get in your way, it may be beneficial to talk with a licensed mental health professional.

Consider this your toolkit to get started. Read through the common blocks and notice which ones cause you to struggle. Start with a mindset shift, adapt it for you, memorize it, and repeat it to yourself when you are struggling. Then, begin to implement the suggested strategies to help move forward towards improved mental health. For additional support in overcoming these mental blocks, we highly recommend working individually with a dietitian, therapist, or health coach. See page 272 for additional resources.

Common Blocks When Getting Started

Procrastination

What it is: Putting off meal planning, cooking, or eating until hunger becomes urgent.

Mindset shift: "Planning meals saves future-me from stress."

Strategies to overcome:
- Use a visual meal planner or a phone app to send you reminders.
- Plan 1–2 meals at a time instead of a full week to reduce feeling overwhelmed.
- Pair your task with something fun – go to your favorite coffee shop to plan your meals or put on your favorite TV show or music in the background as you cook.
- Keep quick, nutritious snacks on hand to eat if needed.

Inconsistent Meal Patterns

What it is: Irregular eating schedules that can worsen energy and mood issues by creating extreme hunger, which can then lead to compensatory overeating.

Mindset shift: "Eating regularly stabilizes my energy."

Strategies to overcome:
- Choose to eat something even if it's not perfect.
- Set alarms for meals and snacks, or schedule them into your day on your calendar.
- Use meal replacements like protein shakes or Grab & Go Meals on busy days.
- Keep easy, quick, nutritious snacks on hand to eat if unable to eat a full meal.

Last-Minute Schedule Changes

What it is: Your schedule changes after you've made your meal plan, and you have less time than you previously planned.

Mindset shift: "My meal plan can be flexible to work around my life."

Strategies to overcome:
- Schedule take-out or Grab & Go Meals into your meal plan so you can switch your plan from different days if something changes at the last minute.
- Avoid over-planning; leave some days blank on your plan for last-minute changes.
- Practice self-compassion as progress is more important than perfection.
- See pages 36–37 for examples and ideas to accommodate schedule changes.

Common Blocks When Getting Started

Overwhelmed by Grocery Shopping

What it is: Feeling overwhelmed in the grocery store, leading to buying random items or forgetting essentials.

Mindset shift: "A list simplifies my trip."

Strategies to overcome:
- Shop online for groceries or use curbside pickup to reduce environmental overstimulation.
- If possible, go to the grocery store at non-peak times, such as mornings, late evenings, or weekdays.
- Organize your shopping list by section of the store or the path in the store that you shop. Cross off items as you get them.
- Keep a running shopping list in the kitchen (or digitally) and add items you need when you think of them, rather than trying to remember when in the store.
- Keep frozen meat and vegetables, dried fruits, grains, and canned foods on hand to delay going to the grocery store a day if you are too busy.

Emotional Eating

What it is: Using food as a coping mechanism for stress or emotions, especially when not physically hungry. This can affect energy levels and emotional well-being by not addressing the underlying issue.

Mindset shift: "It's okay to have emotions, I can feel and cope with them."

Strategies to overcome:
- Practice mindfulness before eating.
- Get in tune with your body's hunger and fullness cues.
- Develop other coping mechanisms for emotional support such as journaling, walking, or deep breathing. See pages 267-270 for more tips.
- Work with a therapist to develop additional coping mechanisms and find the root cause of cravings and underlying unmet needs.

Troubleshooting Guide for Common Challenges in Mental Health

Common Blocks When Getting Started

Unsure How Much to Eat

What it is: Over- or undereating at a meal or snack resulting in feeling overly full afterwards, or feeling hungry within 1–2 hours.

Mindset shift: "My body knows how much I need to eat, and I can learn to listen to its cues."

Strategies to overcome:
- Focus on developing and tuning into hunger and fullness cues with mindful eating exercises or looking into the Intuitive Eating framework.
- Create an eating environment with few distractions to help notice your body cues.
- Avoid creating rules around food, like banning a food, which can lead to compensatory eating in response to this restriction.
- Eat regularly throughout the day, every 3–4 hours starting in the morning to avoid becoming overly hungry.
- Use the "Healthy Plate" method outlined in Section 2 to create a balanced plate with nutrients such as fat, fiber, and protein to support satiety between meals.
- Consider working with a registered dietitian to help you develop mindful eating skills. See resources on page 272.

Cost of Food

What it is: The cost of groceries makes healthy eating difficult.

Mindset shift: "Planning ahead and using my resources can make healthy eating more affordable."

Strategies to overcome:
- Choose vegetables in season for lower cost or use frozen or canned vegetables.
- Find a local CSA (Community Supported Agriculture) for affordable fresh produce from local farms.
- Incorporate vegetarian proteins, like beans or tofu, or use meat as a component of a meal rather than the main dish.
- Buy in bulk when prices are low, then portion the food and freeze it for later.
- Incorporate low-cost whole grains as part of your meal.
- See resources for food insecurity on page 272 if needed.

Common Blocks When Getting Started

Lack of Cooking Experience

What it is: Not having been taught how to cook and learning this new skill on your own.

Mindset shift: "Things feel hard when they are new, but cooking will get easier the more I practice."

Strategies to overcome:
- Practice self-compassion. Everyone starts somewhere!
- Start with simple, well-written recipes.
- Before cooking, read through the entire recipe and set out all the ingredients you need to help reduce feeling overwhelmed.
- Invite a trusted friend or loved one to cook with you who is more familiar with cooking, who can help answer questions or teach you cooking techniques.
- Attend a virtual or local cooking class in your area.
- See the Prep Guide for each meal plan to know what order to cook the recipes.
- Search the Internet to find videos for how to prep unfamiliar ingredients.

Fear of Judgment

What it is: Worries about what others may think of what or how much you are eating, resulting in disconnecting from body cues and over- or under-eating.

Mindset shift: "I deserve to feel nourished and satisfied. My food choices reflect my needs, not others' opinions."

Strategies to overcome:
- Work through rejecting the "diet mentality," making peace with food, and challenging the "food rules" as part of your food healing journey.
- Practice self-compassion when eating.
- Cook alone or with safe people when you are first starting your food healing journey.
- Set boundaries, prepare responses, and focus on your own plate when eating with others.
- Notice how you filter comments and if you are projecting your own fears.

Common Blocks When Getting Started

No Routine With Meal Planning

What it is: Struggling to shop, cook, and eat consistently because you don't meal plan regularly.

Mindset shift: "Scheduling time to make my meal plan saves me time in the long run."

Strategies to overcome:
- Consider what tools you've used to start other new habits and use those to start meal planning. For example, if you use a calendar to organize your schedule, write your planned meals on it.
- Plan meals with your friend or partner.
- Add a time block on your calendar to meal plan each week.
- Work with a registered dietitian, therapist, or life coach to learn skills.
- Simplify meal planning. Instead of planning every meal, choose 2–3 recipes per week to cook.

Different Dietary Needs

What it is: Different dietary needs, food sensitivities, and preferences make meal planning and cooking difficult and time-consuming.

Mindset shift: "With small changes and strategies, I can make meals that work for everyone."

Strategies to overcome:
- Follow the dietary needs for the whole family instead of making separate meals.
- Choose cuisines that naturally support the dietary needs, such as Asian dishes for dairy-free or Mexican dishes for gluten-free.
- Keep easy substitutions on hand for the person with the restriction, such as corn tortillas instead of flour for gluten-free or vegan meatballs instead of beef.
- Use recipes that use single ingredients, such as individual spices instead of a seasoning packet, that are easier to modify for dietary needs.
- Keep ready-to-eat alternatives on hand if unable to adapt the menu, like frozen meals or meal replacements.

Common Blocks When Getting Started

Lack of Time

What it is: Busy schedules interfere with mealtimes and meal prep, so purchased ingredients go to waste and instead of cooking, meals are purchased as take-out or from fast food.

Mindset shift: "Making time to meal plan, shop, and cook will save me time and money in the long run."

Strategies to overcome:
- Plan meals one week at a time using the method outlined in Section 2 to minimize trips to the grocery store.
- Use slow-cooker meals for busy days so that dinner will be ready when you get home.
- Keep 30-minute meal options on hand for quick meals in the evening.
- Schedule in "no-cook" dinner nights, such as "snack dinner," simple sandwiches with a pre-made salad, or Grab & Go Meals.
- If it's within your budget, "buy back" your time by hiring people to do some tasks, like using grocery delivery or purchasing already-prepared vegetables.

Cooking for One

What it is: Preparing food for only one person, making it difficult to cook certain recipes without wasting food or leading to low motivation without others to cook for.

Mindset shift: "I can make simple meals for myself because I deserve to be nourished."

Strategies to overcome:
- Use recipes made for 1–2 servings to prevent food waste or leftover fatigue.
- Make recipes that freeze well. Portion leftovers as individual frozen dinners for variety later.
- Try a "meal swap" with a friend or coworker who is also cooking for one; you both make a meal and bring the leftovers for the other person, so nobody gets bored.

Troubleshooting Guide for Common Challenges in Mental Health

Common Blocks When Getting Started

Picky Eaters

What it is: Eaters who refuse food because they don't like what is served.

Mindset shift: "It's my job to provide a nourishing meal and safe experience, and it's my picky eater's job to decide if and how much to eat."

Strategies to overcome:
- Follow the "division of responsibility" for both kids and adults.
  - The meal planner chooses the menu, time of the meal, and where it's served.
  - The picky eater chooses if and how much of the regular menu to try.
  - Adults and older children have the option of making different food, but this responsibility does not fall on the meal planner.
  - See www.EllynSatterInstitute.org for more picky eating resources.
- Serve a "safe food," which is something the picky eater is known to like, within the prepared meal. This can help reduce stress and anxiety around eating, which can lead to them trying more foods. This can be helpful for adults, too.
- Keep mealtime pleasant and fun without pressure or commenting on what people are eating. Consider adding music, conversion, and table games.
- Use neutral food language, like noticing flavors, colors, and textures, instead of labeling food "like," "dislike," "good," or "bad."

Additional Tips for Picky Children and Teens:
- Avoid bribes and threats, such as requiring your child to finish part of their meal before getting something else or rewarding good behavior with candy.
- Use change language when talking about food, such as, "I don't like it yet."
- Model trying new foods and narrate the process out loud. Talk through your curiosity, your fears, and the senses you notice when you eat a new food.
- Use age-appropriate language to discuss nutrition, focusing on adding in nutrients you need rather than avoiding certain foods or ingredients.
- Try a gentle food progression for very picky eaters. For example, start with fruit snacks, then introduce a new shape of fruit snacks, then switch to fruit leather, then advance to dried fruit before finally trying fresh fruit.
- For very selective eaters or for children with growth concerns, consider working with a food therapist and/or a pediatric dietitian.
- Focus on exposure to foods rather than worrying if your picky eater eats them.

Common Blocks With ADHD

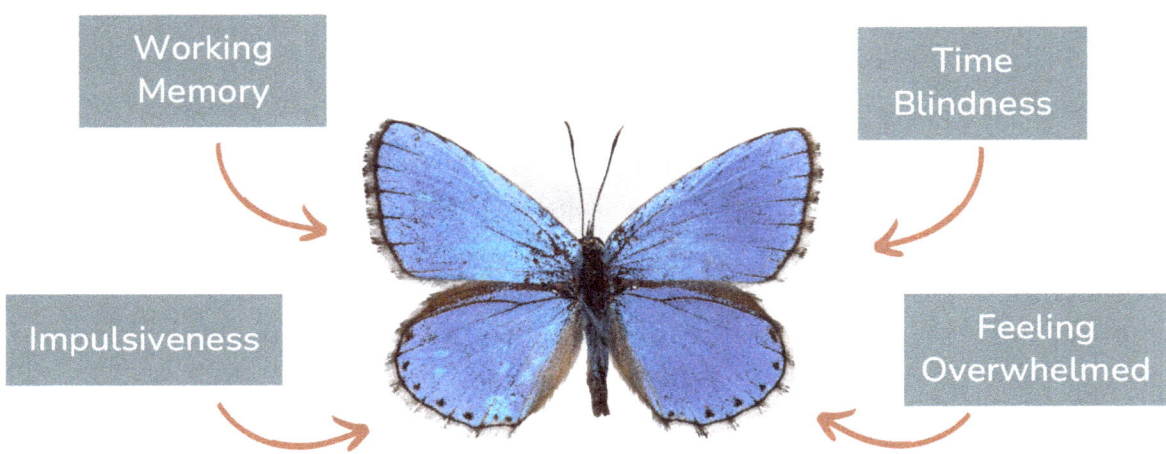

Working Memory

Time Blindness

Impulsiveness

Feeling Overwhelmed

Attention-deficit/hyperactivity disorder, or ADHD, is a common mental health disorder among children and adults. Some of the most challenging tasks for people with ADHD include executive functions such as planning and working memory, which can make it difficult to organize recipes, manage food inventory, and plan meals. Additionally, your appetite can be reduced by hyperfocus in ADHD or by medications used in treatment leading to unbalanced eating patterns.

If you have ADHD, you may struggle with the sense that everything feels equally important. This sense of "equal urgency" can lead to difficulty with organizational skills, including prioritizing tasks and time management. Two things tend to happen. You may try multitasking too many things at once, which can backfire and cause you to feel overwhelmed or to forget things – like missing an ingredient in a recipe or forgetting to turn on the oven. Or you may choose the task that is most apparent, rather than the one that is most important or time sensitive.

When schedules change unexpectedly, it's common to struggle to adjust your meal plan accordingly. The necessary skills like time management, decision making, and mental flexibility are often especially difficult at the end of the day. If there are too many things to juggle – like managing emotions, meal planning around eating preferences or dietary needs, and concerns about forgetting something – you might find yourself distracted and avoiding the problem rather than working through it.

These challenges can affect the way you meal plan, prepare and cook food, and even how you consume food. If you have ADHD, find examples in the following pages of common barriers, as well as inspiration for how to shift your mindset.

Common Blocks With ADHD

Clinical definition: ADHD includes a persistent pattern of inattention and/or hyperactivity-impulsivity that interferes with functioning or development, with symptoms present before age 12. The diagnosis may occur in adulthood, but symptoms will have been present as a child in two or more settings.
Symptoms include failing to pay close attention to details; making careless mistakes in schoolwork, at work, or during other activities; difficulty with hyperactivity, focus, impulse control, and executive functions, such as time management, emotional regulation, task initiation, and planning.

Parts of the brain involved: prefrontal cortex, basal ganglia, and limbic system

Neurotransmitters involved: dopamine and norepinephrine

Critical nutrients: L-theanine, omega-3 fatty acids, vitamin B12, choline, vitamin D, iron, magnesium

Impactful Food Additions for ADHD

Pumpkin seeds: add to salads, enjoy as part of trail mix, or add to granola
Green tea: drink green tea or matcha, try green tea mochi for dessert
Salmon or tuna: try packets for ease, serve on salad, crackers, or sandwiches
Eggs: hard-boil, fry, or scramble eggs for a snack or breakfast; add to sandwiches, top roasted vegetables to make an easy hash, or add to salads
Chia seeds: make pudding, add to smoothies, or baked goods
Nutritional yeast: sub for Parmesan cheese, try on pasta, popcorn, or salad
Edamame: enjoy steamed with salt, incorporate into salads, or add as a topping to meals; find dried edamame to enjoy as a snack
Red meat: enjoy as a component of the meal, such as in tacos, soups, or stews; serve as an entrée once per week
Leafy greens: add kale, spinach, or Swiss chard to soups, stews, stir-fry, smoothies, sandwiches, or salads

Common Blocks With ADHD

Easily Distracted

What it is: Difficulty completing tasks related to starting a meal but getting distracted, losing interest before it's done, or forgetting you're cooking and things start to burn.

Mindset shift: "Tools I use to help me focus can help me stay engaged while cooking."

Strategies to overcome:
- Choose simple meals with few steps, easy ingredients, and fewer pans to reduce feeling overwhelmed and minimize cleanup.
- Use convenient foods like frozen or pre-chopped veggies to speed cooking.
- Use one cooking area or method: use only the oven or the stove instead of both.
- Use "set and forget" appliances, such as a slow cooker, for part of the meal.
- Look at the Prep Guide for each meal in Section 3 to start recipes in the right order so food is ready to eat at the same time.
- Use timers and alarms to stay on track. Break cooking into steps with pauses between tasks to reset your focus.
- Add something enjoyable while cooking, such as listening to audiobooks, podcasts, or music to keep you from getting bored.
- Instead of full food prep, gather ingredients in containers for each day to help use ingredients more quickly and avoid forgetting part of the recipe.

Impulsiveness

What it is: Making quick decisions for immediate gratification that don't align with your long-term goals or values, such as buying take-out instead of cooking.

Mindset shift: "Staying on track will help me meet my long-term goals."

Strategies to overcome:
- Pre-chop veggies or prepare snacks for quick options to reduce your reliance on convenience foods when you are very hungry.
- Keep shelf-stable car snacks if a bit hungry before getting home and cooking meals (eg, trail mix, meat sticks, peanut butter crackers, protein bars).
- Map out a different route home so you don't drive by take-out restaurants.
- Only pay cash at restaurants or fast food and limit the cash you carry.
- Make a slow-cooker meal in the morning or prep ingredients ahead of time so dinner is practically ready when you get home.

Common Blocks With ADHD

Lower Working Memory

What it is: Difficulty remembering information while carrying out a task, usually related to the task. This can result in trouble remembering ingredients, if it has been used, forgetting what you just read, missing a cooking step, or getting distracted by the next step in the recipe while the previous step is not yet complete.

Mindset shift:
- "I can remember items needed with supportive tools and can practice flexibility if I forget something – let's see how creative I can be!"

Strategies to overcome:
- Use apps that have recipes using a "cooking mode" to focus on one step at a time.
- Set out the ingredients before starting to cook to visually remind you to use them.
- Use an app with an ingredient list generator to take to the grocery store.
- Keep a running grocery list on your phone or in a visible spot and check it before heading to the store. If possible, allow your family to add items to the list.
- Substitute ingredients or simply leave them out of the recipe. Most spices can be left out; many vegetables, grains, and proteins can be easily substituted.

Overstimulation

What it is: Feeling amped up, from either external stimulations like sounds or crowds, or internal stimulation of tasks and thoughts, leading to feeling rushed or hurried.

Mindset shift: "I can be aware of overstimulation and use tools to reset and calm."

Strategies to overcome:
- Take a "time out" for yourself with a 5-minute meditation or breathing exercise.
- Find a "sanctuary space," such as a quiet room, closet, or your car, where you can step away for a few minutes and collect yourself in silence.
- If you know the day will be overstimulating, plan a slow-cooker or frozen meal.
- Practice self-regulating activities regularly so you can access these in times of overstimulation. Try these examples or see page 268 for additional resources.
  - Calming: butterfly taps, box breathing, quick visualization, soothing hug
  - Releasing: loud singing, dancing, body shake, lion's breath/roar, acting silly

Common Blocks With ADHD

Novelty-Seeking Behavior or Low Tolerance for Repetition

<u>What it is:</u> Seeking excitement and interest with new experiences. This can lead to boredom with foods or eating out rather than cooking at home.

<u>Mindset shift:</u> "Rotation and small tweaks keep things interesting."

<u>Strategies to overcome:</u>
- Add a new topping to favorite foods, such as nuts, crackers, sprinkles, or dressing.
- Try different cultural spices or recipes.
- Use a different wrapping instead of sandwiches: tortillas, pitas, or croissants.
- Search online, use an app, or try a meal subscription delivery for new ideas.

Decision Paralysis or Decision Fatigue

<u>What it is:</u> Feeling overwhelmed from too many food choices or recipes, making it hard to start.

<u>Mindset shift:</u> "A choice doesn't have to be perfect to be good."

<u>Strategies to overcome:</u>
- Allow others to help with the decision-making process. Ask your family, or use a meal planning app, favorite blog, or recipe subscription for inspiration.
- Make choosing easier by limiting options with a "meal theme" (eg, pasta Monday) or cultural flavor, then choose from those.
- Keep frozen meals on hand that you enjoy if you feel overwhelmed.

Difficulty With Executive Functions

<u>What it is:</u> Struggling with planning, organizing ingredients, or following recipes.

<u>Mindset shift:</u> "Simple meals still nourish me."

<u>Strategies to overcome:</u>
- Use meal kits, grocery delivery services, or apps to help plan and grocery shop.
- Focus on assembling meals rather than cooking (eg, salad kits or wraps).
- Start with recipes you're familiar with, then add one recipe at a time when ready.
- Choose easier recipes with fewer ingredients and simple instructions.
- Organize recipes into one location instead of using several cookbooks or websites.
- Review the recipe and gather all ingredients before starting to cook.

Troubleshooting Guide for Common Challenges in Mental Health

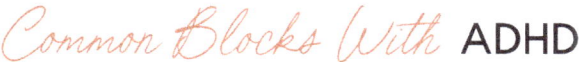 *Common Blocks With* ADHD

Time Blindness

What it is: Losing track of time, often through hyperfocus, or doing 'one more thing,' such as thinking there is time for one more errand resulting in getting home later than expected before beginning meals. Another example is checking a quick email, but staying on your computer or phone much longer than anticipated.

Mindset shift: "Exact timing isn't necessary, but a routine may help me."

Strategies to overcome:
- On your weekly meal plan, write down the start time of when you need to make the meal so that you don't have to calculate it in the moment.
- Set up a routine that helps you to begin cooking so that it becomes automatic. For example, when you come home from work put ingredients on the counter for dinner to return to after changing from work clothes, then begin cooking.
- If your schedule is disrupted or you lose track of time and don't have time to make your originally-planned meal, reschedule the original meal to avoid food waste and instead choose a quick-prep, frozen, or Grab & Go Meal.

Feeling Overwhelmed

What it is: Finding it hard to complete recipes with several steps, especially if they require multitasking, most often with multi-step recipes and clean up.

Mindset shift: "Simplifying recipes doesn't mean I'm failing. I'm making it easier for me and meeting my needs."

Strategies to overcome:
- Choose recipes with few ingredients, few steps, or one-pan meals.
- When you find a recipe you like, bookmark it and repeat it in your rotation.
- Use pre-chopped or frozen ingredients.
- Add small meal prep steps early in the day or the day before. For example, move frozen meat to the refrigerator to thaw or set out canned ingredients to be ready for cooking the next day.
- Use "habit stacking" to prompt you to remember to do small meal prep for the next day's plan. For example, in the evening while packing lunch for the next day, also set up ingredients for dinner the following day.

Common Blocks With Anxiety

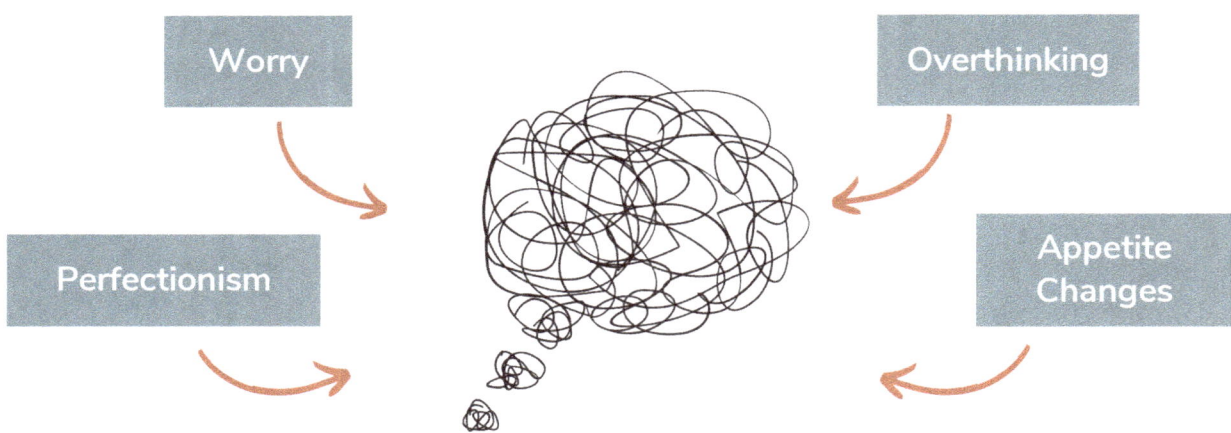

Anxiety symptoms can make routine tasks such as meal planning and eating feel overwhelming. If you struggle with anxiety, you may find yourself worrying about what to eat, how much to eat, and whether the food you prepare is "right." This fear of making a mistake or not being able to cook properly can lead to procrastination or skipping meals altogether. Many people with anxiety feel stuck in a cycle of overthinking, leading to decision paralysis and frustration with not being able to complete the task at hand.

An anxious brain can directly impact digestion via the vagus nerve, which is the main connection between the gut's enteric nervous system and the brain. Anxiety can trigger the sympathetic "fight or flight" nervous system to go into effect, which shifts nutrients and hormones away from digestion. This can lead to symptoms of an upset stomach, reduced appetite, and irregular bowel movements. Coping strategies like deep breathing can help the brain and body shift back into the parasympathetic "rest and digest" nervous system to reduce these symptoms and improve digestion.

The physical symptoms of anxiety, like muscle tension, restlessness, or difficulty relaxing, can also make it harder to enjoy the process of cooking and eating.
To overcome these challenges, focus on taking small steps, be kind to yourself, and remember that it's okay to ask for help. You don't have to have everything figured out right away. Simply focusing on what feels manageable can make a big difference.

Common mental blocks are listed in the following pages that may arise when thinking about food, meals, and the process of cooking. Try implementing some of these mindset shifts and strategies to help you feel more at ease.

Common Blocks With Anxiety

<u>Clinical definition:</u> Anxiety is characterized by excessive worry, fear, or apprehension about a number of events or activities. A diagnosis of an anxiety disorder is made when symptoms occur on more days than not for at least 6 months, are difficult to control, and cause significant distress or impairment. Symptoms include physical tension, restlessness, or feeling on edge; being easily fatigued; difficulty concentrating or mind going blank; irritability; muscle tension; and sleep disturbance. There are different types of anxiety, and not all are described here. We recommend to have an evaluation and diagnosis by a licensed professional for more clarity.

<u>Parts of the brain involved:</u> heightened activity in the limbic system, particularly the amygdala

<u>Neurotransmitters involved:</u> GABA, serotonin, and norepinephrine

<u>Critical nutrients:</u> L-theanine, omega-3 fatty acids, prebiotic fiber, vitamins B1, B2, B5, B6, B9, B12, C, D, E, magnesium, selenium, zinc

Impactful Food Additions for Anxiety

<u>Green tea:</u> drink green tea or matcha; try green tea mochi for dessert
<u>Salmon or tuna:</u> use pre-seasoned packets on salad, crackers, or sandwiches
<u>Oats:</u> enjoy oatmeal for breakfast topped with flax or hemp seeds and berries, add to pancakes or muffins, enjoy in granola to top yogurt or eat as cereal
<u>Greek yogurt:</u> top with almonds, walnuts, and berries for a snack or breakfast; use in place of sour cream or mayonnaise in recipes
<u>Eggs:</u> hard-boil, fry, or scramble eggs for a snack or breakfast; add to sandwiches, top roasted vegetables to make an easy hash, or add to salads
<u>Beans and lentils:</u> add black beans, chickpeas, or lentils to soup, chili, tacos, or salads; use canned beans for convenience
<u>Leafy greens:</u> add kale, spinach, or Swiss chard to soups, stews, stir-fry, smoothies, sandwiches, or salads
<u>Fruit:</u> enjoy bananas, oranges, or dried cranberries for a snack or breakfast
<u>Brazil nuts:</u> eat 1-2 Brazil nuts as a snack a few times a week
<u>Avocado:</u> smash and spread on toast, add to smoothies, enjoy as a topping to sandwiches or in salads, or make into guacamole

Common Blocks With Anxiety

Perfectionism

What it is: Worry about making a meal "perfect," leading to avoidance or procrastination, which can be related to nutrition, taste, or cooking ability.

Mindset shift: "Eating something 'good enough' is better than not eating at all."

Strategies to overcome:
- Move away from tracking or counting points, calories, macronutrients, or portion sizes. Instead, focus on the balance of meals.
- When individual meals aren't perfectly balanced, "zoom out" to consider the balance of the day or week as a whole.
- Cook in smaller batches to practice, reminding yourself that mistakes are opportunities to learn.
- Remember that "fed is best" is still true for adults – eating anything is better than not eating at all. Being underfed can increase the symptoms of anxiety.
- Avoid comparisons with others and remember nobody's meals are always perfectly balanced or cooked. Remember you're only seeing what someone is willing to show you, and often not the challenges in the background.

Fear of New Recipes

What it is: Excessive worry around cooking new foods or using new or different cooking techniques, leading to repetitive meals or skipping cooking altogether.

Mindset shift: "Everyone starts as a beginner. Trying new things builds confidence."

Strategies to overcome:
- Start with what you know and build from there. Instead of making a whole new meal, make something you are comfortable with and add a new easy side dish.
- Only plan to make one new meal per week and slowly build up your repertoire.
- Read through a new recipe completely before starting to cook.
- Plan extra time when making a new recipe and schedule it on a day when you have enough energy to work through the unknowns of a new recipe.
- Use a meal delivery kit designed to help new cooks learn or take a local cooking class to improve your skills and confidence.

Common Blocks With Anxiety

Sensory Sensitivity

What it is: Discomfort with certain textures, smells, or flavors of foods, which can make cooking or eating challenging.

Mindset shift: "I can try new things with safety because I don't have to eat them."

Strategies to overcome:
- Plan meals around food you know you like (called "safe foods"), especially when adding in new foods.
- Focus on different types of exposures to new foods and include all the senses:
  - Sight: What colors, textures, and patterns do you see in the food?
  - Smell: Can you pick out different spices? Does it smell sweet or savory?
  - Touch: How does the food feel in your hands? How does it feel in your mouth?
  - Sound: Is the food crunchy, smooth, or squeaky against your teeth?
  - Taste: What spices do you notice? Is the food sour, sweet, salty, bitter, tangy, spicy, or a combination? Does the taste change as you chew and swallow?
- Adapt recipes when specific needs are present, such as skipping a strong spice in a recipe, chopping foods into smaller pieces, or substituting vegetables.
- Work with a food therapist or dietitian for support. See resources on page 272.

Fear of Cooking Mistakes

What it is: Worry about burning food, undercooking, other cooking errors, or the meal not turning out as hoped, causing stress around meal preparation.

Mindset shift: "It's okay to make mistakes. They're part of learning."

Strategies to overcome:
- Practice cooking recipes in a low-pressure environment, when you have plenty of time, don't feel stressed, and are cooking for people you feel comfortable with.
- Use recipes like soups or casseroles that can't easily be "ruined."
- Start with simple, easy meals with few ingredients. See the Grab & Go Meals and options on page 38 for ideas.
- Use well-written recipes. If a recipe doesn't make sense to you when you read it, try to find a different one.

Common Blocks With Anxiety

Worry About Waste

What it is: Heightened concern about food going to waste, leading to overthinking how much to cook or eat.

Mindset shift: "Experimenting with food is an investment in myself."

Strategies to overcome:
- Buy frozen, canned, or shelf-stable foods to lengthen the time they can be used.
  - Vegetables with a long shelf life include onions, potatoes, carrots, sweet potatoes, winter squash, or cabbage.
  - Fruits with a long shelf life include oranges, apples, clementines, or underripe produce.
- Choose recipes that work well as leftovers, or that you can freeze if there are large portions.
- Cook a smaller portion, then include non-perishable foods to fill in the meal, such as bread, crackers, canned/frozen fruit, or canned/frozen vegetables.
- Move foods that are nearing their expiration to the same place in your refrigerator so you can easily find and remember to use them.
- When shopping, look for the freshest vegetables (good coloring, no wilting, appropriate firmness) and meats with 'best by' dates a week out to give you flexibility as to when to cook.
- Freeze extra meat, vegetables, or fruit before they expire or go bad, if you end up not using them in your original plan.

Common Blocks With Depression

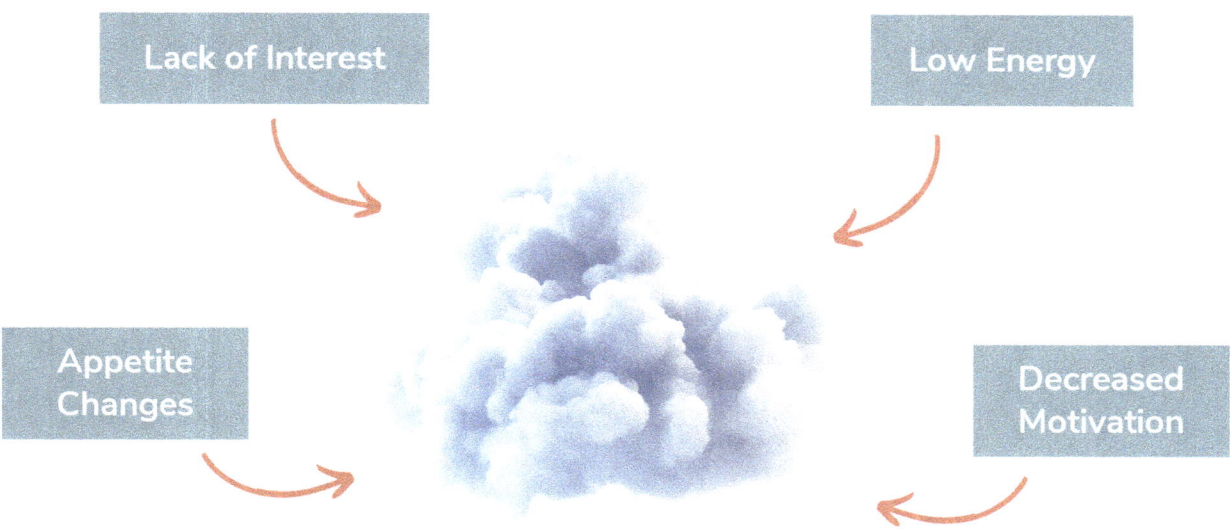

Lack of Interest

Low Energy

Appetite Changes

Decreased Motivation

Depression can cause emotional, cognitive, and physical challenges that make meal planning, grocery shopping, and cooking more difficult. Common symptoms of depression include feelings of worthlessness, hopelessness, and low energy which can make it hard to get out of bed, let alone cook yourself a meal. You might find yourself lacking interest or motivation to do activities you usually enjoy, such as finding interesting recipes or trying new foods. Sometimes even small tasks like deciding what snack to eat can feel overwhelming. The mental exhaustion that comes with depression often makes nourishing yourself more challenging.

You might also experience difficulty concentrating and have memory issues, making it difficult to follow multi-step recipe instructions and remember what you need at the grocery store. Depression symptoms can lead to avoidance of social situations and instead of attending events with friends involving food, you might find yourself opting to stay home – leading to more isolation and fewer opportunities to enjoy food. Appetite changes are also common in depression and can contribute to over- or undereating. The cumulative effect of all these symptoms often results in unplanned weight loss or gain.

Although these blocks are common in depression, there are mindset shifts and strategies that can help you overcome them. Find the ones you identify with most and take small steps to work on them one at a time.

Common Blocks With Depression

<u>Clinical definition:</u> Depression includes 5 or more of these symptoms, with consideration to the duration and severity, and should be diagnosed by a licensed professional:
- Feeling hopeless or empty most of the day
- Less interest in activities that were previously found enjoyable
- Significant weight loss or gain, including a change in appetite
- Insomnia or hypersomnia (sleeping too little or too much)
- Loss of energy or feeling tired
- Feelings of guilt or worthlessness; excessive or inappropriate guilt
- Thoughts of suicide or death

<u>Parts of the brain involved:</u> amygdala, hippocampus, prefrontal cortex, basal ganglia

<u>Neurotransmitters involved:</u> serotonin, dopamine, norepinephrine, and GABA

<u>Critical nutrients:</u> L-theanine, creatine, omega-3 fatty acids, prebiotic fiber, vitamins B1, B2, B6, B9, B12, C, D, K, calcium, iron, magnesium, selenium, zinc, beta-carotene, lycopene, anthocyanins, isoflavones

Impactful Food Additions for Depression

<u>Salmon or tuna:</u> use pre-seasoned packets on salad, crackers, or sandwiches
<u>Beans and lentils:</u> add black beans, chickpeas, or lentils to soup, chili, tacos, or salads; use canned beans for convenience
<u>Walnuts, almonds, and pecans:</u> add to salads, enjoy in trail mix, pair with chocolate, or choose flavored nuts as a snack
<u>Leafy greens:</u> add kale, spinach, or Swiss chard to soups, stews, stir-fry, smoothies, sandwiches, or salads
<u>Hummus:</u> use as a dip for pita chips or veggies; add to sandwiches or wraps
<u>Avocado:</u> smash and spread on toast, add to smoothies, enjoy as a topping to sandwiches or in salads, or make into guacamole
<u>Eggs:</u> hard-boil, fry, or scramble eggs for a snack or breakfast; add to sandwiches, top roasted vegetables to make an easy hash, or add to salads
<u>Fruit:</u> enjoy bananas, oranges, or strawberries for a snack or breakfast
<u>Brazil nuts:</u> eat 1-2 Brazil nuts as a snack a few times a week

Common Blocks With Depression

Energy & Fatigue

What it is: Feeling too tired to cook, eat, or even think about meal preparation.

Mindset shift: "Small steps count as progress."

Strategies to overcome:
- Focus on no-cook or minimal-prep meals like sandwiches, salads, canned soup, or pre-made frozen options.
- Accept help when offered and ask for help before you need it. Find a friend and create a "safe word" so that if you text them, they know to bring food to you, so you have something to eat.
- Serve "snack dinner" with ready-to-eat protein, carbs, and veggies. See the Grab & Go Meals and the options on page 38 for balanced ideas with minimal prep.
- Schedule take-out into your meal plan so you can flip-flop your timing of meals if you are more tired than expected and go out to eat without going over budget.
- Keep a list of nourishing fast-food options as a back-up plan.

Decreased Motivation

What it is: Struggling to find the drive to make a meal, especially if eating feels unappealing.

Mindset shift: "Feeding myself is a form of self-care."

Strategies to overcome:
- Pair cooking and eating with something enjoyable, like listening to music or a podcast to make the activity feel more fun.
- Remember that every meal is not going to have all your favorite foods, but you can add foods you like.
- "Fed is best" is still true for adults – eating anything is better than not eating at all.
- Consider meal replacement options, frozen dinners, or other very easy ways of adding nourishment. For example, try a protein shake with an apple on the side or a protein bar with baby carrots.
- See the Grab & Go Meals and the options on page 38 for balanced ideas with minimal prep.

Common Blocks With Depression

Feeling Overwhelmed

What it is: Even simple tasks like washing vegetables or boiling water feel difficult, making it difficult to prepare and cook food.

Mindset shift: "One step at a time makes the task manageable. I can ask for help if needed."

Strategies to overcome:
- Break down tasks into smaller steps and focus on one at a time.
- Do some tasks when you have more energy, such as meal planning on a different day than when you plan to cook.
- Ask for help <u>before</u> you need it. Find a friend and create a "safe word" so that if you text them, they know to bring food to you, so you have something to eat.
- Ask a friend to "body double" and call or video chat while completing your task to have someone to help motivate or create some accountability.

Appetite Changes

What it is: Decreased hunger cues, lack of interest in food, or cravings only for comfort foods, which can lead to less nutritious eating.

Mindset shift: "Even if I don't feel physically hungry, eating regularly will help my brain and body have more energy and function better."

Strategies to overcome:
- Include comfort foods in your meal plan and keep easy, nutritious options on hand to add in. For example:
  - If you love mac & cheese, add canned green beans on the side.
  - If enjoy a quesadilla, add a side of black beans with taco seasoning.
  - If you are craving ramen noodles, add in a hard-boiled egg or choose a protein and veggie or fruit to go on the side.
- If your low appetite is related to the lack of interest in food, consider small meals or snacks to spark appetite.
- Schedule meals with a friend to enjoy the social part of eating.

Troubleshooting Guide for Common Challenges in Mental Health

Common Blocks With Depression

Negative Self-Talk

What it is: Thoughts like "I can't do this," or "It's not worth it," make cooking feel even harder.

Mindset shift: Choose an affirmation that challenges your negative thought but feels true and believable to you.
- "I am still learning, I can start small."
- "Just because I have a thought does not make it true."
- "I have done other hard things."
- "This is part of my journey."
- "I don't have to do it all. I just have to do the next thing."

Strategies to overcome:
- Start small: don't cook the meal, just open the recipe. Don't prep all the ingredients, just focus on getting out what you need first. Repeat until the meal is done.
- Use affirmations and self-compassion techniques, such as talking to yourself as you would a close friend.
- Acknowledge small wins, like preparing one part of a meal or adding something nutritious.
- Consider speaking with a therapist if negative thoughts don't improve.

Common Blocks With Cognitive Impairment

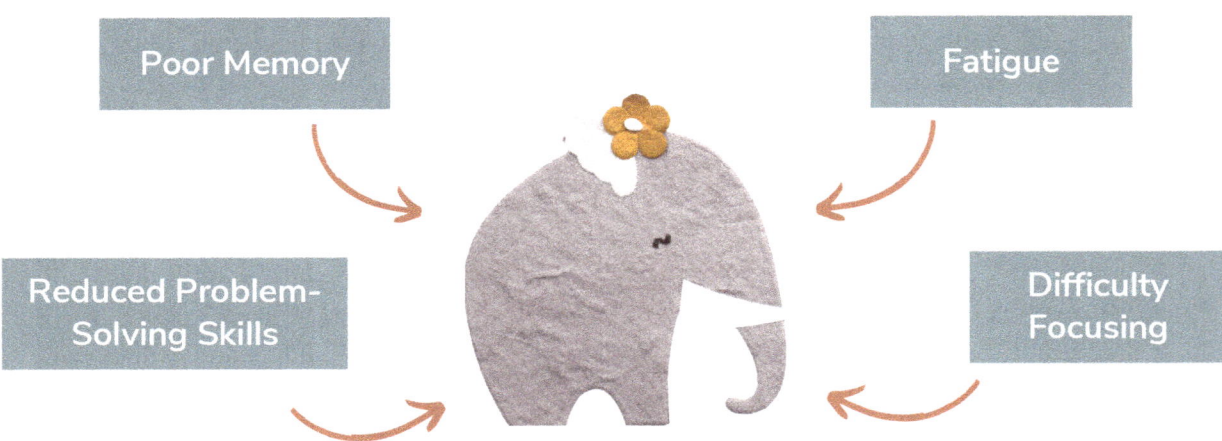

Poor Memory

Fatigue

Reduced Problem-Solving Skills

Difficulty Focusing

Cognitive function refers to a person's mental processes, ranging from learning, memory, judgment, and more. Cognitive impairment refers to any difficulty with cognition, either from the normal aging process, traumatic brain injury, or other neurological changes. This often causes challenges with meal planning, grocery shopping, and multi-step cooking due to difficulty with tasks that require focus, problem-solving, or retaining new information.

If you have cognitive impairment, you might find it easier to use convenience foods or eat snacks rather than making a nutrient-dense meal, especially if you struggle with following recipes or using appliances safely. It can become more difficult to identify food safety issues, like if a food is fully cooked or if it has spoiled. Grocery shopping can be challenging if you can't remember what you need to buy or what ingredients you have at home. You might find your hunger and fullness cues are reduced. When this happens alongside poor memory, you might accidentally skip meals or eat a meal twice because you forgot.

Additionally, if you have difficulty in group settings, such as having trouble following conversations or recognizing social cues, this might lead you to avoid eating with others. If you begin to withdraw from social events around food, this can further reduce your enjoyment of eating and overall mental wellness.

The cumulative result of these effects from cognitive impairment can lead to a lack of variety in your diet and poor nutrition over time. If you or a loved one suffers from any level of cognitive impairment, use these strategies for common blocks to meal planning, preparation, and eating to improve nutrition and quality of life.

Common Blocks With Cognitive Impairment

Clinical definition: Cognitive impairment disrupts a person's ability to think, remember, and use judgement. Symptoms include memory loss; trouble concentrating, completing tasks, and problem solving; understanding and following instructions.

Parts of the brain involved: hippocampus, prefrontal cortex, and amygdala

Neurotransmitters involved: glutamate, dopamine, and acetylcholine

Critical nutrients: L-theanine, creatine, omega-3 fatty acids, vitamins B2, B3, B5, B9, B12, C, D, E, K, choline, selenium, iron, zinc

Impactful Food Additions for Cognitive Function

Green tea: drink green tea or matcha; try green tea mochi for dessert
Salmon or tuna: use pre-seasoned packets on salad, crackers, or on sandwiches
Trail mix: add walnuts, almonds, sunflower or pumpkin seeds along with dried cherries, blueberries, or cranberries
Eggs: hard-boil, fry, or scramble eggs for a snack or breakfast; add to sandwiches, top roasted vegetables to make an easy hash, or add to salads
Avocado: smash and spread on toast, add to smoothies, enjoy as a topping to sandwiches or in salads, or make into guacamole
Beans and lentils: add black beans, chickpeas, or lentils to soup, chili, tacos, or salads; use canned beans for convenience
Leafy greens: add kale, spinach, or Swiss chard to soups, stews, stir-fry, smoothies, sandwiches, or salads
Fresh vegetables: raw broccoli, peppers, or cauliflower with hummus
Brazil nuts: eat 1-2 Brazil nuts as a snack a few times a week

 Supplemental creatine may be uniquely impactful for cognitive function, especially for those following a vegetarian, vegan, or low-meat diet, if you have a history of traumatic brain injury, or have chronic sleep deprivation. Read more about creatine on pages 181–182.

Common Blocks With Cognitive Impairment

Unintentional Weight Loss

What it is: Reduced awareness of hunger cues, resulting in a lack of motivation to eat and unintentional weight loss.

Mindset shift: "I may need to eat even if I don't feel physically hungry, to maintain my health and strength, and can use strategies to help me remember to eat regularly."

Strategies to overcome:
- Use alarms, visual meal schedules, or a whiteboard with daily meal reminders.
- In the morning, set out non-perishable snacks for the day on the table or counter so you can see if you've consumed them or not.
- Use a written meal plan to keep track of which recipes to cook each day.
- Serve small, nutrient-dense meals, especially if feeling full quickly after a meal.
- Incorporate your favorite foods into meals and snacks to increase your enjoyment.
- Eat with others in a social environment when possible.

Trouble Following Cooking Steps

What it is: Becoming confused or overwhelmed by multiple steps in a recipe.

Mindset shift: "Easy meals can meet my needs and be delicious."

Strategies to overcome:
- Choose simple recipes with fewer ingredients and steps.
- Use pre-prepared meal kits or pre-made meals instead of cooking from scratch every day.
- Keep quick options on hand to make a meal without needing to cook. See the Grab & Go Meals and examples on page 38 for ideas.

Common Blocks With Cognitive Impairment

Difficulty With Grocery Shopping

What it is: Forgetting needed items when buying food or ingredients, feeling overwhelmed in the grocery store, having difficulty walking or carrying items, or struggling with decision-making around food.

Mindset shift: "There are tools I can use to make grocery shopping easier."

Strategies to overcome:
- Use a grocery list organized by category to make shopping easier, spend less time in the store, and take fewer steps.
- If possible, shop at off-peak store hours, such as in the mornings, on weekdays, or late in the evening.
- Use an electric shopping cart to reduce the amount of walking.
- Use grocery delivery or pick-up services instead of going into the store.

Unsafe or Challenging Food Preparation

What it is: Forgetting to turn off appliances, struggling with knife and stovetop safety, and/or experiencing an inability to recognize spoiled food.

Mindset shift: "Simpler meals can be quicker, less stressful, and safer."

Strategies to overcome:
- Use pre-cut, frozen, or canned ingredients that don't require the use of knives.
- Set timers to remind you that an appliance is turned on or use slow cookers or appliances that turn off automatically.
- Make a habit of looking around the kitchen before leaving the room or the house to check that appliances are turned off.
- Label leftovers with dates and clean the refrigerator regularly.
- Store perishable items in clear containers where they are easy to see.

Common Blocks With Cognitive Impairment

Social Isolation

What it is: Eating alone can decrease motivation to prepare and enjoy meals.

Mindset shift: "I still deserve nourishment when I'm cooking for just me, and I can schedule times to eat with others because I enjoy it."

Strategies to overcome:
- Schedule shared meals with family or friends. If they live far away, use virtual mealtime calls for social interaction.
- Join groups where meals are part of the activity or meet a group member before or after an event for a shared meal.
- Keep single-serving meals on hand to use when eating at home alone.
- When eating alone, add enjoyment to the meal by reading a favorite book, setting the table nicely, or eating outside on a nice day.

Struggles With Hydration

What it is: Decreased sensation of thirst, taking diuretic medication, or forgetting to drink enough fluids, leading to dehydration.

Mindset shift: "Drinking enough fluids is essential for health."

Strategies to overcome:
- Keep a water bottle nearby and take a drink when you see it.
- Incorporate hydrating foods like fruits and soups into your meal plan.
- Add beverages you enjoy, such as flavored or sparkling water, or add lemon and lime juice to water.
- Drink decaffeinated options, when possible, to reduce diuretic effects.
- Add an electrolyte mix to water to improve hydration (use with caution if on a low sodium diet).

Coping With Emotions *in Healthy Ways*

Everyone uses coping mechanisms to navigate emotions, and food is one of the most common and socially-acceptable options in our culture. Whether happy or sad, we often celebrate or commiserate with food. Improving your mental health and healing your relationship with food is not only about including the right nutrients, but also about responding to your emotions in a supportive way. If you have bad days when all you want to do is eat – or avoid eating – identifying other ways to meet your underlying needs is essential for your mental and physical health.

There is nothing inherently wrong with using food to navigate big emotions, but eating for reasons besides hunger can cause other challenges if it's overused as a coping mechanism. Sometimes using food to cope is a distraction from navigating and solving root cause issues. When this happens, it can feel like eating is never enough and cravings are never satisfied, leading to overeating and discomfort. This often results in dissatisfaction with food and body, and sometimes can lead to disordered eating patterns.

Instead of trying to avoid eating as a coping mechanism, we encourage you to expand your options for coping strategies using the examples provided in the following pages. Focus on healing root causes of painful emotions, and make sure you have plenty of tools to use when you encounter a difficult situation. With this approach, you will naturally rely less on food as a coping mechanism because you will spend your energy using other options.

This is not an exhaustive list of coping strategies, but rather a place to start. Incorporating layers of coping, including preventative strategies, is key to helping you feel your best. If possible, we recommend working with a licensed therapist to understand root causes of challenges, implement coping strategies, and develop a comprehensive treatment plan. You can find recommended resources on page 272.

Fear

- Identify if the fear is rational or not
- Practice "safe place" visualization
- Seek reassurance from trusted people
- Use exposure therapy techniques for mild fears
- Shift focus to what you can control

Loneliness

- Call or text a friend or family member
- Engage in online or local communities with shared interests
- Go to a public place: a library or café
- Find ways to enjoy your own presence: self-care, explore hobbies
- Volunteer or do acts of kindness

Coping With Emotions *in Healthy Ways*

Feeling Anxious

- Write down your worries and challenge anxious thoughts
- Use somatic practices such as deep breathing or grounding techniques
  - <u>4-7-8 deep breathing:</u> breathe in for 4 counts, hold for 7 counts, breathe out for 8 counts; repeat this for several minutes
  - <u>Box breathing:</u> breathe in for 4 counts, hold for 4 counts, breathe out for 4 counts, hold for 4 counts; repeat this for several minutes
  - <u>5-4-3-2-1 grounding technique:</u> name 5 things you see, 4 things you are touching, 3 things you hear, 2 things you smell, and 1 thing you taste
- Use relaxation techniques such as progressive muscle relaxation, wave visualization, cloud visualization, or river visualization where you watch thoughts pass by on a wave, cloud, or a slow river
- Incorporate relaxing exercise, including taking a gentle walk or yoga
- Reduce caffeine and stimulants, or switch from coffee or energy drinks to a different form of caffeine, such as matcha or green tea
- Reduce or eliminate substance use such as alcohol, nicotine, or others
- Consider using an app such as Headspace®, Calm®, or Insight Timer® for beginning meditation and breathing practices

Feeling Overwhelmed

- Use the "brain dump" method to get thoughts on paper and write down everything you are thinking or worried about
- Break tasks into smaller, manageable steps
- Prioritize what truly needs to be done
- Use the Pomodoro Technique to complete overwhelming tasks: set a timer for 25 minutes and work without distraction, then take 5-minute breaks in between working sets
- Reduce sensory overload with a quiet, calming space
- Ask for help and delegate when possible

Troubleshooting Guide for Common Challenges in Mental Health

Coping With Emotions *in Healthy Ways*

Boredom

- Keep a list of tasks to accomplish or activities you enjoy to help remind yourself of options when you are feeling bored
- Engage in a new or forgotten hobby
- Listen to a podcast or audiobook
- Do a small productive task like organizing, cleaning, or decluttering
- Move your body with stretching or a dance break
- Experiment with new meal ideas instead of mindless snacking

Inadequacy

- Recognize and challenge self-comparisons
- Write a list of your accomplishments
- Set small, realistic goals and celebrate progress
- Engage in positive self-talk with affirmations or journaling
- Learn a new skill or practice self-growth
- Share your feelings with a trusted friend who can help encourage positive self-image

Anger

- Release physical energy with exercise, pillow slams, lion's breaths, or yelling safely
- Journal or write a letter you don't send
- Use music, writing, or art to express your emotions
- Practice feeling anger in your body (often tension) then releasing it
- Listen to loud music to feel and release then soothing music to calm
- Practice breathing techniques

Guilt

- Identify what's within your control and release what isn't
- Offer a sincere apology if needed and make amends
- Write a self-forgiveness letter
- Challenge self-criticism and reframe your thoughts
- Think of how you would speak to a loved one who has made a mistake and has done what is needed for apology and amends

Coping With Emotions *in Healthy Ways*

Embarrassment

- Reframe the situation with humor, perspective, or as a learning moment
- Use self-compassion – remember everyone makes mistakes
- Remind yourself that it's temporary
- Distract yourself with a fun activity
- Remember that people forget moments quickly
- Engage in self-soothing techniques
- Find a supportive person to talk to
- Engage in an activity that restores your confidence

Insecurity

- Challenge negative self-talk
- List qualities that make you unique and valuable
- Dress in a way that makes you feel confident
- Spend time with positive, uplifting people
- Engage in activities that reinforce your strengths
- Reduce your time on social media
- Volunteer for causes important to you to help reframe your perspective

Sadness

- Practice self-compassion, speak to yourself like a friend
- Listen to uplifting music or a comforting playlist
- Allow yourself to feel your emotions, reminding yourself that it's okay to feel sad
- Journal your feelings or write a letter to yourself, helping you to understand and process some emotions
- Get fresh air, go for a walk, or do some gentle yoga
- Spend time in sunlight if available

Resentment

- Recognize unmet expectations or boundaries
- Practice gratitude for relationships or for things that are good in life
- Practice asking/advocating for your needs to be met in safe environments
- Practice self-reflection
- Explore writing about feelings connected to resentment
- Engage in mindfulness to stay present
- Consider seeking therapy or professional guidance

Continuing *Your Journey*

The human brain is a complex organ, and it's literally made up of the nutrients we eat. Nutrition is foundational for health and allows every other tool you have — from meditation to medication — to work more effectively. We hope the knowledge and skills you've learned in these pages help you build a nutritional foundation for mental health, using this guide to inform your decisions about food and supplements.

We want to thank you for taking the time to invest in your health and well-being. Nutrition is so much more than organizing your meals. It's a way to nurture your body, support your mental health, celebrate events, experience culture, and commune with the people in your life whom you love.

There is no one "right" way to eat, plan your meals, or decide what supplements you need. This journey is about finding what works for you — for your tastes, your schedule, and your needs. Progress, not perfection, is the goal.

As you move forward, we encourage you to continue listening to your body, honor your cravings, and give yourself grace. Use this information to ask questions of your mental health team and advocate for yourself. Your mental health is worth every ounce of effort you put into caring for yourself, one meal at a time.

This journey does not end here. For continued support, we've listed our favorite resources on the next page. You can also find us on Instagram @the.brain.plate, @nutrimindpllc, and @peasandhoppiness for ongoing information, support, and community.

Here's to balanced plates, peaceful minds, and meals that nourish both body and soul!

With gratitude,

Amanda & Ann

Amanda and Ann

Additional Resources

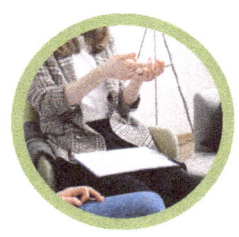

Mental Health Resources

Work with Amanda Ashcraft*: www.Nutrimind.org

Find a licensed therapist and psychiatrist near you:
www.psychologytoday.com

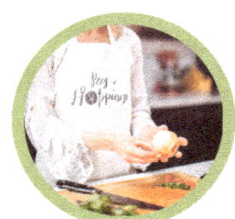

Meal Planning App & Cooking Resources

The Peas and Hoppy Meal Guides - Meal Planning App or work
with Ann Kent*: www.PeasAndHoppiness.com

Find a registered dietitian near you: DietitianDirectory.com or
www.EatRight.org/find-a-nutrition-expert

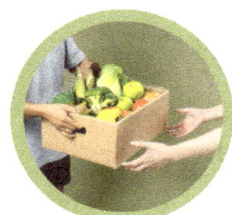

Nutrition Resources

Find an Intuitive Eating counselor near you:
www.IntuitiveEating.org/certified-counselors

Resources for Parents & Kids: www.EllynSatterInstitute.org

Resources for Eating Disorders: www.NationalEatingDisorders.org

Resources for Food Insecurity: www.feedingamerica.org

Resources for Integrative Medicine Doctor: awcim.arizona.edu

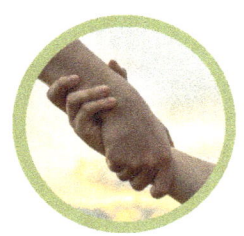

Emergent Needs

Suicide Hotline: Call 988 or go to FindAHelpline.com

If you are in immediate danger, please call 911 or go to your
nearest emergency department.

**Find links to these resources
and more at TheBrainPlate.com**

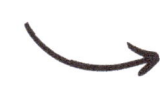

*Subject to licensure laws

References

- Adan, R. A., van der Beek, E. M., Buitelaar, J. K., et al. (2011). Nutritional psychiatry: Towards improving mental health by what you eat. *European Neuropsychopharmacology, 21*(12), 841–848. https://doi.org/10.1016/j.euroneuro.2011.07.008
- American Heart Association. (2024, August 23). Fish and omega-3 fatty acids. https://www.heart.org/en/healthy-living/healthy-eating/eat-smart/fats/fish-and-omega-3-fatty-acids
- American Psychological Association. (2019). Clinical practice guideline for the treatment of depression across three age cohorts. Retrieved from https://www.apa.org/depression-guideline
- Australian Government Department of Health. (2022). Kava – Drug Facts. Alcohol and Drug Foundation. https://adf.org.au/drug-facts/kava/
- Calder, P. C. (2013). Omega-3 polyunsaturated fatty acids and inflammatory processes: Nutrition or pharmacology? *British Journal of Clinical Pharmacology, 75*(3), 645–662. https://doi.org/10.1111/j.1365-2125.2012.04374.x
- Covington, M. B. (2004). Omega-3 fatty acids. American Family Physician, 70(1), 133–140. Retrieved from https://www.aafp.org/pubs/afp/issues/2004/0701/p133.html
- Davidson, M., & McEwen, B. S. (2012). Social influences on neuroplasticity: Stress and interventions to promote well-being. *Nature Neuroscience, 15*(5), 689–695. https://doi.org/10.1038/nn.3093
- Demelash, S. (2017). The role of micronutrient for depressed patients. *Journal of Neuropsychopharmacology & Mental Health, 2*(01) 1-4. https://doi.org/10.4172/2472-095X.1000116
- Examine. (n.d.). Independent scientific information on supplements & nutrition. Retrieved May 21, 2025, from https://examine.com/
- Fernstrom, J. D. (2013). Role of precursor availability in control of monoamine biosynthesis in brain. *Physiological Reviews, 63*(2), 484–546. https://doi.org/10.1152/physrev.1983.63.2.484
- Gasperi, V., Sibilano, M., Savini, I., & Catani, M. V. (2019). Niacin in the central nervous system: An update of biological aspects and clinical applications. *International Journal of Molecular Sciences, 20*(4), 974. https://doi.org/10.3390/ijms20040974
- Harvard T.H. Chan School of Public Health. (n.d.). Nutrition and mental health. https://www.hsph.harvard.edu/nutritionsource/nutrition-and-mental-health/
- Healthline. (2023). Lavender for anxiety: Uses, effects, and how to use it. https://www.healthline.com/health/anxiety/lavender-for-anxiety
- Healthline. (2023). Rhodiola rosea: Benefits, side effects, dosage, and more. https://www.healthline.com/nutrition/rhodiola-rosea
- Ji, K., Sun, M., Li, L., Hong, Y., Yang, S., & Wu, Y. (2024). Association between vitamin B2 intake and cognitive performance among older adults: A cross-sectional study from NHANES. *Scientific Reports, 14*(1), 21930. https://doi.org/10.1038/s41598-024-72949-0
- Kelaiditis, C. F., Gibson, E. L., & Dyall, S. C. (2023). Effects of long-chain omega-3 polyunsaturated fatty acids on reducing anxiety and/or depression in adults: A systematic review and meta-analysis of randomised controlled trials. Prostaglandins, Leukotrienes and Essential Fatty Acids, 192, 102572. https://doi.org/10.1016/j.plefa.2023.102572
- Kennedy, D. O. (2016). B vitamins and the brain: Mechanisms, dose and efficacy—A review. *Nutrients, 8*(2), 68. https://doi.org/10.3390/nu8020068
- Kennedy, D. O., Scholey, A. B., Tildesley, N. T. J., Perry, E. K., & Wesnes, K. A. (2002). Modulation of mood and cognitive performance following acute administration of Melissa officinalis (lemon balm). *Pharmacology Biochemistry and Behavior, 72*(4), 953–964. https://doi.org/10.1016/S0091-3057(02)00777-3
- Kris-Etherton, P. M., Petersen, K. S., Hibbeln, J. R., et al. (2021). Nutrition and behavioral health disorders: Depression and anxiety. *Nutrition Reviews, 79*(3), 247–260. https://doi.org/10.1093/nutrit/nuaa025
- Kyrou, I., & Tsigos, C. (2009). Stress hormones: Physiological stress and regulation of metabolism. *Current Opinion in Pharmacology, 9*(6), 787–793. https://doi.org/10.1016/j.coph.2009.08.007
- Lewis, J. E., Tiozzo, E., Melillo, A. B., Leonard, S., Chen, L., Mendez, A., Woolger, J. M., & Konefal, J. (2013). The effect of methylated vitamin B complex on depressive and anxiety symptoms and quality of life in adults with depression. ISRN Psychiatry, 2013, 1-7. https://doi.org/10.1155/2013/621453
- Li, J., Wang, J., Wang, M., Zheng, L., Cen, Q., Wang, F., Zhu, L., Pang, R., & Zhang, A. (2023). Bifidobacterium: a probiotic for the prevention and treatment of depression. Frontiers in microbiology, 14, 1174800. https://doi.org/10.3389/fmicb.2023.1174800

References

- Liu, C., Xie, X., Wang, Y., et al. (2022). Magnesium intake and risk of depression: A meta-analysis. Journal of Affective Disorders, 312, 187–193. https://doi.org/10.1016/j.jad.2022.06.025
- Markova, N., Bazhenova, N., Anthony, D. C., Vignisse, J., Svistunov, A., Lesch, K. P., Bettendorff, L., & Strekalova, T. (2017). Thiamine and benfotiamine improve cognition and ameliorate GSK-3β-associated stress-induced behaviours in mice. Progress in Neuro-Psychopharmacology and Biological Psychiatry, 75, 148–156. https://doi.org/10.1016/j.pnpbp.2016.11.001
- Mayo Clinic. (2023). Melatonin side effects: What's safe? https://www.mayoclinic.org/healthy-lifestyle/adult-health/expert-answers/melatonin-side-effects/faq-20057874
- McCabe, D., Lisy, K., Lockwood, C., & Colbeck, M. (2017). The impact of essential fatty acid, B vitamins, vitamin C, magnesium and zinc supplementation on stress levels in women: A systematic review. JBI Database of Systematic Reviews and Implementation Reports, 15(2), 402–453. https://doi.org/10.11124/JBISRIR-2016-002965
- MedlinePlus. (2023).
  - Ashwagandha. U.S. National Library of Medicine. https://medlineplus.gov/druginfo/natural/953.html
  - Chaga. U.S. National Library of Medicine. https://medlineplus.gov/druginfo/natural/905.html
- Memorial Sloan Kettering Cancer Center. (2023). Rhodiola. https://www.mskcc.org/cancer-care/integrative-medicine/herbs/rhodiola
- Mocking, R. J., Harmsen, I., Assies, J., Koeter, M. W., Ruhé, H. G., & Schene, A. H. (2016). Meta-analysis and meta-regression of omega-3 polyunsaturated fatty acid supplementation for major depressive disorder. Translational Psychiatry, 6(3), e756. https://doi.org/10.1038/tp.2016.29
- Mount Sinai. (2023). Passionflower. https://www.mountsinai.org/health-library/herb/passionflower
- Muscaritoli, M. (2021). The impact of nutrients on mental health and well-being: Insights from the literature. Frontiers in Nutrition, 8. https://doi.org/10.3389/fnut.2021.656290
- National Center for Complementary and Integrative Health (NCCIH). (2022).
  - Ashwagandha. National Institutes of Health. https://www.nccih.nih.gov/health/ashwagandha
  - Kava. National Institutes of Health. https://www.nccih.nih.gov/health/kava
  - Lavender. National Institutes of Health. https://www.nccih.nih.gov/health/lavender
  - Passionflower. National Institutes of Health. https://www.nccih.nih.gov/health/passionflower
  - Rhodiola. National Institutes of Health. https://www.nccih.nih.gov/health/rhodiola
  - St. John's Wort. National Institutes of Health. https://www.nccih.nih.gov/health/st-johns-wort
  - St. John's Wort and depression: In-depth. National Institutes of Health. https://www.nccih.nih.gov/health/st-johns-wort-and-depression-in-depth
  - Valerian. National Institutes of Health. https://www.nccih.nih.gov/health/valerian
- National Institutes of Health, Office of Dietary Supplements. (2023).
  - Ashwagandha: Fact sheet for health professionals. https://ods.od.nih.gov/factsheets/Ashwagandha-HealthProfessional/
  - Niacin: Fact sheet for health professionals. https://ods.od.nih.gov/factsheets/Niacin-HealthProfessional/
  - Thiamin: Fact sheet for health professionals. https://ods.od.nih.gov/factsheets/Thiamin-HealthProfessional/
  - Valerian: Fact sheet for health professionals. https://ods.od.nih.gov/factsheets/Valerian-HealthProfessional/
  - Vitamin B6: Fact sheet for health professionals. https://ods.od.nih.gov/factsheets/VitaminB6-HealthProfessional/
  - Vitamin B12: Fact sheet for health professionals. https://ods.od.nih.gov/factsheets/VitaminB12-HealthProfessional/
  - Vitamin D: Fact sheet for health professionals. https://ods.od.nih.gov/factsheets/VitaminD-HealthProfessional/
  - Vitamin E: Fact sheet for health professionals. https://ods.od.nih.gov/factsheets/VitaminE-HealthProfessional/
  - Vitamin K: Fact sheet for health professionals. https://ods.od.nih.gov/factsheets/VitaminK-HealthProfessional/
- National Research Council (US) Committee on Military Nutrition Research. (1999). Thiamin, riboflavin, niacin, vitamin B6, vitamin B12, and choline. In The role of dietary supplements for physically active people. National Academies Press. https://www.ncbi.nlm.nih.gov/books/NBK114331/
- Oregon State University, Linus Pauling Institute. (2023). Vitamin K: Micronutrient information center. https://lpi.oregonstate.edu/mic/vitamins/vitamin-K

References

- Palmer, A. C., Hossain, M. I., Ali, H., Ayesha, K., Shaikh, S., Islam, M. T., et al. (2025). Protein supplementation delivered alone or in combination with presumptive azithromycin treatment for enteric pathogens did not improve linear growth in Bangladeshi infants: Results of a cluster-randomized controlled trial. American Journal of Clinical Nutrition, 121(3), 597–609. https://doi.org/10.1016/j.ajcnut.2024.12.027
- Qaseem A, Barry MJ, Kansagara D; Clinical Guidelines Committee of the American College of Physicians. Nonpharmacologic Versus Pharmacologic Treatment of Adult Patients With Major Depressive Disorder: A Clinical Practice Guideline From the American College of Physicians. Ann Intern Med. 2016 Mar 1;164(5):350-9. doi: 10.7326/M15-2570. Epub 2016 Feb 9. PMID: 26857948.
- Rabheru, R., Langan, A., Merriweather, J., Connolly, B., Whelan, K., & Bear, D. E. (2025). Reporting of nutritional screening, status, and intake in trials of nutritional and physical rehabilitation following critical illness: A systematic review. American Journal of Clinical Nutrition, 121(3), 703–723. https://doi.org/10.1016/j.ajcnut.2024.12.028
- Sarris, J., Ravindran, A., Yatham, L. N., Marx, W., Rucklidge, J. J., McIntyre, R. S., Akhondzadeh, S., Benedetti, F., Caneo, C., Cramer, H., Cribb, L., de Manincor, M., Dean, O., Deslandes, A. C., Freeman, M. P., Gangadhar, B., Harvey, B. H., Kasper, S., Lake, J., … Berk, M. (2022). Clinician guidelines for the treatment of psychiatric disorders with nutraceuticals and phytoceuticals: The World Federation of Societies of Biological Psychiatry (WFSBP) and Canadian network for mood and Anxiety Treatments (CANMAT) taskforce. The World Journal of Biological Psychiatry, 23(6), 424–455. https://doi.org/10.1080/15622975.2021.2013041
- Sateia, M. J., Buysse, D. J., Krystal, A. D., Neubauer, D. N., & Heald, J. L. (2017). Clinical Practice Guideline for the Pharmacologic Treatment of Chronic Insomnia in Adults: An American Academy of Sleep Medicine Clinical Practice Guideline. Journal of Clinical Sleep Medicine, 13(2), 307–349. https://doi.org/10.5664/jcsm.6470
- Sleep Foundation. (2023). Melatonin: How it works, when to take it, and side effects. https://www.sleepfoundation.org/melatonin
- Su, K. P., Matsuoka, Y., & Pae, C. U. (2015). Omega-3 polyunsaturated fatty acids in prevention of mood and anxiety disorders. Clinical Psychopharmacology and Neuroscience, 13(2), 129–137. https://doi.org/10.9758/cpn.2015.13.2.12
- Su, K. P., Tseng, P. T., Lin, P. Y., Okubo, R., Chen, T. Y., Chen, Y. W., & Matsuoka, Y. J. (2018). Association of use of omega-3 polyunsaturated fatty acids with changes in severity of anxiety symptoms: A systematic review and meta-analysis. JAMA Network Open, 1(5). https://doi.org/10.1001/jamanetworkopen.2018.2327
- Therapeutic Research Center. (n.d.). Natural Medicines [Monographs on alpha-linolenic acid (ALA), ashwagandha, calcium, chaga, choline, cordyceps, creatine, docosahexaenoic acid (DHA), eicosapentaenoic acid (EPA), folic acid, German chamomile, ginkgo, iron, kava, lavender, lemon balm, lion's mane mushroom, magnesium, melatonin, niacin, pantothenic acid, Panax ginseng, passion flower, Reishi mushroom, riboflavin, Rhodiola, saffron, SAMe, selenium, St. John's wort, thiamine, theanine, turmeric, valerian, vitamin B6, vitamin B12, vitamin C, vitamin D, vitamin E, vitamin K, and zinc]. Natural Medicines. Retrieved July 30, 2025, from https://naturalmedicines.therapeuticresearch.com/
- Wani, A. L., Bhat, S. A., & Ara, A. (2015). Omega-3 fatty acids and the treatment of depression: A review of scientific evidence. Integrative Medicine Research, 4(3), 132–141. https://doi.org/10.1016/j.imr.2015.07.003
- WebMD. (2023).
  - Chaga: Uses, side effects, and more. https://www.webmd.com/vitamins/ai/ingredientmono-1474/chaga
  - Cordyceps: Benefits and uses. https://www.webmd.com/vitamins/ai/ingredientmono-602/cordyceps
  - Lion's Mane mushroom: Benefits, side effects, and more. https://www.webmd.com/vitamins/ai/ingredientmono-1536/lions-mane-mushroom
  - Niacin (oral) - Uses, side effects, and more. https://www.webmd.com/drugs/2/drug-58193/niacin-time-oral/details
- Xie, Y., Li, S., Wu, D., Wang, Y., Chen, J., Duan, L., Li, S., & Li, Y. (2024). Vitamin K: Infection, inflammation, and auto-immunity. Journal of Inflammation Research, 17, 1147–1160. https://doi.org/10.2147/JIR.S445806
- Yoo, M., Kim, S. M., Lee, J., Kim, H.-J., & Park, S. J. (2024). Glycine transporter 1 (GlyT1) is a novel therapeutic target for Alzheimer's disease. Alzheimer's & Dementia: Translational Research & Clinical Interventions, 10(1), e70101. https://doi.org/10.1002/trc2.70101
- Zhang, Y., Ding, J., & Liang, J. (2022). Associations of dietary vitamin A and beta-carotene intake with depression: A meta-analysis of observational studies. Frontiers in Nutrition, 9. https://doi.org/10.3389/fnut.2022.881139

Recipe Index

Index

Index

Cod 40–42, 183, 185, 201
Coffee 208–209, 214, 216, 239, 268
Cordyceps – see *Functional mushrooms*
Cortisol 8–9, 17–18, 197, 218, 233
Cucumber 38, 92, 99, 119, 122, 126, 138, 141–142, 158

D

Dairy or milk alternatives 174–175, 181, 187, 195, 200, 203, 207, 209, 212,
  Coconut milk 41–44, 111–113, 202, 208–209
  Dairy milk 38, 40, 65, 70, 85, 96, 130, 149–150, 164–165, 187–188, 197, 201, 207, 209, 225
  Milk alternatives 38, 65, 70, 82, 85, 96, 165, 207
  Yogurt 38, 40, 51, 57, 61, 68–71, 95–98, 129, 149–150, 157, 159, 178, 188, 191, 194, 197, 201, 253
Depression 11, 22, 26, 180–182, 185–186, 190, 192, 194–195, 198–200, 202–204, 206–216, 218, 220–221, 223–224, 226–228, 231–235, 257–261
DHA – see *Omega-3 fatty acids*
Diabetes 7, 8, 192, 194, 203, 209; see also *Blood glucose* and *Insulin*
Digestion (digestive system) 8–11, 14–15, 20, 168, 183, 189, 199, 208, 210–211, 224, 235, 252
Dopamine – see *Neurotransmitters*
Dried Fruit 38, 93, 133, 188, 208, 240, 245

E

Egg 38, 40, 65–66, 71–72, 74–75, 77, 79, 85, 95, 128–129, 131, 134, 157–158, 160–161, 178, 195, 197, 200–201, 203, 212, 225, 247, 253, 258, 260, 263
Electrolytes 6–7, 18, 173, 266
Endorphins 17, 231
Energy 2, 6–8, 10, 15, 17–19, 26, 30–34, 164, 168, 177–179, 181, 187, 193–195, 197, 200, 208–209, 211, 216, 239–240, 254, 257–260, 267, 269

Enteric nervous system 8–10, 14–16, 189, 192, 252
EPA – see *Omega-3 fatty acids*
Epinephrine – see *Neurotransmitters*
Executive function 22, 32, 201, 246–247, 250

F

Fat 2, 10–11, 14, 18–19, 22, 27–28, 32, 43, 52, 113, 129, 167, 174, 176–177, 182–187, 190, 194, 196–197, 200–206, 209, 215, 220, 241, 247, 253, 258, 263
Fatigue 9, 26, 32, 182, 200, 202–203, 211–212, 231, 234, 244, 250, 253, 259
Fiber (includes prebiotic fiber) 10, 12, 20, 28, 32, 38, 70, 102, 167, 177, 187–192, 208–209, 241, 253, 258
Flaxseeds – see *Seeds*
Focus 11, 17–18, 180, 194–195, 208, 246–251, 262
Folate – see *Vitamin B9*
Food and Drug Association (FDA) 19, 170, 172, 180, 186, 216–217, 219, 222–224, 230, 233, 235
Free radical 19, 20, 195, 205
Frontal lobe 13
Functional mushrooms 227–229

G

Gamma-aminobutyric acid (GABA) – see *Neurotransmitters*
Generally Recognized As Safe (GRAS) 19, 219, 223–224, 230, 233, 235
Gingko Biloba 221
Ginseng 220
Glutamate – see *Neurotransmitters*
Grab & Go Recipe – see *Recipes Index*
Green Beans 38, 71, 86, 89, 260
Gut Health 6, 10, 12, 189–192

H

Heart (heart health) – see *cardiovascular system*
Hemp seeds – see *Seeds*
Histamine 18, 198
Homeostasis 6–8, 15, 17–18

Hormones 2, 6–8, 10–12, 17–18, 178, 183, 190, 193, 197, 207, 220, 225–226, 232, 252; see also *Cortisol, Dopamine, Epinephrine, GABA, Insulin, Norepinephrine, Oxytocin, Serotonin*
Hypothalamic-pituitary-adrenal axis (HPA axis) 14, 189, 192, 218, 233
Hypothalamus 14, 18, 203

I

Iron 12, 168, 174–175, 196, 207–208, 213, 247, 258, 263
  Cast iron 56, 101, 115, 118, 121, 146
Inflammation 9–10, 17, 181, 183–186, 192–193, 195–196, 200, 202–203, 205–206, 212, 214–215, 227, 235
Insoluble fiber – see *Fiber*
Insulin 8, 17–18, 209, 220

K

Kale 47, 54, 83–84, 134, 148–150, 247, 253, 258

L

L-theanine 12, 179–180, 210, 247, 253, 258, 263
Lavender 223
Lemon Balm 224, 230
Lentils 38, 40, 49–51, 78, 81, 95, 178, 188, 199, 207–209, 212–213, 253, 258, 263
Lion's mane – see *Functional mushrooms*
Limbic system 13, 18, 223, 247, 253, 258

M

Magnesium 2, 12, 174–175, 209–211, 247, 253, 258
Macronutrients 2–3, 19, 27, 177, 254, see also *Carbohydrates, Fats,* and *Proteins*
Memory 13–14, 17–18, 22, 32, 180–182, 194–195, 197–201, 206, 208, 211, 214, 220–222, 224, 227–228, 234–235, 246, 249, 257, 262–263

Index

Index